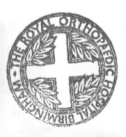

Carpal Tunnel Syndrome and Other Disorders of the Median Nerve

Carpal Tunnel Syndrome and Other Disorders of the Median Nerve

Richard B. Rosenbaum, M.D.
Department of Medicine, Providence Hospital
Department of Neurology, Good Samaritan Hospital
Clinical Professor of Neurology
Oregon Health Sciences University
Portland, Oregon

José L. Ochoa, M.D., Ph.D., D.Sc.
Neuromuscular Unit
Good Samaritan Hospital
Professor of Neurology and Neurosurgery
Oregon Health Sciences University
Portland, Oregon

Eugenia Vásquez Bermudez, Illustrator

Butterworth-Heinemann

Boston London Oxford Singapore Sydney Toronto Wellington

Every effort has been made to ensure that the drug dosage schedules within this text are accurate and conform to standards accepted at time of publication. However, as treatment recommendations vary in the light of continuing research and clinical experience, the reader is advised to verify drug dosage schedules herein with information found on product information sheets. This is especially true in cases of new or infrequently used drugs.

Recognizing the importance of preserving what has been written, it is the policy of Butterworth-Heinemann to have the books it publishes printed on acid-free paper, and we exert our best efforts to that end.

Library of Congress Cataloging-in-Publication Data

Rosenbaum, Richard B., 1946–
    Carpal tunnel syndrome and other disorders of the median nerve /
Richard B. Rosenbaum, José L. Ochoa : Eugenia Vásquez Bermudez,
illustrator.
        p.   cm.
    Includes bibliographical references and index.
    ISBN 0-7506-9229-4 (alk. paper)
    1. Carpal tunnel syndrome.   2. Median nerve—Diseases.   I. Ochoa,
José.   II. Title.
    [DNLM: 1. Carpal Tunnel Syndrome.   2. Median Nerve—pathology.
WL 500 R8125c]
RC422.C26R67   1993
616.8'7—dc20
DNLM/DLC
for Library of Congress   92-49623
                                                                      CIP

British Library Cataloguing-in-Publication Data.
A catalogue record for this book is available from the British Library.

Butterworth-Heinemann
80 Montvale Avenue
Stoneham, MA 02180

10   9   8   7   6   5   4   3   2

Printed in the United States of America

To our wives, children, and parents

Contents

Foreword

Roger Gilliatt was preparing a foreword for this book just before his untimely death. We shall miss his wisdom and example.

Acknowledgments

We thank the following colleagues for their invaluable encouragement and suggestions: Morris Button, Mario Campero, Catherine Ellison, Gary Franklin, George Goodman, Paul Kohnen, Paolo Marchettini, Christopher J. Morgan, Peter A. Nathan, Beverly Phillipson, Stephen F. Quinn, Patrick Radecki, James T. Rosenbaum, Lois O. Rosenbaum, Robert A. Rosenbaum, Thomas J. Rosenbaum, Renato Verdugo, Richard Wernick, Asa Wilbourn, and David Yarnitsky.

Our thanks also to our office staffs for their long hours of assistance.

Introduction

Has medicine become so complex that we need a separate book for each nerve in the body?

Long before carpal tunnel syndrome began to draw attention in the media, at social gatherings, and in factories and offices around the country, physicians had been regularly attentive to it in their patients. As neurologists, we see hundreds of cases each year. Despite this ever-growing clinical experience, patients with carpal tunnel syndrome can be a challenge to diagnose and treat. Behind the generation of this book was a desire to synthesize the recorded knowledge about this prevalent syndrome and to answer some of the questions raised by our patients and our colleagues. Toward this end, we reviewed well over 2,000 articles and books on carpal tunnel syndrome. Of course, every answer raises additional questions, but we hope that the present monograph addresses the important clinical considerations.

There is abundant literature on carpal tunnel syndrome because of the prevalence of this condition and because of the relative ease of study of the median nerve. Median nerve compression at the wrist is an archetype for other focal compression neuropathies. It also has unique features that distinguish it from other focal nerve compressions, such as the anatomic interrelationships of the nerve within the bony carpal canal and the effects of wrist posture and tendon movement on the median nerve.

Carpal tunnel syndrome is by definition a clinical condition manifested by signs and symptoms. Many people, if investigated in detail, exhibit subclinical evidence of median nerve dysfunction in the carpal tunnel. The clinician must be wary of relying solely on diagnostic tests that demonstrate subclinical pathology and that potentially lead to overdiagnosis and overtreatment of median nerve dysfunction.

The excellent clinical description by Kremer et al. (1953, 590–1) has not been surpassed:

The usual complaint is then of attacks of painful tingling in one or both hands at night, sufficient to wake the sufferer after a few hours' sleep. The pain and paraesthesiae are usually described as "burning" or "agonising," and a deep-seated ache may spread up the forearm to the elbow. The ache is severest on the inner aspect of the forearm and more rarely may be felt in muscles as high as the shoulder. With the pain and tingling there is a subjective feeling of uselessness in the fingers, which are sometimes described as swollen; yet on inspection little or no swelling is apparent. Relief may be obtained by hanging the arm out of bed or shaking or rubbing the hand; but, as symptoms increase, the patients often get out of bed and walk about until eased.

There is still no substitute for evaluating patients by taking a history and conducting a physical examination. The clinician must attend carefully to the timing, location, and nature of symptoms, distinguishing pains, paresthesias, and motor phenomena. Separation of carpal tunnel syndrome from other neurologic conditions, differential diagnosis in relation to other musculoskeletal disorders, and consideration of the possibility of an underlying medical condition all start with the initial clinical evaluation. Often the clinical examination is sufficient to yield a confident diagnosis of carpal tunnel syndrome and to guide initial conservative treatment without further laboratory, electrophysiologic, or imaging evaluation.

Carpal tunnel syndrome is a focal, usually chronic compression neuropathy. The pathophysiology of carpal tunnel syndrome is intriguingly complex. Important determinants include:

1. Individual variation in size and contents of the carpal tunnel.
2. Pathologic change that occurs in connective tissue within the carpal tunnel, such as edema and fibrosis of flexor synovium.
3. Variable pressure within the carpal tunnel, affected steadily by canal anatomy and connective tissue pathology and dynamically by changes in wrist posture and hand use and by shifts in distribution of body fluid.
4. Eventual chronic focal mechanical compression of the median nerve, leading first to damage in the myelin of large-caliber fibers.
5. Transient episodes of compression and ischemia of the median nerve, resulting in spontaneous firing of sensory fibers and evoking the intermittent paresthesias that are so characteristic of the syndrome.
6. Variable susceptibility to compression of individual fibers within the median nerve based on nerve fiber diameter and myelination and also, to some extent, on fascicular arrangement of the nerve; in myelinated fibers, conduction block occurs earlier than axonal interruption; small-caliber nerve fibers are relatively resistant to compression and ischemia.

Each of these aspects of pathophysiology is discussed in one or more of the chapters that follow. In every patient it is helpful to attempt to clarify the interaction of these mechanisms and to consider the pathophysiology of the patient's symptoms.

Since a syndrome is by definition a collection of signs and symptoms, strictly speaking, *symptomatic carpal tunnel syndrome* is redundant. There may be subclinical focal nerve pathology at the carpal tunnel, but *asymptomatic carpal tunnel syndrome* is nonexistent (or refers to that small group of patients who develop physical signs of carpal tunnel syndrome without ever becoming aware of the symptoms). Yet the pathogenesis of carpal tunnel syndrome begins before any symptoms develop. We have very little information about the range of carpal tunnel sizes in the population and about whether the risk of developing carpal tunnel syndrome varies with canal size. We know little about the cause or reversibility of pathology in the flexor tendon synovium.

The early pathologic changes in large myelinated fibers are often asymptomatic. Physiologic dysfunction of a portion of these fibers is often clinically undetectable. In many individuals, median nerve compression apparently may reach this stage, but may never proceed to become a clinical problem.

Methods for neurophysiologic investigation of carpal tunnel syndrome have become more and more sensitive and may detect abnormalities in large-caliber myelinated fibers before symptoms develop. Nerve conduction techniques will necessarily show occasional "false-negative" and/or "false-positive" results. Nerve conduction testing is a diagnostic aid but cannot replace clinical diagnostic judgment. Attributing an atypical assortment of sensorimotor symptoms in the upper limb to carpal tunnel syndrome based on nerve conduction tests but not on appropriate clinical evidence of the syndrome remains, unfortunately, a common error.

Understanding the pathophysiology of carpal tunnel syndrome helps in planning treatment and in evaluating the results of carpal tunnel surgery. In some patients the appearance of symptoms, especially the paresthesias from spontaneous neuronal firing, announces that the underlying pathology has reached a symptomatic stage, and surgical treatment eventually becomes necessary. In other patients, such as women who develop carpal tunnel syndrome during pregnancy, the early symptoms and the assumed underlying pathology are totally reversible.

In most patients who undergo carpal tunnel surgery, the symptoms are completely relieved after section of the flexor retinaculum, even though some asymptomatic pathologic changes in the median nerve may remain without eliciting symptoms.

Evidence of interruption of the axons of myelinated fibers or of dysfunction of small-caliber fibers is an indication for more aggressive therapy and also a clue that recovery of neuronal function may be gradual or incomplete following successful therapy.

We have emphasized both pathophysiologic and clinical findings. Analysis of patients from both a clinical and pathophysiologic viewpoint often helps in diagnosis of difficult cases and planning therapy.

REFERENCE

Kremer M, Gilliatt RW, Golding JSR, Wilson TG. Acroparaesthesiae in the carpal-tunnel syndrome. Lancet 1953; 2: 590–95.

1

Anatomy of the Median Nerve

Figure 1.1 depicts the formation, course, and branching of the median nerve. Thorough understanding of median neuropathies requires a detailed awareness of the anatomy of the median nerve. Knowledge of the relationships between the nerve and surrounding bone and connective tissues is important to the study of entrapment neuropathies. The newer imaging techniques, such as computed tomography (CT) and magnetic resonance imaging (MRI), are being applied to the median nerve so that topography of the nerve's relationships can now be studied noninvasively. Anomalous nerve courses and patterns of innervation sometimes cause atypical clinical presentations and can often be demonstrated by combining anatomic knowledge with clinical and laboratory testing. Particular anatomic arrangements of nerve fascicles may account for the clinical presentation of partial nerve injuries.

Sunderland (1978) reviews the anatomy of the nerve in exquisite detail, based on dissection of 200 cadaver arms.

MEDIAN NERVE FORMATION

The median nerve is formed from nerve roots C5 to T1, as shown in Figure 1.2. The C5, C6, and C7 roots contribute to the lateral cord of the brachial plexus, whereas the C8 and T1 roots contribute to the medial cord of the plexus. Fibers from the medial and lateral cords of the plexus join to form the median nerve.

A number of uncommon anomalies can affect the nerve roots and proximal median nerve (Kerr 1918; Kaplan and Spinner 1980). For example:

1. The median nerve may lack fibers from the C5 or T1 roots.
2. The median nerve and lateral and medial cords may follow a variety of patterns in relation to the axillary artery.
3. The connection from the lateral cord to the median nerve may consist of one or multiple discrete bundles.
4. The median and musculocutaneous nerves may unite by proximal anastomoses or even be fused.

1

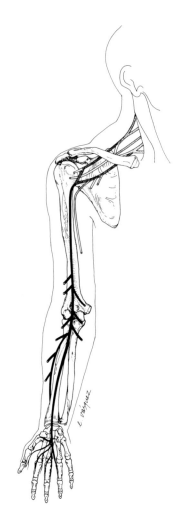

Figure 1.1 The median nerve.

MEDIAN NERVE BRANCHES

The median nerve gives off a number of motor branches in the forearm, as illustrated in Figure 1.3. Often more than one branch goes to an individual muscle. The number of branches per muscle may vary, and the order of branching is not constant (Sunderland 1978). Typically the initial branches, usually two to four, are to the pronator teres. Subsequent branches are to the flexor carpi radialis, the palmaris longus (this muscle is not always present), and the flexor digitorum superficialis.

In the antecubital space and forearm, nerve branches also supply elbow and radioulnar joints and the brachial artery.

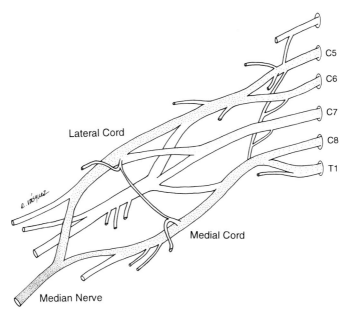

Figure 1.2 Formation of the median nerve from nerve roots C5 to T1 forming the lateral and medial cords of the brachial plexus.

Anterior Interosseous Nerve

The anterior interosseous nerve takes origin from the median nerve distal to the muscular branches in the forearm (Figure 1.4). The anterior interosseous

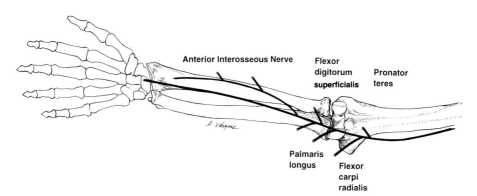

Figure 1.3 Motor branches of the median nerve in the forearm. The order of muscular branches and the number of branches per muscle vary among individuals.

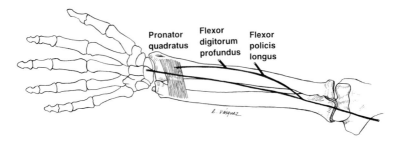

Figure 1.4 Motor branches of the anterior interosseous nerve.

nerve is a predominantly motor trunk that innervates the flexor pollicis longus, pronator quadratus, and part of the flexor digitorum profundus (FDP) muscles. The anterior interosseous nerve innervates the FDP for the index finger almost always, the FDP for the middle finger about half the time, and the FDP to the ring or little fingers rarely (Sunderland 1978). The ulnar nerve provides the remainder of the FDP innervation. The anterior interosseous nerve carries no cutaneous innervation; its deep sensory branches supply the radiocarpal and carpal-carpal joints and probably its forearm muscles.

Palmar Cutaneous Branch of the Median Nerve

The palmar cutaneous branch leaves the radial side of the median nerve 5 to 8 cm proximal to the distal wrist crease, runs parallel to the median nerve, crossing over the navicular tubercle, to reach the thenar eminence (Carroll and Green 1972; Sunderland 1978). This nerve is purely sensory, innervating the skin of the proximal palm and thenar eminence. These areas may receive overlapping innervation from the digital branches of the median nerve, the anterior branch of the lateral cutaneous nerve of the forearm, the superficial radial nerve, the medial cutaneous nerve of the forearm, and the ulnar nerve. Interruption of the palmar cutaneous branch does not always cause discernible sensory loss because of this overlapping pattern.

Hobbs et al. (1990) dissected the median palmar cutaneous nerves in the hands of 25 cadavers. The nerve was present and arose from the lateral aspect of the median nerve in all 25 hands. Although the nerve displayed a variety of branching patterns, no terminal branch extended more than 1 cm medial to a line drawn through the center of the middle finger. Figure 1.5 shows the typical extent of the terminal branches of the median palmar cutaneous nerve.

Recurrent Thenar Motor Branch of the Median Nerve

The three final branches of the median nerve take origin within or distal to the carpal tunnel. The recurrent thenar motor branch supplies the median-innervated thenar muscles. In the typical pattern, the recurrent motor branch supplies the abductor pollicis brevis, opponens pollicis, and flexor pollicis brevis.

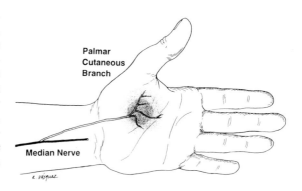

Figure 1.5 Palmar cutaneous branch of the median nerve. The *shaded area* shows the typical distribution of sensory cutaneous innervation. (Redrawn with permission of the publisher from Carroll RE, Green DP. The significance of the palmar cutaneous nerve at the wrist. Clin Orthop 1972; 83:24–28.)

However, such pattern occurs in only about one third of hands (Rowntree 1949). Figure 1.6 shows the distribution of the variations on this pattern. The most common variation is supply of the flexor pollicis brevis by the ulnar nerve or by both the median and ulnar nerves (Forrest 1967). Extremes of variation include ulnar supply of every thenar muscle and median supply of all hand intrinsic muscles. In the latter case, the rare *all median hand*, the innervation of those hand intrinsics that are normally ulnar innervated is via a Martin-Gruber anastomosis (Marinacci 1964a). Some of the variations may be explained by communications *(Riche-Cannieu anastomosis)* in the palm between the deep branch of the ulnar nerve and the median nerve and its branches (Figure 1.7) (Sunderland 1978; Kaplan and Spinner 1980). Mannerfelt (1966) and Falconer and Spinner (1985) dissected 19 hands and found six instances of Riche-Cannieu anastomosis. Harness and Sekeles (1971) found ulnar-median anastomoses in 27 of 35 hands and described a number of variations in the connections. Very rarely, an anastomotic branch from the radial nerve to the median nerve may innervate the abductor pollicis brevis, or the musculocutaneous nerve may contribute fibers to muscles also innervated by the median nerve (Marinacci 1964b; Schultz and Kaplan 1984).

Another rare pattern is for the median nerve to innervate the hypothenar muscles via an anomalous branch that arises from the median nerve in the carpal tunnel (Seradge and Seradge 1990).

Digital Nerves

Figure 1.8 illustrates the usual pattern of digital branches of the median nerve. The radial side of each finger is supplied by a "radial" proper digital nerve; the ulnar side of each finger by an "ulnar" proper digital nerve. The terminology is confusing because *ulnar* and *radial* in this context refer to the medial and lateral sides of the finger in these branches of the *median* nerve. At each web space, the proper digital nerves for adjacent fingers usually join to form a common digital nerve in the palm. Typically, the radial proper digital nerve of the thumb and first three common digital nerves arise from the median nerve.

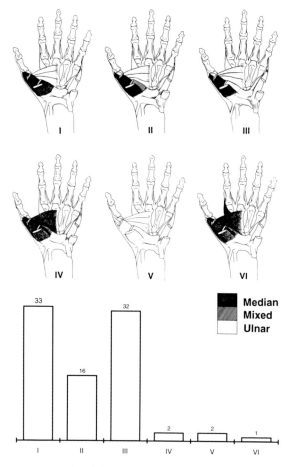

Figure 1.6 Variations in supply of the thenar muscles by the ulnar and median nerves. As shown by the bar graph, the classic pattern of median innervation of abductor pollicis brevis, opponens pollicis, and flexor pollicis brevis is present in only about one third of hands. (Redrawn with permission of the publisher and author from Rowntree T. Anomalous innervation of the hand muscles. J Bone Joint Surg 1949:31B:505–10.)

Each proper digital nerve carries cutaneous sensory fibers from the volar fingertip and from the ipsilateral half of the volar and lateral finger and distal dorsal finger. Those fibers from the dorsal aspect of the finger usually join the proper digital nerves proximal to the proximal interphalangeal joint, except for the thumb where the distal dorsal sensory fibers usually join the superficial radial nerve (Wallace and Coupland 1975). The digital nerves also carry sensory fibers from the finger joints and flexor tendons (Schultz et al. 1984; Pesson et al. 1991).

Sensory integrity of the tip of the thumb is very important to hand function, and surgeons have extensively studied the anatomy of the digital nerves to the

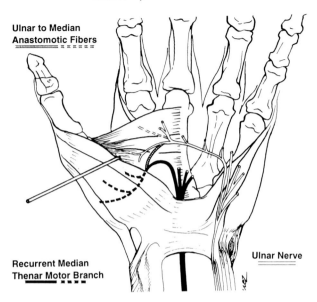

Ulnar to Median Anastomotic Fibers

Recurrent Median Thenar Motor Branch

Ulnar Nerve

Figure 1.7 Fibers may pass from ulnar to the median nerve in the palm via the Riche-Cannieu anastamosis. (Redrawn with permission of the publisher from Kaplan EB, Spinner M. Normal and anomalous innervation patterns in the upper extremity. In: Omer Jr GE, Spinner, M, eds. Management of peripheral nerve problems. Philadelphia: WB Saunders.

thumb to facilitate microscopic repair (Hirasawa et al. 1985). In the distal phalanx of the thumb, each proper digital nerve divides into three terminal branches, which are protected under subcutaneous tissue (Chow 1980).

Fibers from the ulnar and radial digital nerves may overlap at the fingertip so that damage to a single proper digital nerve may cause ipsilateral sensory loss on one side of the proximal finger but spare sensation on the fingertip (Dellon 1981).

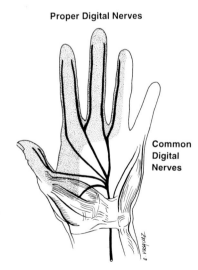

Proper Digital Nerves

Common Digital Nerves

Figure 1.8 The common digital nerves in the palm divide to form the proper digital nerves to each finger. The shaded area represents the usual area of median nerve cutaneous sensory innervation. The recurrent thenar motor branch of the median nerve is also shown in the diagram.

The median cutaneous sensory patterns have been mapped in man by careful study of patients with median, ulnar, or radial nerve injuries, using a camel hair brush to find the areas of sensory loss (Stopford 1918). Figure 1.9 shows the usual pattern and the limits of variation. The typical pattern is present in about three quarters of patients: The median digital nerves supply the palmar surfaces of the thumb, index, middle, and lateral one half of the ring fingers. The digital nerves also supply the dorsal tips of the index, middle, and lateral side of the ring finger at least as far proximally as the distal interphalangeal joints and sometimes over part of the middle phalanges.

Many individuals have variations from the usual sensory pattern. Frequent-

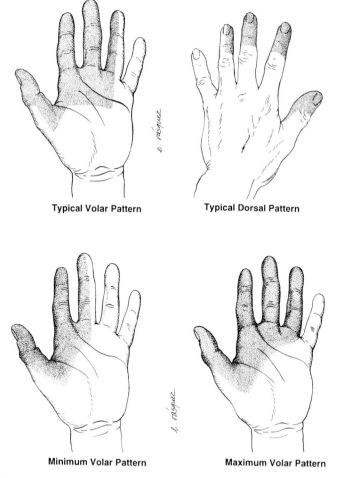

Typical Volar Pattern   **Typical Dorsal Pattern**

Minimum Volar Pattern   **Maximum Volar Pattern**

Figure 1.9 Variations of median cutaneous sensory innervation of the hands. (Redrawn with permission of the publisher from Stopford JSB. The variation in distribution of the cutaneous nerves of the hand and digits. J Anat 1918;53:14–25.)

ly, areas of innervation overlap, so that injury to an individual nerve causes an area of sensory loss smaller than predicted by classical anatomic charts. Crossover with the cutaneous innervation of the ulnar and superficial radial nerves is common.

The most common variation is supply of the lateral aspect of the ring finger by the ulnar nerve. At times this area has both median and ulnar innervation. In one cadaver study, 80% of palms showed a communication between the ulnar nerve and the median-innervated digital nerves, either the radial proper digital to the ring finger or the third common digital nerve (Figure 1.10) (Meals and Shaner 1983). This anastomosis explains the ulnar innervation of the lateral ring finger or even medial middle finger in some individuals.

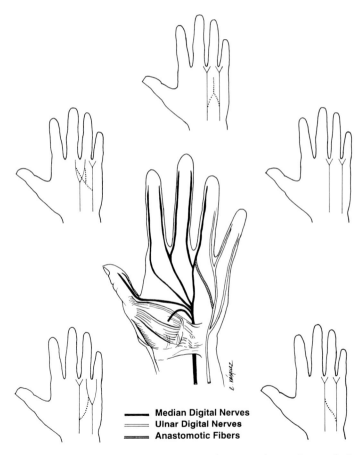

	Median Digital Nerves
	Ulnar Digital Nerves
	Anastomotic Fibers

Figure 1.10 Anastomotic fibers may communicate between the median and ulnar digital nerves. Examples of some variations are shown. (Reproduced with permission of the publisher from Meals RA, Shaner M. Variations in digital sensory patterns: a study of the ulnar nerve–median nerve palmar communicating branch. J Hand Surg 1983;8:411–14.

Another area of variation is the volar thumb, where radial overlap of the usual median territory is common (Fetrow 1970). Sensory innervation of the volar surface of the other digits via the superficial radial nerve is exceedingly rare (Bergman et al. 1970).

In the average median nerve, two thirds of the fascicular cross-sectional area is destined for the digital nerves (Sunderland 1978). On average a proper digital nerve is composed of 9 to 15 fascicles and contains 1,500 to 3,000 or more myelinated fibers (Bonnel et al. 1989).

Median Nerve Branches to the Lumbricals

The terminal motor branches of the median nerve typically innervate the lumbricals of the index and middle fingers, whereas the ulnar nerve innervates the lumbricals of the ring and little fingers (Sunderland 1978). The motor branch to the first lumbrical usually arises from the radial proper digital nerve of the index finger; the motor branch to the second lumbrical usually arises from the common digital nerve of the second intermetacarpal space (Schultz and Kaplan 1984). This pattern is found in about one half of hands. The most common variation is partial median innervation of the lumbrical of the ring finger. Rarer variations are median innervation of the lumbrical of the little finger and ulnar innervation of the lumbrical of the index finger.

Median Nerve Autonomic Innervation

The digital nerves also carry sudomotor and vasomotor sympathetic fibers to skin and blood vessels. There is wide variation in the relative contributions of ulnar and median nerves to the sympathetic supply of the superficial arterial arch of the palm (Meals and Shaner 1983). On the palmar surface of the hand, the cutaneous sensory distribution of the median nerve matches the cutaneous vaso-motor distribution of median sympathetic fibers (Woollard and Phillips 1932). The median sympathetic vasomotor pattern can be documented by thermography following local anesthetic nerve blocks. Colorplates 10.1, 16.2, and 16.4 are hand thermograms obtained after local anesthetic block of the median nerve. On the dorsum of the hand, the pattern of warming demonstrated by thermography after median nerve block matches the radial cutaneous sensory pattern; the thermo-gram of the dorsum of the hand is unaffected by radial nerve block (Verdugo, Campero, and Ochoa, unpublished).

Sweat glands are supplied by sympathetic sudomotor fibers that accompany sensory fibers. Fingerprinting followed by ninhydrin staining can be used to document cutaneous sympathetic sudomotor supply to the fingers. This technique can be combined with local anesthetic nerve blocks to document variations in cutaneous innervation. The results parallel those found by examining sensation in patients after nerve injuries (Fetrow 1970).

Table 1.1 summarizes the contributions of individual cervical nerve roots to

Table 1.1 Nerve root contributions to the median nerve

	Lateral Cord		Medial Cord	
	C6 Root	C7 Root	C8 Root	T1 Root
Muscular branches in the forearm				
Pronator teres	x	X		
Flexor carpi radialis	x	X	x	
Palmaris longus		x	X	x
Flexor digitorum superficialis		x	X	X
Anterior interosseous nerve branches				
Flexor pollicis longus		x	X	X
Flexor digitorum profundus		x	X	X
Pronator quadratus		x	X	X
Hand intrinsic muscles				
Abductor pollicis brevis			X	x
Opponens pollicis			X	x
Flexor pollicis brevis			X	X
Lumbricals		x	X	X

X = Major contributing roots.

x = Minor contributing roots.

(After Haymaker and Woodhall 1953.)

the innervation of each muscle supplied by the median nerve. Contributions vary from individual to individual. Kendall and McCreary (1983) discuss some of the disagreements among different authorities regarding the radicular supply of each muscle. Note that the medial cord of the brachial plexus from the C8 and T1 roots provides the motor supply of the thenar hand muscles and most of the motor supply to the anterior interosseous nerve. In contrast, the lateral cord of the brachial plexus—from the C5, C6, and C7 roots—provides motor fibers to pronator teres and flexor carpi radialis, and part of the motor supply to palmaris longus and finger flexors. The lateral cord is the usual pathway for median nerve sensory fibers supplying the skin of the hand.

TOPOGRAPHIC RELATIONSHIPS
Upper Arm

In the upper arm the median nerve travels with the brachial artery in a neurovascular bundle. The course is along the medial aspect of the arm and relatively superficial, particularly as the bundle leaves the axilla and again in the antecubital fossa. In the axilla the median nerve is near the ulnar and musculocutaneous nerves and the medial cutaneous nerves of the arm and the forearm. By midhumerus the median nerve-brachial artery bundle is well separated from these other nerves.

Antecubital Space and Proximal Forearm

The median nerve crosses the antecubital fossa to enter the proximal forearm. In doing so, it may pass under one or two fibrous arches, which are potential sites of nerve compression (see Figure 17.5) (Dellon 1986). Johnson et al. (1979) found at least one fibrous arch in 75% of cadaver arms. These relationships, discussed in more detail in the following paragraphs, are of particular interest in considering the pronator syndrome and other forms of median nerve compression in the forearm (see Chapter 17).

The Ligament of Struthers

In about 1% of the population, the median nerve enters the antecubital space by passing under a ligament running from the medial epicondyle and medial intermuscular septum to the distal anterior medial humerus (see Figure 17.7). When this ligament (the *ligament of Struthers*) is present, it usually attaches proximally to the humerus at an anomalous bony supracondylar spur 1 to 6 cm above the elbow. The supracondylar spur is present in less than 4% of the population and may vary in prominence (Kessel and Rang 1966). At times the spur is easily palpable; at the other extreme, the ligament may arise from the humerus without a visible spur (Suranyi 1983). Alternatively, the supracondylar spur may be present without a corresponding ligament (Dellon and Mackinnon 1987). When the ligament is present, the median nerve runs beneath it in a neurovascular bundle. The brachial artery may run within the bundle; alternatively, the brachial artery may divide proximal to the bundle so that only the ulnar artery runs with the median nerve under the ligament (Gessini et al. 1983).

Lacertus Fibrosus

The median nerve passes through the antecubital space beneath the lacertus fibrosus (also called the aponeurosis of the biceps brachii), a fascial band that runs from the biceps tendon medially toward the proximal ulna (see Figure 17.6) (Martinelli et al. 1982). The lacertus fibrosus is continuous with the origin of the humeral head of the pronator teres muscle.

Humeral Origin of Pronator Teres

The relationship of the median nerve to the pronator teres muscle is variable (Beaton and Anson 1939; Dellon 1986; Dellon and Mackinnon 1987). One source of variation depends on the site of origin of the humeral head of the pronator teres. In the common pattern, the pronator teres originates at the medial epicondyle or within 2 cm of it, and the median nerve remains uniformly cylindrical as it passes beneath the humeral head of the pronator.

One variant is origin of the pronator teres 2 cm or more proximal to the epicondyle (Dellon and Mackinnon 1987). In this configuration the fascial edge of the pronator teres crosses the median nerve proximal to the elbow flexion crease so that the nerve is potentially compressed with elbow extension or forearm pronation. Dellon (1986) found this variant in 11 of 64 cadavers studied; when this variant was present, there was sometimes a groove or segmental narrowing in the median nerves where the pronator mass crossed.

Heads of Pronator Teres

Typically, the median nerve passes between the deep (ulnar) head and superficial (humeral) head of the pronator teres. Possible variations include absence of the deep head, passage of the nerve deep to both heads, or penetration of the nerve through the superficial head. In one series, only 83% of cadaver arms showed the typical pattern (Beaton and Anson 1939).

Flexor Digitorum Superficialis

Once past the pronator teres, the median nerve courses deep to the flexor digitorum superficialis, which also may vary in its origin. Along this course many individuals have an idiosyncratic arrangement of fibrous bands that may arise from the pronator teres, flexor carpi radialis, and flexor digitorum superficialis muscles and that have the potential for nerve compression (see Figure 17.5) (Johnson and Spinner 1989).

Forearm—Anterior Interosseous Nerve

The anterior interosseous nerve originates from the median nerve. In over 90% of people the branching occurs distal to the pronator teres, 5 to 8 cm distal to the lateral epicondyle (Spinner 1970; Chidgey and Szabo 1989). If the branching occurs proximal to the pronator teres, the anterior interosseous and median nerves usually remain parallel in their course past the heads of pronator teres (Megele 1988).

The anterior interosseous nerve may be crossed in the forearm by several anatomic structures: an accessory head of the flexor pollicis longus (Gantzer's muscle; see Figure 17.3), ulnar collateral vessels, an accessory muscle from the flexor digitorum superficialis to the flexor pollicis longus, the deep tendinous head of the pronator teres, or a fibrous arch (Spinner and Schreiber 1969). The anterior interosseous nerve may originate from either the posterior or the radial aspect of the median nerve and is more susceptible to compression when originating from the radial aspect (Dellon 1986).

Distal Forearm

In the forearm the median nerve is sheltered by the flexor digitorum superficialis until the nerve is about 5 cm proximal to the wrist (Sunderland 1978).

The Carpal Tunnel

Robbins (1963) reviewed the anatomy of the carpal tunnel in detail based on dissection of seven cadavers. In vivo data on carpal tunnel anatomy is now available from CT (Zucker-Pinchoff et al. 1981; Cone et al. 1983; Jessurun et al. 1987) and MRI (Middleton et al. 1987; Mesgarzadeh et al. 1989; Zeiss et al. 1989) studies (see Figures 1.11–1.13).

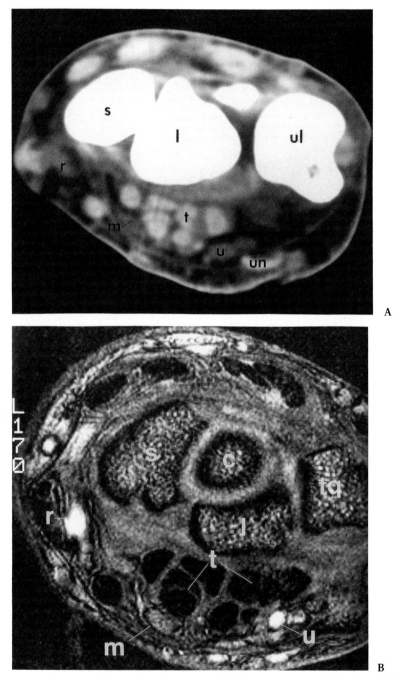

Figure 1.11 Normal CT (**A**) and MR (**B**) images of the proximal carpal tunnel (right hand, palm down, thumb to the left). *c*, capitate; *l*, lunate; *m*, median nerve; *r*, radial artery; *s*, scaphoid; *t*, flexor tendons; *tq*, triquetrum; *u*, ulnar artery; *ul*, ulna; *un*, ulnar nerve. (Images courtesy of Dr. Stephen F. Quinn.)

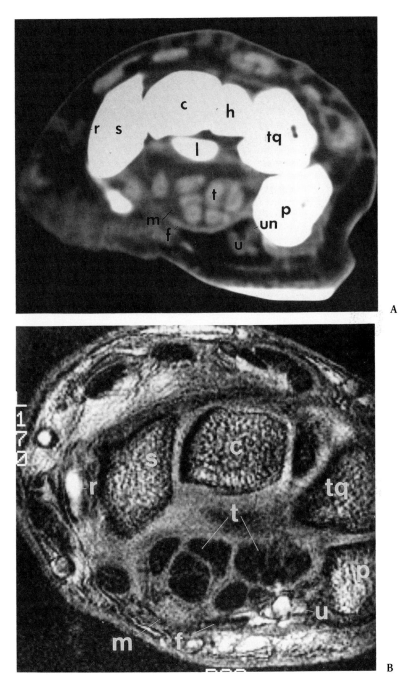

Figure 1.12 Normal CT (**A**) and MR (**B**) images of the midcarpal tunnel (right hand, palm down, thumb to the left). *c*, capitate; *f*, flexor retinaculum; *h*, hamate; *l*, lunate; *m*, median nerve; *p*, pisiform; *r*, radial artery; *s*, scaphoid; *t*, flexor tendons; *tq*, triquetrum; *u*, ulnar artery; *un*, ulnar nerve. (Images courtesy of Dr. Stephen F. Quinn.)

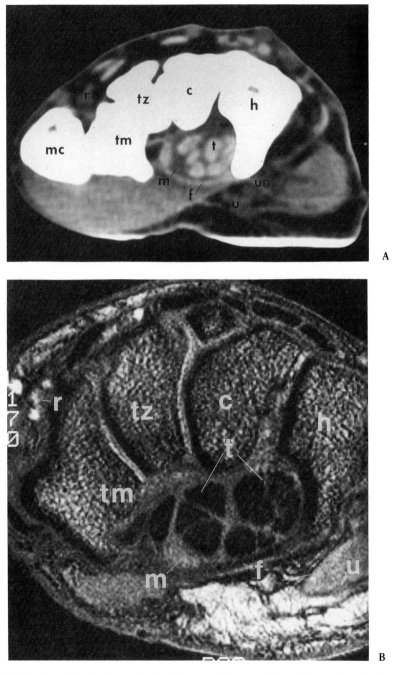

Figure 1.13 Normal CT (**A**) and MR (**B**) images of the distal carpal tunnel at the level of the hook of the hamate (right hand, palm down, thumb to the left). *c,* capitate; *f,* flexor retinaculum; *h,* hamate; *m,* median nerve; *mc,* first metacarpal; *r,* radial artery; *t,* flexor tendons; *tm,* trapezium; *tz,* trapezoid; *u,* ulnar artery; *un,* ulnar nerve. (Images courtesy of Dr. Stephen F. Quinn.)

Carpal Bones

The tunnel is formed by the eight carpal bones and is roofed by the flexor retinaculum or transverse carpal ligament. The bones form a roughly C-shaped arcade in two sets of four bones. Proximally, the four bones, naming from radial side to ulnar side, are the scaphoid (navicular), lunate, triquetrum, and pisiform. The volar portion of the lunate projects into the tunnel. The distal four bones, from radial to ulnar, are the trapezium and trapezoid (alternative names—greater and lesser multangular), capitate, and hamate. The bones are covered and joined by ligaments on their dorsal and volar surfaces.

Cailliet (1982) provides a clear discussion of the anatomy of hand and wrist bones and ligaments that is important to understanding musculoskeletal hand disorders other than median neuropathies.

Flexor Retinaculum

The flexor retinaculum (also known as the transverse carpal ligament) attaches to the hook of the hamate and the pisiform on the ulnar side of the hand and to the navicular tubercle, trapezium, and sometimes the radial styloid on the radial side to close the oval-shaped tunnel. The proximal border of the flexor retinaculum aligns roughly with the distal wrist crease. The flexor retinaculum extends distally to the bases of the metacarpals, where it blends into the palmar fascia. The flexor retinaculum ranges from 1 to 2 mm in thickness. Its greatest thickness is over the distal two thirds of the capitate. At this point, 2 to 2.5 cm from its proximal origin, the tunnel has its smallest cross-sectional area. Proximally, the attachment of the flexor retinaculum to the pisiform allows for intermittent laxity of the ligament because the pisiform is a mobile, sesamoid bone (Cailliet, 1982). The pisiform becomes fixed when the flexor carpi ulnaris tendon is taut. Distally, the flexor retinaculum maintains more constant tension. Zbrodowski and Gajisin (1988) describe additional details of the anatomy and blood supply of the flexor retinaculum.

Flexor Tendons

Dorsally, the four tendons of the flexor digitorum profundus overlie the carpal bones. The four tendons of the flexor digitorum superficialis occupy the volar, medial portion of the tunnel. The flexor pollicis longus tendon is in the volar, lateral position. The tendon of the flexor carpi radialis adjoins the dorsal lateral border of the tunnel; the flexor retinaculum divides as it makes its radial attachments to form a separate passage outside the carpal tunnel for this tendon.

Median Nerve in the Carpal Tunnel

The median nerve is normally just dorsal to the flexor retinaculum, superficial to the flexor pollicis longus tendon laterally and the flexor digitorum superficialis tendons medially. As the nerve enters the tunnel, it is shaped as a flattened ellipse with its anterior-posterior diameter roughly one half of its medial-lateral diameter (Tanzer 1959; Middleton et al. 1987). Its dimensions may increase slightly between the proximal and distal ends of the tunnel.

A very unusual occurrence is for a loop of the median nerve to leave the nerve in the carpal tunnel, pierce the flexor retinaculum, then rejoin the nerve distally (Davlin et al. 1991).

Recurrent Thenar Motor Branch of the Median Nerve

The recurrent motor branch to the thenar muscles varies in its departure from the median nerve and in its relationship to the flexor retinaculum (Figure 1.14) (Poisel 1974; Lanz 1977; Falconer and Spinner 1985). The recurrent motor branch typically leaves the median nerve distal to the flexor retinaculum, then curves back to reach the thenar muscles. However, the recurrent motor branch may leave the median nerve within the carpal tunnel, then either pierce the flexor retinaculum or cross the distal edge of the flexor retinaculum before curving back to the muscles. The origin of this branch usually, but not invariably, is from the radial side of the median nerve. Commonly, a single recurrent motor branch divides into three terminal branches to the abductor pollicis brevis, opponens

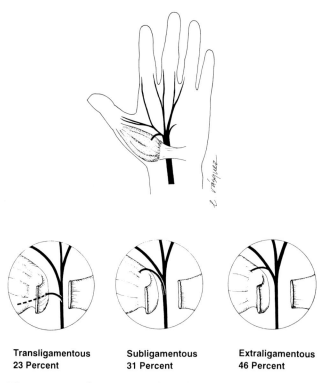

| Transligamentous | Subligamentous | Extraligamentous |
| 23 Percent | 31 Percent | 46 Percent |

Figure 1.14   The recurrent thenar motor branch varies in its course. The three most common patterns are shown. (Redrawn with permission of the publisher from Lanz U. Anatomical variations of the median nerve in the carpal tunnel. J Hand Surg 1977;2:44–53; incidence data from Poisel 1974.

pollicis, and flexor pollicis brevis; however, a number of variations are known (Lanz 1977; Mumford et al. 1987). Examples of rare anomalies are a pair of motor branches and a proximal accessory motor branch originating from the median nerve proximal to the carpal tunnel. Accessory thenar motor branches may also arise distally in the tunnel.

Variations in Canal Contents

A number of variations in the anatomy of the contents of the carpal tunnel are known (Tountas et al. 1987). Incidence of these variations differs from series to series and is, as expected, higher in cadaver studies than in surgical series, because the former allow a more thorough search for variations.

Extra structures within the tunnel, or anomalous arrangements of normal structures, may compromise volume available for the median nerve and increase the possibility of nerve compression. A persistent median artery may enter the tunnel with the median nerve, and at times, the nerve divides around the artery. The lumbrical muscles typically originate off the flexor digitorum profundus tendons distal to the tunnel, but on occasion, lumbrical muscles may be within the tunnel. Tendons of flexor digitorum superficialis or flexor pollicis longus occasionally interpose between the median nerve and flexor retinaculum. Chapter 6 reviews anomalous contents of the carpal canal that have been reported in patients with carpal tunnel syndrome.

Digital Nerve Relationships

Sunderland (1978) and Schultz and Kaplan (1984) provide detailed descriptions of the courses of the digital nerves. The two medial common digital branches of the median nerve travel into the palm between metacarpals accompanied by flexor tendons and blood vessels. At the metacarpal heads, a "digital tunnel" is formed by deep and superficial metacarpal ligaments connecting adjoining metacarpals. The digital nerves are particularly vulnerable to entrapment or traumatic injury at this point. In the fingers, each proper digital nerve runs in a neurovascular bundle with the digital artery and a small venous plexus lateral to the tendon sheath (Eaton 1968).

INTRANEURAL ANATOMY

The median nerve has the histologic arrangement typical of a peripheral nerve (Figure 1.15) (Sunderland 1991). The nerve consists of multiple nerve fiber fascicles loosely bound by the collagenous epineurium. An extensive network of arterioles, venules, and lymphatics provides circulation within the epineurium. In the median nerve the ratio of connective tissue to neural tissue varies, so that fascicles may occupy from 25% to 71% of the cross-sectional area of the nerve (Sunderland 1978). This ratio changes from person to person and also along the course of an individual nerve.

Each fascicle is encased in a tighter cellular and connective tissue sheath, the

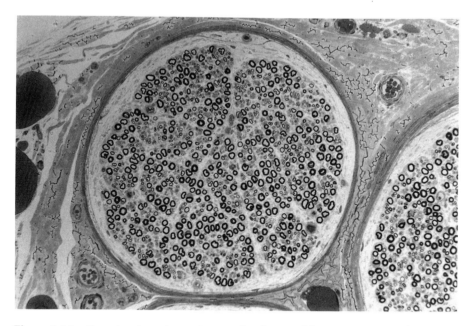

Figure 1.15 Cross section photomicrograph of normal human nerve trunk, showing abundant large- and small-caliber myelinated fibers scattered randomly in the endoeurium. Unmyelinated fibers are not properly discerned by optic microscopy. The structure of endoneurial capillaries appears normal. A perineurial sheath defines the fascicle. Maximum diameter of myelinated fibers = 15 μm.

perineurium. Capillaries are the chief blood vessels within the fascicular endoneurium. Sunderland (1945, 1978) provides extensive data on the intraneural topography of median nerve fascicles. Figure 1.16 is an example of the fascicular anatomy of the nerve shortly before its terminal branching. Sunderland (1945, 1978) and Bonnel et al. (1980, Bonnel 1981) found abundant intermingling of fascicles as the nerve courses from neck to hand and variation in the number of fascicles along the course of the nerve. Sunderland assumed that these fascicular changes implied extensive nerve fiber crossover.

Sunderland's description of intraneural anatomy is based on serial sections of a single median nerve that do not allow tracing of individual nerve fibers along the fascicles. A computer-aided study of serial sections of 30 median nerves suggests that fascicular integrity is maintained over long portions of the nerve (Watchmaker et al. 1991). Microelectrode studies of median and ulnar nerve function suggest that despite interfascicular connections, each fascicle maintains a substantial degree of independence in fiber contents. Tactile stimulation of the fingers elicits electrical responses in individual fascicles at the wrist corresponding to the sensory distribution of single or adjacent digital nerves (Hagbarth et al. 1970). Microstimulation of median nerve fascicles in the distal upper arm shows

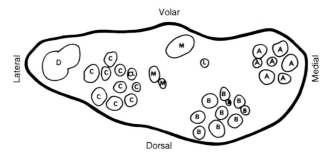

Figure 1.16 Fascicular anatomy of the median nerve at the distal end of the carpal tunnel. *A,* cutaneous fibers from the third interspace; *B,* cutaneous fibers from the second interspace; *C,* cutaneous fibers from the first interspace; *D,* cutaneous fibers from the radial side of the thumb; *L,* lumbrical fibers; *M,* thenar muscle fibers. (Reprinted with permission of the publishers from Sunderland S. The intraneural topography of the radial, median and ulnar nerves. Brain 1945;68:243–98; and Sunderland S. The median nerve. Anatomical and physiological considerations. In: Nerves and nerve injuries. 2nd ed. Edinburgh: Churchill Livingstone, 1978; 674.)

that most of the cutaneous sensory fibers within a fascicle at this level innervate the cutaneous territory of a single digital nerve (Schady et al. 1983; Marchettini et al. 1990). Much of the organization of the nerve into distinct motor and sensory territories occurs at the level of the brachial plexus, rather than through interfascicular connections.

The fascicles destined for a nerve branch are distinctly separate from other fascicles for some distance before actual branching occurs. For example, at the level of the cords of the brachial plexus, fascicles containing fibers for the anterior interosseous nerve are distinct from those pertaining to the rest of the median nerve. (Sunderland 1945). The fascicles destined for the anterior interosseous nerve run on the dorsal medial aspect of the median nerve as it travels through the antecubital space, and these fascicles can be microdissected free as a nerve bundle with its own epineurium separate from the remainder of the median nerve 93 mm or more proximal to the medial humeral epicondyle (Jabaley et al. 1980).

Analysis of distal partial nerve injuries supports the anatomic and microelectrode data on fascicular arrangement (Perotto and Delagi 1979). There is much individual variation in the arrangement of fascicles within the nerve. For example, in partial nerve injuries at the wrist studied by Perotto and Delagi (1979), fascicles to lumbricals appeared more dorsally located than predicted by Sunderland. Therefore, it is difficult to predict the nature of the neurologic deficit caused by injury to only a portion of the nerve (Bonnel et al. 1980).

At first glance, this intraneural detail seems of little practical import; however, variations in fascicular anatomy are among the factors that determine the probability of neural regeneration after transection and suture. In theory, the arrangement of fascicles and connective tissue within the nerve has an effect on the nerve's susceptibility to compression, but we are unaware of data linking individual variations in intraneural topography to the risk of development of carpal tunnel syndrome or other compression neuropathies in humans.

VASCULAR SUPPLY OF THE MEDIAN NERVE

In the axilla and upper arm, the median nerve receives its blood supply from the accompanying axillary and brachial arteries. In the forearm and hand, the vascular supply is variable but fits into three basic patterns (Pecket et al. 1973). The common pattern, found in 70% of cadavers studied, is for the radial and ulnar arteries to supply the median nerve via multiple anastomotic branches that feed a small artery adjoining the anterior surface of the nerve. In the palm, the nerve and its branches receive blood from the superficial arterial arch.

In 10% of cadavers, a persistent median artery arises from the brachial artery and accompanies the median nerve in the forearm and through the carpal tunnel. The median artery is usually present only in the fetus. When a well-developed median artery persists, anastomoses between the radial and ulnar arteries are poorly developed, and the superficial palmar arterial arch is absent.

Some 20% of cadavers exhibit an intermediate pattern: The median artery is present but often incompletely developed, and the superficial palmar arch and other contributions from the radial and ulnar arteries are also present.

VARIATIONS OF MEDIAN NERVE BRANCHING
Martin-Gruber Anastomosis

The most common, clinically relevant variation in hand and forearm in-innervation is crossing of nerve fibers from the median nerve to the ulnar nerve in the forearm (Figure 1.17), which is commonly called the Martin-Gruber anastomosis. Incidence has been reported to be 10% to 40% of median nerves (Thomson 1893; Mannerfelt, 1966). This anastomosis was present in 15% of normal fetuses (Srinivasan and Rhodes 1981). The crossing fibers may supply hypothenar, thenar, or interosseous muscles; the adductor pollicis and first dorsal interosseous are the muscles most likely to receive innervation via a Martin-Gruber anastomosis (Spinner 1978). Usually the crossing fibers originate from the distal anterior interosseus nerve rather than from the median nerve proper, but a number of other branching patterns are described:

1. branching from the proximal anterior interosseous nerve to the ulnar nerve
2. branching directly from median to ulnar nerve
3. branching from the median branch to flexor digitorum superficialis
4. branching from the anterior interosseous nerve to the branch of the ulnar nerve innervating the flexor digitorum profundus
5. branching from the anterior interosseous nerve, then bifurcating to join the ulnar nerve at more than one site (Thomson 1893; Sriniva-san and Rhodes 1981)

A survey of the incidence of the Martin-Gruber anastomosis using nerve

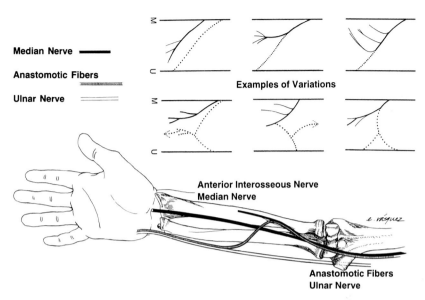

Figure 1.17 The fibers of Martin-Gruber anastomosis carry fibers from the median nerve to the ulnar nerve in the forearm. In the most common pattern, the median nerve fibers travel with the anterior interosseous nerve. A number of other known variations are shown. (Redrawn with permission of the publisher from Srinivasan R, Rhodes J. The median-ulnar anastomosis (Martin-Gruber) in normal and congenitally abnormal fetuses. Arch Neurol 1981;38:418–19.)

conduction tests suggests that the anomaly is inherited as an autosomal dominant trait in some families (Crutchfield and Gutmann 1980).

The Martin-Gruber anastomosis usually carries motor but not sensory fibers (Valls-Sole 1991). However, in one case, sensory conduction studies with stimulation of the middle or little finger and recording over the median and ulnar nerves showed that some sensory fibers from both of these fingers left the hand with the ulnar nerve and crossed to the median nerve in the forearm (Santoro et al. 1983).

The Martin-Gruber anastomosis may lead to unusual sparing of muscles after proximal ulnar nerve injuries or, conversely, to unexpectedly widespread denervation after proximal median nerve injuries (Marinacci 1964a). For example, a patient with leprosy developed a combination of complete distal median and proximal ulnar neuropathies (Brandsma et al. 1986). Median-innervated thenar muscles and ulnar-innervated forearm muscles were paretic, but, because of a Martin-Gruber anastomosis, there was sparing of some intrinsic hand muscles, whose nerve fibers crossed the antecubital space with the median nerve and then crossed the wrist with the ulnar nerve.

Electromyographic detection of the Martin-Gruber anastomosis and its potential effects in the presence of carpal tunnel syndrome are covered in Chapter 7.

Ulnar-to-Median Crossovers

Ulnar-to-median crossovers in the forearm are extremely rare. Marinacci (1964b) described a case of median nerve transection in the forearm with denervation of median-innervated forearm muscles but preservation of all hand intrinsic muscles. Nerve stimulation showed that nerve fibers destined for thenar muscles traveled with the ulnar nerve at the elbow but crossed the wrist at the usual location for the median nerve. Ulnar-to-median anastomosis in the forearm has also been noted as an incidental finding on nerve conduction studies (Streib 1979).

At times, minor anomalies can be clarified by clever use of nerve blocks and nerve conduction testing. Hopf (1990) reported a case of ulnar-to-median sensory crossover in the forearm. After ulnar nerve block at the elbow, the patient had sensory loss not only in the little finger and ulnar side of the ring finger but also in the radial side of the ring finger and ulnar side of the middle finger. Electrical stimulation of the digital nerves on the radial side of the ring finger or ulnar side of the middle finger elicited a sensory nerve action potential over the median nerve at the wrist (but not in the antecubital space) and over the ulnar nerve at the elbow (but not at the wrist). The patient had no evidence of crossover of motor fibers.

Collision studies of sensory conduction in another patient with the same anomalous sensory pattern suggested that in some patients the nerve fibers to the radial side of the ring finger and ulnar side of the middle finger took a different anomalous course, traveling with the ulnar nerve across the wrist and through the forearm (Valls-Sole 1991).

Ulnar-to-median communications in the palm, including digital nerve connections and crossover of motor fibers via Riche-Cannieu anastomosis, have been discussed earlier in this chapter.

REFERENCES

Beaton LE, Anson BJ. The relation of the median nerve to the pronator teres muscle. Anat Rec 1939;7:23–26.

Bergman FO, Blom SEG, Senström SJ. Radical excision of a fibro-fatty proliferation of the median nerve, with no neurological loss symptoms. Plast Reconstr Surg 1970;46:375–80.

Bonnel F. Fascicular organization of the peripheral nerves. Int J Microsurg 1981;3:85–92.

Bonnel F, Foucher G, Saint-Andre J-M. Histologic structure of the palmar digital nerves of the hand and its application to nerve grafting. J Hand Surg 1989;14A:874–81.

Bonnel F, Mailhe P, Allieu Y, Rabischong P. Bases anatomiques de la chirurgie fasciculaire du nerf médian au poignet. Ann Chir 1980;9:707–10.

Brandsma JW, Birke JA, Sims DS Jr. The Martin-Gruber innervated hand. J Hand Surg 1986;11A:536–39.

Cailliet R. Hand pain and impairment. 3rd ed. Philadelphia: FA Davis, 1982.

Carroll RE, Green DP. The significance of the palmar cutaneous nerve at the wrist. Clin Orthop 1972;83:24–28.

Chidgey LK, Szabo RM. Anterior interosseous nerve palsy. In: Szabo RM, ed. Nerve compression syndromes: diagnosis and treatment. Thorofare, NJ: Slack, 1989;153–62.

Chow SP. Digital nerves in the terminal phalangeal region of the thumb. Hand 1980;12:193–96.

Cone RO, Sabo R, Resnick D, Gelberman R, Taleisnik J, Gilula LA. Computed tomography of the normal soft tissues of the wrist. Invest Radiol 1983;18:546–51.

Crutchfield CA, Gutmann L. Hereditary aspects of median-ulnar nerve communications. J Neurol Neurosurg Psychiatry 1980;43:53–55.

Davlin LB, Aulicino PL, Bergfield TG. Sensory neural loop of the median nerve at the carpal tunnel. J Hand Surg 1991;16A:863–65.

Dellon AL. Evaluation of sensibility and re-education of sensation in the hand. Baltimore: Williams & Wilkins, 1981.

Dellon AL. Musculotendinous variations about the medial humeral epicondyle. J Hand Surg 1986;11B:175–81.

Dellon AL, Mackinnon SE. Musculoaponeurotic variations along the course of the median nerve in the proximal forearm. J Hand Surg 1987;12B:359–63.

Eaton RG. The digital neurovascular bundle. Clin Orthop 1968;61:176–85.

Falconer D, Spinner M. Anatomic variations in the motor and sensory supply of the thumb. Clin Orthop 1985;195:83–96.

Fetrow KO. Practical and important variations in sensory nerve supply to the hand. Hand 1970;2:178–84.

Forrest WJ. Motor innervation of human thenar and hypothenar muscles in 25 hands: a study combining electromyography and percutaneous nerve stimulation. Can J Surg 1967;10:196–99.

Gessini L, Jandolo B, Pietrangeli A. Entrapment neuropathies of the median nerve at and above the elbow. Surg Neurol 1983;19:112–16.

Hagbarth K-E, Hongell A, Hallin RG, Torebjörk HE. Afferent impulses in median nerve fascicles evoked by tactile stimuli of the human hand. Brain Res 1970;24:423–42.

Harness D, Sekeles E. The double anastomotic innervation of thenar muscles. J Anat 1971;109:461–66.

Haymaker W, Woodhall B. Peripheral nerve injuries. 2nd ed. Philadelphia: WB Saunders, 1953.

Hirasawa Y, Sakakida K, Tokioka T, Ohta Y. An investigation of the digital nerves of the thumb. Clin Orthop 1985;198:191–96.

Hobbs RA, Magnussen PA, Tonkin MA. Palmar cutaneous branch of the median nerve. J Hand Surg 1990;15A:38–43.

Hopf HC. Forearm ulnar-to-median nerve anastomosis of sensory axons. Muscle Nerve 1990;13:654–56.

Jabaley ME, Wallace WH, Heckler FR. Internal topography of major nerves of the forearm and hand: a current view. J Hand Surg 1980;5:1–18.

Jessurun W, Hillen B, Zonneveld F, Huffstadt AJ, Beks JW, Overbeek W. Anatomical relations in the carpal tunnel: a computed tomographic study. J Hand Surg 1987;12B:64–67.

Johnson RK, Spinner M. Median nerve compression in the forearm: the pronator tunnel syndrome. In: Szabo RM, ed. Nerve compression syndromes: diagnosis and treatment. Thorofare, NJ: Slack, 1989;137–52.

Johnson RK, Spinner M, Shrewsbury MM. Median nerve entrapment syndrome in the proximal forearm. J Hand Surg 1979;4:48–51.

Kaplan EB, Spinner M. Normal and anomalous innervation patterns in the upper extremity. In: Omer GE Jr, Spinner M, eds. Management of peripheral nerve problems. Philadelphia: WB Saunders, 1980;75–99.

Kendall FP, McCreary EK. Muscles testing and function. 3rd ed. Baltimore: Williams & Wilkins, 1983.

Kerr AT. The brachial plexus of nerves in man, the variations in its formation and branches. Am J Anat 1918;23:285–395.

Kessel L, Rang M. Supracondylar spur of the humerus. J Bone Joint Surg 1966;48B:765–69.

Lanz U. Anatomical variations of the median nerve in the carpal tunnel. J Hand Surg 1977;2:44–53.

Mannerfelt L. Studies on the hand in ulnar nerve paralysis. Acta Orthop Scand 1966;S87:1–176.

Marchettini P, Cline M, Ochoa JL. Innervation territories for touch and pain afferents of single fascicles of the human ulnar nerve. Brain 1990;113:1491–1500.

Marinacci AA. Diagnosis of "all median hand." Bull Los Angeles Neurol Soc 1964a;29:191–97.

Marinacci AA. The problem of unusual anomalous innervation of hand muscles. Bull Los Angeles Neurol Soc 1964b;29:133–42.

Martinelli P, Gabellini AS, Poppi M, Gallassi R, Pozzati E. Pronator syndrome due to thickened bicipital aponeurosis. J Neurol Neurosurg Psychiatry 1982;45:181–82.

Meals RA, Shaner M. Variations in digital sensory patterns: a study of the ulnar nerve–median nerve palmar communicating branch. J Hand Surg 1983;8:411–14.

Megele R. Anterior interosseous nerve syndrome with atypical nerve course in relation to the pronator teres. Acta Neurochir (Wien) 1988;91:144–46.

Mesgarzadeh M, Schneck CD, Bonakdarpour A. Carpal tunnel: MR imaging part I: normal anatomy. Radiology 1989;171:743–48.

Middleton WD, Kneeland JB, Kellman GM, Cates JD, Sanger JR, Jesmanowicz A, Froncisz W, Hyde JS. MR imaging of the carpal tunnel: normal anatomy and preliminary findings in the carpal tunnel syndrome. AJR 1987;148:307–16.

Mumford J, Morecraft R, Blair WF. Anatomy of the thenar branch of the median nerve. J Hand Surg 1987;12A:361–65.

Pecket P, Gloobe H, Nathan H. Variations in the arteries of the median nerve. With special considerations on the ischemic factor in the carpal tunnel syndrome (CTS). Clin Orthop 1973;97:144–47.

Perotto AO, Delagi EF. Funicular localization in partial median nerve injury at the wrists. Arch Phys Med Rehabil 1979;60:165–69.

Pesson CM, Finney TP, Depaolo CJ, Dabezies EJ, Zimny ML. Anatomical demonstration of the nerve-supply to the flexor tendon. J Hand Surg 1991;16B:92–93.

Poisel S. Ursprung und Verlauf des Ramus muscularis des Nervus digitalis palmaris communis I (N. medianus). Chir praxis 1974;18:471–74.

Robbins H. Anatomical study of the median nerve in the carpal tunnel and etiologies of the carpal-tunnel syndrome. J Bone Joint Surg 1963;45A:953–66.

Rowntree T. Anomalous innervation of the hand muscles. J Bone Joint Surg 1949;31B:505–10.

Santoro L, Rosato R, Caruso G. Median-ulnar nerve communications: electrophysiological demonstration of motor and sensory fibre cross-over. J Neurol 1983;229:227–35.

Schady W, Ochoa JL, Torebjörk HE, Chen LS. Peripheral projections of fascicles in the human median nerve. Brain 1983;106:745–60.

Schultz RJ, Kaplan EB. Nerve supply to the muscles and skin of the hand. In: Spinner M, ed. Kaplan's functional and surgical anatomy of the hand. 3rd ed. Philadelphia: JB Lippincott, 1984;222–43.

Schultz RJ, Krishnamurthy S, Johnston AD. A gross anatomic and histologic study of the innervation of the proximal interphalangeal joint. J Hand Surg 1984;9A:669–74.

Seradge H, Seradge E. Median innervated hypothenar muscle: anomalous branch of median nerve in the carpal tunnel. J Hand Surg 1990;15A:356–59.

Spinner M. The anterior interosseous-nerve syndrome, with special attention to its variations. J Bone Joint Surg 1970;52A:84–94.

Spinner M. Injuries to the major branches of peripheral nerves of the forearm. 2nd ed. Philadelphia: WB Saunders, 1978.

Spinner M, Schreiber SN. Anterior interosseous-nerve paralysis as a complication of supracondylar fractures of the humerus in children. J Bone Joint Surg 1969;51A:1584–90.

Srinivasan R, Rhodes J. The median-ulnar anastomosis (Martin-Gruber) in normal and congenitally abnormal fetuses. Arch Neurol 1981;38:418–19.

Stopford JSB. The variation in distribution of the cutaneous nerves of the hand and digits. J Anat 1918;53:14–25.

Streib EW. Ulnar-to-median nerve anastomosis in the forearm: electromyographic studies. Neurology 1979;29:1534–37.

Sunderland S. The intraneural topography of the radial, median and ulnar nerves. Brain 1945;68:243–98.

Sunderland S. The median nerve. Anatomical and physiological considerations. In: Nerves and nerve injuries. 2nd ed. Edinburgh: Churchill Livingstone, 1978;656–90.

Sunderland S. Nerve injuries and their repair. Edinburgh: Churchill Livingstone, 1991.

Suranyi L. Median nerve compression by Struther's ligament. J Neurol Neurosurg Psychiatry 1983;46:1047–49.

Tanzer RC. The carpal-tunnel syndrome. J Bone Joint Surg 1959;41A:626–34.

Thomson A. Third annual report of the committee of collective investigation of the anatomical society of Great Britain and Ireland for the year 1891–92. Anat Physiol 1893;27:192–94.

Tountas CP, Bihrle DM, MacDonald CJ, Bergman RA. Variations of the median nerve in the carpal canal. J Hand Surg 1987;12A:708–12.

Valls-Sole J. Martin-Gruber anastomosis and unusual sensory innervation of the fingers: report of a case. Muscle Nerve 1991;14:1099–1102.

Wallace WA, Coupland RE. Variations in the nerves of the thumb and index finger. J Bone Joint Surg 1975;57A:491–94.

Watchmaker GP, Gumucio CA, Crandall RE, Vannier MA, Weeks PM. Fascicular topography of the median nerve: a computer based study to identify branching patterns. J Hand Surg 1991;16A:53–59.

Woollard HH, Phillips R. The distribution of sympathetic fibres in the extremities. J Anat 1932;67:18–26.

Zbrodowski A, Gajisin S. The blood supply of the flexor retinaculum. J Hand Surg 1988;13B:35–39.

Zeiss J, Skie M, Ebraheim N, Jackson WT. Anatomic relations between the median nerve and flexor tendons in the carpal tunnel: MR evaluation in normal volunteers. AJR 1989;153:533–36.

Zucker-Pinchoff B, Hermann G, Srinivasan R. Computed tomography of the carpal tunnel: a radioanatomical study. J Comput Assist Tomogr 1981;5:525–28.

2

Historical Understanding of Carpal Tunnel Syndrome

Modern understanding of carpal tunnel syndrome has evolved from a variety of clinical and pathologic observations on median nerve injury following wrist trauma, thenar atrophy as a consequence of median neuropathy, and the results of surgical decompression of the median nerve in the carpal tunnel. A unifying insight was the recognition that acroparesthesia, a common, well-known symptom, was often the first manifestation of median nerve compression and could be relieved by carpal tunnel surgery.

MEDIAN NEUROPATHY FOLLOWING WRIST FRACTURE

Paget (1865 p. 50) is frequently credited with one of the first descriptions of median neuropathy caused by nerve compression at the wrist; his patient developed median neuropathy after distal radial fracture:

> A man was at Guy's Hospital, who, in consequence of a fracture at the lower end of the radius, repaired by an excessive quantity of new bone, suffered compression of the median nerve. He had ulceration of the thumb, and fore and middle fingers, which resisted various treatment, and was cured only by so binding the wrist that the parts of the palmar aspect being relaxed, the pressure on the nerve was removed. So long as this was done, the ulcers became and remained well; but as soon as the man was allowed to use his hand, the pressure on the nerves was renewed, and the ulceration of the parts supplied by them returned.

Lewis and Miller (1922) reported an extensive series of traumatic nerve injuries. They included one patient with distal median neuropathy, manifest by thenar atrophy and hypoesthesia in the median nerve distribution, who became symptomatic 18 years after a reverse Colles' fracture. The distal radial fragment was displaced anteriorly. In their literature review, they found three other cases of median neuropathy after radial fractures: Bouilly in 1884, De Rouville in 1905, and Gensoul, in 1836.

Abbott and Saunders (1933) classified the types of median nerve injuries that may be associated with distal radial fractures. Type 1, direct injury to the median nerve in the forearm by fractured bone, was very rare. The more common problem was type 2, secondary compression of the median nerve against the proximal edge of the flexor retinaculum by the displaced fracture. Type 3 was delayed median neuropathy appearing as a late sequel after distal radial fracture. Type 4 was median nerve compression exacerbated by treatment of the radial fracture by fixation in palmar flexion.

Zachary (1945) described two patients who developed median neuropathy as a late sequel of fractures. One patient had had a scaphoid fracture, whereas the other patient had a malunited Colles' fracture. Both presented with partial thenar atrophy with minimal median sensory disturbance. In both cases, median nerve compression in the carpal tunnel was identified as the cause, and both patients were treated with section of the flexor retinaculum. Zachary explained the sparing of flexor pollicis brevis in his patients by the ulnar innervation of this muscle in some individuals and the paucity of sensory findings by selective vulnerability of different median nerve fibers to trauma. He noted that motor recovery could occur after surgery; the patient who had had symptoms for 15 months, but not the patient who had had thenar paralysis for 14 years, recovered thenar strength postoperatively.

THENAR ATROPHY

Hunt (1911) described a case of thenar atrophy to the American Neurological Association in 1909 and published this case and two others. His patients had atrophy of thenar muscles innervated by the median nerve and no abnormalities on sensory examination. Each patient had done repetitive gripping, and Hunt hypothesized damage to the recurrent motor branch of the median nerve. Note, however, that at least two of his patients went through a period of intermittent hand paresthesia prior to development of the motor signs; today we would probably diagnose these patients as having severe carpal tunnel syndrome.

Marie and Foix (1913) described the autopsy results in an 80-year-old woman with bilateral isolated thenar atrophy. They noted normal bulk of the ulnar-innervated thumb adductor and thinning of the median nerve beneath the flexor retinaculum *(ligament annulaire)* with thickening of the median nerve in the distal forearm proximal to the site of constriction. With myelin stains, they demonstrated attenuation of the myelin sheath in the constricted portion of the nerve, suggesting that transection of the flexor retinaculum might have been appropriate treatment if the diagnosis had been made in life. Mumenthaler (1984) has provided an English translation of this remarkable paper.

Brouwer (1920) described 15 patients with isolated partial atrophy of thenar muscles. He attributed the localized atrophy to phylogenetic congenital "inferiority" of the thenar muscles with a possible causative role of overuse of the affected muscles.

Moersch (1938) reported a woman with bilateral progressive thenar wasting or atrophy. He hypothesized damage to the recurrent thenar motor branch by direct trauma or irritation. He noted that some patients with thenar atrophy also had median sensory symptoms, and he suggested that the median nerve in these patients might be compressed by the flexor retinaculum.

Wartenberg (1939) provided an extensive review of early theories on isolated thenar atrophy. He cited the work of Marie and Foix (1913) and Moersch (1938) on the possible pathogenetic import of the flexor retinaculum, and he was aware that patients with thenar atrophy might have sensory symptoms. Despite his scholarship, he sided with Brouwer (1920), concluding that partial thenar atrophy resulted from "abiotrophy" rather than from median neuropathy.

ACROPARESTHESIAS

A distinctive clinical syndrome of periodic hand paresthesias has been recognized for well over a century, even though understanding of its relation to the median nerve is a more recent development. Mitchell (1881), in a chapter on disorders of sleep, described transient nocturnal hand paresthesias as "night palsy" or "brachial monoplegia" but included descriptions of patients with more widespread "nocturnal hemiplegia."

Putnam (1880) reported a number of patients with periodically recurring paresthesias of their hands. His clinical description clearly fits that of carpal tunnel syndrome: Hand paresthesias or numbness occurred especially at night or in the early morning, often with associated arm pain. Numbness most prominently affected fingers innervated by the median nerve. The fingers felt stiff at times. Symptoms improved with hanging or shaking the hand. One patient and the mother of another patient noted exacerbation of symptoms during pregnancy. The hands often felt swollen to the patient, but objective swelling was rarely evident. Women were affected much more commonly than men. Putnam hypothesized that the syndrome was caused by alterations of the distal blood supply of nerves.

Ormerod (1883) described 12 women with intermittent nocturnal hand paresthesias. He recognized that his patients' symptoms were different than Raynaud's phenomenon and mentioned the relationship between symptoms and daily hand activities. Sinkler (1884) reported nine similar cases.

Saundby (1885) described some patients with nocturnal hand paresthesias and other patients with paresthesias in hands and feet. He attributed the cause to a stomach disorder and ascribed successful treatment to rhubarb powder, peppermint water, subchloride of mercury, and bromide of potassium. He identified Handfield Jones, who in 1870 diagnosed the syndrome as brachial neuralgia, among his predecessors who had considered this disorder (cited in Saundby 1885).

Schultze is credited with introducing in 1893 the term "acroparesthesia" for this syndrome (cited in Kremer et al., 1953).

Wartenberg (1944) described "brachialgia statica paraesthetica" as a syndrome of nocturnal hand pain and paresthesias waking patients from sleep. He emphasized the absence of objective physical signs and the long, benign, waxing and waning course of the condition. His patients were mostly women, aged 40 to 55 years, who tended to describe their paresthesias as ulnar in distribution. Wartenberg believed the cause to be transient compression of the lower brachial plexus during sleep. Behrman (1945) also attributed acroparesthesia to brachial plexopathy.

Walshe (1945) commented on seeing an increased number of cases of acroparesthesia in women during World War II, which he attributed to women's increased manual activities because of wartime. His patients clearly exhibited the characteristics that we now recognize as carpal tunnel syndrome, including nocturnal paresthesias with generally normal physical examinations. Walshe hypothesized that the cause was pressure on the brachial plexus by a normal first rib.

McArdle, in a lecture in 1949 to the Association of British Neurologists, articulated the relationship between acroparesthesias and median nerve compression in the carpal tunnel (cited in Kremer et al. 1953).

SURGERY FOR CARPAL TUNNEL SYNDROME

Learmonth (1933) reported from the Mayo Clinic that he had sectioned the transverse carpal ligament of a 71-year-old woman with severe median neuropathy complicated by ulcerations of the tips of the index and middle fingers. At surgery the median nerve appeared compressed between the ligament and osteophytes arising from the carpal bones. The ulcers healed postoperatively. Amadio (1992) has reviewed patient records of the Mayo Clinic and traces the clinical experiences that preceded the publication of this case.

Cannon and Love (1946) reported 38 cases with what they termed "tardy median palsy," insidious and progressive median neuropathy. In 9 of these cases they decompressed the median nerve by section of the transverse carpal ligament. They also made transverse incisions in the epineurium. Four of their cases had wrist deformities secondary to old fractures, one had acromegaly, one had a median neuroma in the carpal tunnel, and three showed no clear cause of their carpal tunnel syndrome.

Brain et al. (1947) reported 6 women with typical motor and sensory symptoms of carpal tunnel syndrome. All 6 underwent section of the transverse carpal ligament, with rapid relief of pain and paresthesia.

Kremer et al. (1953) confirmed the relationship between acroparesthesia and carpal tunnel syndrome by successful relief of acroparesthesia after surgical section of the flexor retinaculum.

Interest in carpal tunnel syndrome has been growing over the last four decades. Subsequent chapters cover current knowledge of carpal tunnel syndrome and include references to the evolution of this knowledge. For example, the history of electrodiagnosis of carpal tunnel syndrome is included in Chapter 7, and the history of the understanding of the effect of activity on carpal tunnel syndrome is in Chapter 13.

REFERENCES

Abbott LC, Saunders JBdeCM. Injuries of the median nerve in fractures of the lower end of the radius. Surg Gynecol Obstet 1933;57:507–16.

Amadio PC. The Mayo Clinic and carpal tunnel syndrome. Mayo Clin Proc 1992;67:42–48.

Behrman S. Acroparaesthesia. Proc R Soc Med 1945;38:600–601.

Brain WR, Wright AD, Wilkinson M. Spontaneous compression of both median nerves in the carpal tunnel. Lancet 1947;1:277–82.

Brouwer B. The significance of phylogenetic and ontogenetic studies for the neuropathologist. J Nerv Ment Dis 1920;51:113–37.

Cannon BW, Love JG. Tardy median palsy; median neuritis; median thenar neuritis amenable to surgery. Surgery 1946;20:210–16.

Hunt JR. The thenar and hypothenar types of neural atrophy of the hand. Am J Med Sci 1911;141:224–41.

Kremer M, Gilliatt RW, Golding JSR, Wilson TG. Acroparaesthesiae in the carpal-tunnel syndrome. Lancet 1953;2:595.

Learmonth JR. Treatment of diseases of peripheral nerves. Surg Clin North Am 1933;13:905–13.

Lewis D, Miller EM. Peripheral nerve injuries associated with fractures. Trans Am Surg Assoc 1922;40:489–580.

Marie P, Foix C. Atrophie isolée de l'éminence thénar d'origine névritique: rôle du ligament annulaire antérieur du carpe dans la pathogénie de la lésion. Rev Neurol 1913;26:647–49.

Mitchell SW. Lectures on diseases of the nervous system. Philadelphia: Henry C. Lea's Son, 1881.

Moersch FP. Median thenar neuritis. Proc Staff Mtgs Mayo Clin 1938;13:220–22.

Mumenthaler M. Carpal tunnel syndrome: first description. Neurology 1984;34:921.

Ormerod JA. On a peculiar numbness and paresis of the hands. St Barts Hosp Rep 1883;19:17–26.

Paget J. Lectures on surgical pathology. Philadelphia: Lindsay & Blakiston, 1865. Third American.

Putnam JJ. A series of cases of paraesthesia, mainly of the hands, of periodical recurrence, and possibly of vaso-motor origin. Arch Med 1880;4:147–62.

Saundby R. On a special form of numbness of the extremities. Lancet 1885;2:422–23.

Sinkler W. On a form of numbness of the upper extremities. NY Med J 1884;40:107–108.

Walshe FMR. On "acroparaesthesia" and so-called "neuritis" of the hands and arms in women. Br Med J 1945;2:596–98.

Wartenberg R. Partial thenar atrophy. Arch Neurol Psychiat 1939;42:373–93.

Wartenberg R. Brachialgia statica paresthetica. J Nerv Ment Dis 1944;99:877–87.

Zachary RB. Thenar palsy due to compression of the median nerve. Surg Gynecol Obstet 1945;81:213–17.

3

Carpal Tunnel Syndrome: Clinical Presentation

Carpal tunnel syndrome is defined by a constellation of symptoms and signs of median nerve compression in the carpal canal, and there are a variety of possible clinical presentations. The most common is caused by chronic median nerve compression and presents as acroparesthesias, but less common variants include thenar atrophy without sensory symptoms; acute carpal tunnel syndrome; and atypical profiles of nerve compressive symptoms, particularly in children or the elderly (Spinner et al. 1989).

There is no absolute clinical standard or definitive test for carpal tunnel syndrome. Histopathologic proof of local median nerve disease is not available as a diagnostic resource. Many published series discuss the findings in hundreds of patients with carpal tunnel syndrome without offering a precise definition of the patients eligible for the diagnosis (Yamaguchi et al. 1965; Phalen 1972; Maxwell et al. 1973; Hybbinette and Mannerfelt 1975; Gainer and Nugent 1977; Paine and Polyzoidis 1983). We shall discuss the common symptoms and physical findings in carpal tunnel syndrome before struggling with more rigorous clinical criteria for making the diagnosis.

SYMPTOMS

A carefully taken history is the first step toward diagnosis of carpal tunnel syndrome. Without strong historical support for the diagnosis, reliance on physical examination or on tests such as nerve conduction studies invites error.

Acroparesthesias of the hands are the most common presenting symptoms. A clinical description by Kremer et al. (1953) is quoted in the introduction. Important symptomatic details are the nature, location, and timing of both parethesias and pain.

Paresthesias

Today, patients with carpal tunnel syndrome often come to medical attention early in their illness, when intermittent hand paresthesias are the predominant symptoms. At this early stage, pain may be absent or trivial.

Patients frequently characterize the paresthesias as their hand "going to sleep" and may attribute the symptoms to "cutting off" their circulation. They can sometimes identify arm postures in sleep that seem to incite symptoms. At times the paresthesias are described as clearly following the sensory field of the median nerve, but even anatomically sophisticated patients may report that paresthesias include all the fingers or even seem to favor ulnar-innervated fingers. Paresthesias will at times seem to localize to a single median-innervated finger or to spread into the palm. Diagnosis of carpal tunnel syndrome is not excluded by these atypical patterns but is more likely to be correct when sensory changes are limited to two or three median-innervated digits (Katz and Stirrat 1990).

Early in the illness, sensory symptoms are intermittent. Paresthesias, sometimes accompanied by pain, characteristically interrupt sleep and may also be present on awakening or recur at rest during the day. Patients may sense that their fingers are stiff. Particularly common times of occurrence are while driving a car or holding a telephone receiver. Patients may note that certain hand activities, such as prolonged gripping, cause symptoms, which usually abate shortly after the activity is stopped. In some patients, paresthesias—and pain, when present— are most prominent during repetitive wrist use, and nocturnal hand symptoms are absent or less bothersome (Braun et al. 1989).

Typically, symptoms develop insidiously. Figure 3.1 shows the duration of symptoms before the diagnosis was made in one series (Phalen 1966). By the time

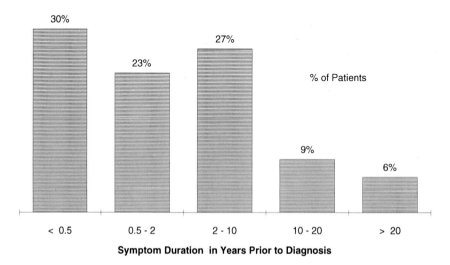

Figure 3.1 Duration of symptoms of carpal tunnel syndrome prior to diagnosis. (Data from Phalen 1966.)

the patient comes to the physician, the frequency of nocturnal awakening has gradually increased. The patient may identify a change in hand activities temporally related to the development of symptoms and even note relief of symptoms on vacations or weekends. The white-collar home handyman may report a reverse pattern, with symptoms only occurring after weekends of work around the house.

In some patients, symptoms are preceded by a change in health such as development of rheumatoid arthritis, appearance of other symptoms of hypothyroidism or diabetes, or occurrence of pregnancy. In the majority of patients, however, the symptoms arise in an otherwise healthy body. Often no recent change in a lifelong pattern of hand and arm use is evident.

With time, sensory symptoms may become constant during the day. In patients who have developed a fixed sensory loss, anatomic reliability of sensory assessment is increased, and the initial nocturnal pattern of positive sensory symptoms may abate.

Proximal Arm Symptoms

While patients typically perceive the paresthesias as localized below the wrist, the accompanying pain often radiates into the forearm or even as proximally as the shoulder. Estimates of the incidence of referral of pain to the shoulder range from 5% to 40% of patients (Cherington 1974). In rare instances, shoulder pain may be the predominant symptom (Kummel and Zazanis 1973). If the patient's sole problem is carpal tunnel syndrome, the pain will appear and disappear along with the paresthesias. Continuous arm pain, or arm pain that occurs independent of episodes of paresthesias, signals the possibility of an alternative or additional cause of arm symptoms.

The intraneural stimulation studies of Torebjörk et al. (1984) provide an experimental parallel for proximal referral of pain in carpal tunnel syndrome. Strong stimulation of median nerve cutaneous fascicles with a microelectrode elicited cutaneous pain in the median-innervated sensory territory. In contrast, stimulation of median nerve motor fascicles elicited deep pain projected to median-innervated muscles. In about one quarter of motor fascicles, stimulation also elicited deep pain referred to the upper arm, axilla, or pectoral regions. Studies of the human ulnar nerve give comparable results (Marchettini et al. 1990).

Two series emphasize clinical clues helpful in assessing the possibility of carpal tunnel syndrome in patients with proximal upper extremity pain. LaBan et al. (1975) described 22 patients who presented with neck and shoulder pain and who had improvement of these symptoms following carpal tunnel release. Invariably, these patients had physical signs of carpal tunnel syndrome, including thenar weakness, and their proximal symptoms often worsened with wrist hyperextension or flexion.

Crymble (1968) described 21 patients who had prominent proximal arm pain that led to initial diagnoses such as cervical radiculopathy or brachial plexopathy. Diagnosis of carpal tunnel syndrome was often delayed in these patients, yet they responded well to carpal tunnel surgery. Crymble emphasized that the patients' proximal pain might be more severe than their distal pain. The important diagnostic details were that in each case the pain extended distally to the hand and forearm, and the patients' distal arm symptoms were, in character and timing, typical for carpal tunnel syndrome. Ochoa (1990) has described a personal experience with an analogous presentation of ulnar neuropathy with proximal symptoms.

In summary, neck, shoulder, or proximal arm pain that is separable from associated distal arm pain and hand paresthesia is rarely, if ever, a symptom of carpal tunnel syndrome. When carpal tunnel syndrome does cause proximal pain, the patient will have accompanying distal arm symptoms and signs.

Hand Pain Diagram

Katz and Stirrat (1990) emphasized the importance of a careful clinical history for establishing the diagnosis of carpal tunnel syndrome and recommended inviting patients to fill out a hand diagram, recording their areas of pain, tingling, numbness, and decreased sensation. In Katz and Stirrat's series, if patients had a classic sensory pattern with sensory symptoms limited to at least two of the thumb, index, and middle fingers, the diagnosis, when established, was invariably carpal tunnel syndrome. The probability of the diagnosis decreased the more the patient's sensory diagram strayed from the classic pattern.

Motor Manifestations

Patients with carpal tunnel syndrome frequently note unreliability of grip. Both muscle weakness and sensory deficits can contribute to this symptom. Patients often complain of dropping objects or of difficulty grasping even before the occurrence of demonstrable weakness and long before the appearance of thenar atrophy. As median nerve damage progresses, thenar weakness may become more pronounced, and thenar atrophy may appear.

On occasion, patients may present with severe thenar atrophy and weakness, with median sensory loss, or both, and deny passing through a stage of intermittent pain and paresthesias that preceded development of fixed neurologic signs. This presentation is more common in patients in their sixties or older. It is unclear whether these patients are heavy sleepers who have slept through the stage of nocturnal paresthesias, stoics who have ignored intermittent hand symptoms, or physiologically distinctive patients who have been spared the characteristic early positive sensory symptoms.

EXAMINATION

Patients being evaluated for carpal tunnel syndrome should have a regional arm and neck examination and a neurologic examination. The examination must be sufficiently thorough to clarify the differential diagnosis, look for causative medical or orthopedic disorders, and consider the possibility of coexisting conditions. Neurologic issues include existence of other mononeuropathies, brachial plexopathy, radiculopathy, myelopathy, or diffuse peripheral neuropathy. At times, wrist and hand examination will give evidence of tenosynovitis, deformity, or injury. The adequacy of vascular supply and the possibility of autonomic, skin, or trophic changes should be considered.

In patients with carpal tunnel syndrome, physical findings will reflect the severity of median nerve dysfunction. In early or mild cases, when symptoms are intermittent, no signs may be present. Conversely, demonstration of neurologic deficits indicates that median nerve injury has passed the initial stages. The incidence of abnormal signs varies from series to series, depending on the examination methods applied and the distribution of severity of cases in the series. Nonetheless, the relative sensitivity of signs follows a reliable pattern among series.

Sensory Examination

The patient with carpal tunnel syndrome almost always describes paresthetic phenomena, yet the sensory examination may be characterized as normal despite the patient's sensory complaints. While most patients have some disturbance of sensation by history, examination demonstrates hypoesthesia in only about 70% of patients in older surgical series (Phalen 1966, 1972; Maxwell et al. 1973; Hybbinette and Mannerfelt 1975). A small number of patients describe "hyperesthesia." Loss of two-point discrimination is a rarer finding. The incidence of changes on sensory examination is lower in most clinics now because patients are coming to medical attention earlier in the course of the syndrome.

Spindler and Dellon (1982) compared a variety of clinical sensory tests in 74 symptomatic hands with carpal tunnel syndrome. They tested pain sensitivity using a 25-gauge needle. Perception of vibration was measured by asking the patient to report the feeling of a 256-Hz tuning fork head touching the fingertip. Two-point discrimination was tested both to a static pressure at one application to the fingertip and as a "moving two-point discrimination" test by dragging the stimuli along the surface of the fingertip. Figure 3.2 shows the sensitivity of the tests in this series. The order of sensitivity was not invariable, so that a total of 66% of hands showed abnormality on some aspect of the sensory exam. In many cases with intermittent symptoms, the vibratory perception test was the only abnormal test of sensation.

The relative sensitivities of sensory tests have a parallel in experimental subjects experiencing acute median nerve compression (Lundborg et al. 1982; Gelberman et al. 1983). Pressure is applied to the volar wrist so that the median nerve is compressed without more generalized vascular compression. Usually, paresthesias appear after a few minutes of compression at pressures greater than 30 mm Hg. The more sensitive sensory tests—monofilament tactile threshold testing or vibration perception threshold—may become abnormal about the time of perception of paresthesias or shortly after paresthesias appear. Abnormal

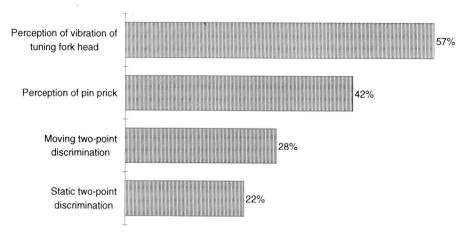

Percentage of Patients with Carpal Tunnel Syndrome in whom Test is Abnormal

Figure 3.2 The sensitivity of sensory tests in patients with carpal tunnel syndrome. (Data from Spindler and Dellon 1982.)

two-point discrimination is a much later manifestation of acute nerve compression.

Sensory abnormalities, when present, may not always follow the traditional median sensory distribution (volar thumb, index, middle, and lateral half of the ring finger) because of the wide range of anatomic variations (see Figure 1.9). Sensation of the volar hand is often blunted over callused skin; examination of sensation on the median-innervated dorsal distal fingers may be particularly helpful (Dawson et al. 1990).

A photograph of the mapped pattern of sensory abnormalities is useful for documenting consistency of examinations and following the patient's clinical course (Figure 3.3).

The skin of the thenar eminence receives its sensory innervation from the recurrent palmar branch of the median nerve. This branch typically leaves the median nerve proximal to the carpal tunnel; so thenar sensory loss may indicate a median neuropathy proximal to the carpal tunnel or an anomalous sensory pattern.

The diagnostic value of sensory testing can be improved by using quantitative sensory testing techniques as discussed in Chapter 9 (Szabo et al. 1984; Borg and Lindblom 1988). The sensitivity can be increased further by using provocative techniques to elicit the sensory abnormalities (Borg and Lindblom 1986; Braun et al. 1989).

Motor Examination

In experimental acute median nerve compression, thenar weakness usually does not occur until sensory loss is marked (Lundborg et al. 1982; Gelberman et al. 1983). Clinically, in chronic median nerve compression, the same pattern is the

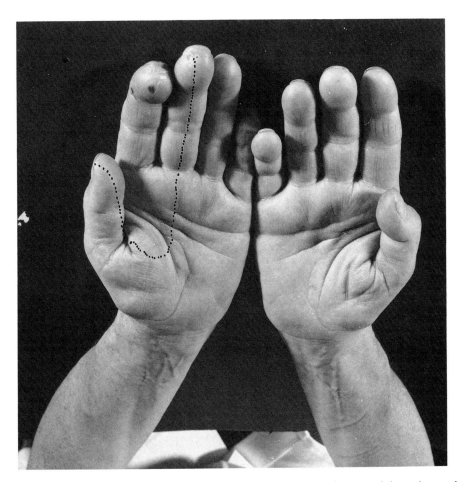

Figure 3.3 Photograph of the sensory deficit in a patient with severe bilateral carpal tunnel syndrome. Note the unusual finding of chronic trophic ulcers on the fingertips.

norm: thenar weakness is rarer than sensory loss, and thenar atrophy is even less common. The muscles that receive median innervation distal to the carpal tunnel are the abductor pollicis brevis (APB), opponens pollicis, flexor pollicis brevis (FPB), and the lumbricals to the index and middle fingers. Figures 3.4–3.6 illustrate examining the strength of the thenar muscles. Weakness of the APB is the most sensitive motor sign of carpal tunnel syndrome. The APB is the least likely of the thenar muscles to receive ulnar innervation. Care should be taken to examine APB strength in relative isolation by ensuring that the thumb is held parallel to the index finger while testing abduction up from the plane of the palm.

The opponens pollicis mediates rotation at the metacarpal-trapezial joint, swinging the thumb medially to meet the little finger. While testing this motion, observe that the movement is occurring at the metacarpal-trapezial joint rather than through action of the FPB at the metacarpal-phalangeal joint. This is

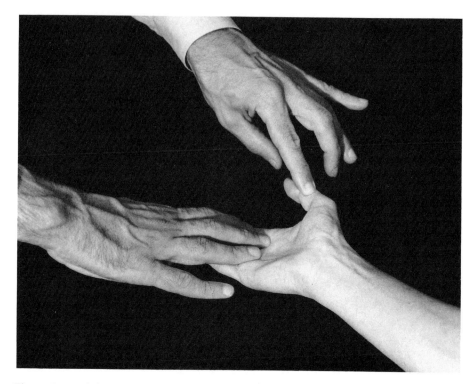

Figure 3.4 Abductor pollicis brevis is tested by assessing strength of thumb movement away from the palm in a plane perpendicular to the plane of the palm.

important because the FPB is more likely than the opponens pollicis to receive innervation from the ulnar nerve and hence may be spared in a median neuropathy.

Lumbricals are difficult to test in isolation. One test for lumbrical weakness is to observe action at the distal interphalangeal (DIP) joints while the metacarpal-phalangeal joints are voluntarily flexed to 90°. If the lumbricals are weak, the DIP joints will not be maintained in extension (Aiache and Delagi 1974). Even if the lumbricals are examined with care, lumbrical strength is often relatively preserved in carpal tunnel syndrome until after thenar muscles are weakened (Desjacques et al. 1980; Yates et al. 1981; Logigian et al. 1987).

Motor examination in the patient with suspected carpal tunnel syndrome should exclude motor manifestations of more widespread neurologic dysfunction such as ulnar neuropathy, proximal median neuropathy, brachial plexopathy, or radiculopathy.

Cutaneous Examination

Patients with carpal tunnel syndrome often describe their hands as swollen, particularly on arising from sleep. The patient's perception of swelling is usually not accompanied by an actual increase in hand volume. Phalen (1966) noted hand

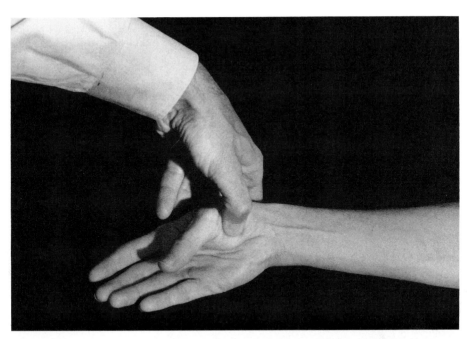

Figure 3.5 The opponens pollicis moves the metacarpal bone of the thumb to touch the little finger; the thumb is rotated so that the thumbnail becomes parallel to the palm.

swelling in only 51 of 654 hands with carpal tunnel syndrome. Even when hand volume is carefully measured, most patients with carpal tunnel syndrome show no significant swelling over the course of the day (Wilson MacDonald et al. 1984).

Phalen (1966) described isolated volar forearm swelling in 11% of his patients. This physical finding has been colloquially called Phalen's "volar hot dog" because of its sausage-like shape (Hodgkins and Grady 1988).

Cutaneous manifestations of carpal tunnel syndrome are varied but quite uncommon. In severe cases, ulcerative, necrotic, or bullous lesions of the skin of the median-innervated fingertips may occur (see Figure 3.3) (Besson et al. 1989). Digital anhydrosis, dorsal digital alopecia, and nail changes have been described and may improve following carpal tunnel release (Aratari et al. 1984). A patient with carpal tunnel syndrome and hand exposure to detergents developed contact dermatitis limited to the median-innervated fingers (Fast et al. 1989). Trophic changes severe enough to lead to finger amputation are extremely rare (Quinlan 1967).

PROVOCATIVE TESTS

Patients with carpal tunnel syndrome typically appear in the physician's examining room with intermittent symptoms and no objective neurologic dysfunction. A number of provocative tests have been used to elicit symptoms or

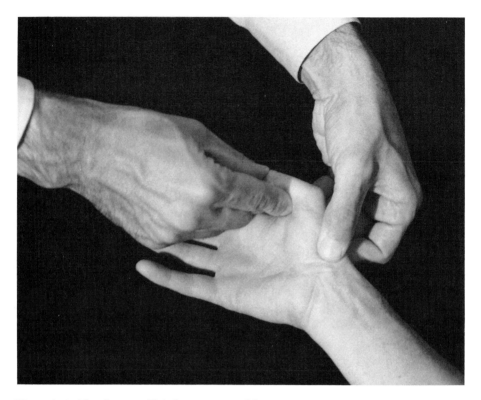

Figure 3.6 The flexor pollicis brevis is tested by assessing the strength of flexion of the metacarpal-phalangeal joint of the thumb. Be wary of trick movements from action of flexor pollicis longus or opponens pollicis.

neurologic abnormalities. Invariably, initial descriptions of these tests are followed by reports showing that the tests are flawed by both false-positive and false-negative results.

Tinel's Sign

Tinel (1915) reported that percussion over a posttraumatic neuroma often elicited tingling sensations *("fourmillement")* perceived in the distribution of the injured nerve. The phenomenon is not limited to posttraumatic neuromas, and Phalen (1966) found this sign present with percussion over the median nerve at the wrist in 73% of his patients. The sign may be elicited over a variety of nerves and so is properly described by location: for example, "a positive Tinel's sign over the median nerve at the wrist." The test is only positive for carpal tunnel syndrome if the percussion over the median nerve at the wrist leads to paresthesias in a median distribution; it should not be confused with percussion tenderness of the wrist. In different series the sensitivity of Tinel's sign in patients with carpal tunnel syndrome has ranged from 65% to 26%, (Golding et al. 1986; Daras et al. 1987).

The high incidence of Tinel's sign in individuals without carpal tunnel syndrome is now widely recognized. The incidence of false positives has been reported from 6% to 45% (Gelmers 1979; Gellman et al. 1986; Golding et al. 1986; Seror 1987b). The incidence of false positives in these series increases parallel to the incidence of true positives. For example, the incidence of positives, both true and false, may be increased by extending the wrist and using a "Queen Square" reflex hammer for the percussion (Mossman and Blau 1987). In the general population, most individuals with a positive Tinel's sign over the median nerve at the wrist will not have carpal tunnel syndrome.

Phalen's Sign

Phalen (1966, 214) described the "wrist flexion test":

The patient is asked to hold the forearms vertically and to allow both hands to drop into complete flexion at the wrist for approximately one minute.

The position is shown in Figure 3.7.

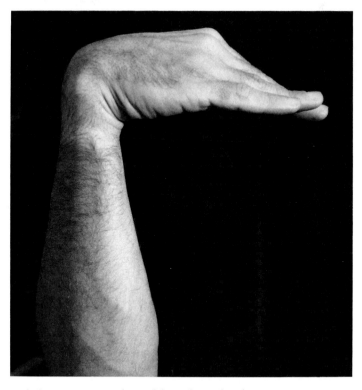

Figure 3.7 Phalen's test is performed by asking the patient to report any symptoms induced by one minute of sustained wrist flexion. This test relies on subjective reporting by the patient and is most helpful if the patient describes induction of paresthesias in the sensory distribution of the median nerve.

A patient with a positive Phalen's sign will report numbness or paresthesias in the distribution of the median nerve within one minute of sustained wrist flexion. Reports of pain alone do not prove median compression, but the test is particularly helpful if the patient reports pain and paresthesias mimicking his or her typical intermittent symptoms. Phalen found the test positive in 74% of hands with carpal tunnel syndrome. He attributed some of the false-negative results to hands that already had "an advanced degree of sensory loss." Other series have found similar sensitivity of the test (Gellman et al. 1986; Seror 1988).

Phalen noted that median paresthesias occur in normal persons if wrist flexion is sustained long enough. False-positive results in Phalen's test are found in 25% of normal hands (Gellman et al. 1986; Seror 1988). As with Tinel's sign, the diagnostic value of Phalen's test is diluted by the high incidence of false negatives in a condition with relatively low prevalence in the general population.

Tourniquet Test

Gilliatt and Wilson (1953, 1954) described the use of forearm ischemia to provoke the symptoms of carpal tunnel syndrome. They reported that following occlusion of forearm blood flow using a pneumatic cuff, patients with carpal tunnel syndrome experienced reproduction of their intermittent symptoms of hand paresthesias or experienced sensory loss in a median distribution. The paresthesias typically developed in 3 minutes or less; sensory loss usually took 5 to 10 minutes to become established. Gilliatt and Wilson stressed that normal subjects often note acroparesthesias with forearm ischemia; distinguishing features in the carpal tunnel syndrome patients were localization of the paresthesias or sensory loss to the median distribution and development of median sensory loss in less than 10 minutes. Patients with other focal neuropathies or radiculopathies may also respond to arm ischemia with sensory loss in a sensory pattern appropriate to their lesion.

In a controlled study using only one minute of forearm ischemia, a false-positive result was found in 40% of control subjects without carpal tunnel syndrome (Gellman et al. 1986). In comparison, 71% of carpal tunnel syndrome patient's had a true positive test after one minute of ischemia.

The "Flick" Sign

Pryse-Phillips (1984) noted that his patients often shook or "flicked" the wrist of the symptomatic hand when describing their attempts to alleviate carpal tunnel syndrome symptoms. He reported a 93% true-positive rate in patients with nerve conduction evidence supporting the diagnosis of carpal tunnel syndrome. The false-positive rate was 5% in patients with other neurogenic symptoms in the hand. Subsequent correspondents found that the sensitivity and specificity of this sign were disappointingly lower in their own patients (Krendel et al. 1986; Seror 1987a; Roquer and Herraiz 1988).

Tethered Median Nerve Stress Test

The tethered median nerve stress test is performed by hyperextending the index finger at the DIP joint with the wrist supinated (LaBan et al. 1986, 1989). A positive test is production of volar forearm pain. In the small series in which this test was described, 18 of 20 patients with carpal tunnel syndrome had positive tests. Confirmatory reports or data on specificity are not available.

Carpal Compression Test

Durkan (1991) described a "carpal compression test" in which the examiner applies pressure of 150 mm Hg directly over the volar wrist for 30 seconds. The test is positive if the patient reports "numbness, pain, or paraesthesias in the distribution of the median nerve." His initial report of high sensitivity and specificity for this test has not been independently confirmed.

Provocative Tests—A Summary

On statistical grounds, based on specificity and sensitivity rates, the provocative tests cannot prove diagnosis of carpal tunnel syndrome in patients with atypical symptomatic presentations. In an occasional instance, however, they can be especially helpful when a provocative maneuver replicates a patient's symptoms or allows a more accurate assessment of localization of sensory symptoms or signs. The results of provocative tests must be interpreted with thoughtful suspicion in patients with varied or widespread somatic aches and pains or in patients who are suggestible.

EPIDEMIOLOGY

Many large clinical series of patients with carpal tunnel syndrome provide a consistent description of the demographics of carpal tunnel syndrome patients (Yamaguchi et al. 1965; Phalen 1966; Maxwell et al. 1973; Birkbeck and Beer 1975; Hybbinette and Mannerfelt 1975; Gainer and Nugent 1977; Tountas et al. 1983). Some 70% of patients are women, and 30% are men. The proportion of male patients may be higher in some work-related settings (Tountas et al. 1983; Franklin et al. 1990).

About one half of patients have bilateral carpal tunnel syndrome. Of those with unilateral symptoms, the dominant hand is more frequently affected. For example, Gainer and Nugent (1977) found that the dominant hand was predominantly affected two thirds of the time. Reinstein (1981) confirmed this finding in both right- and left-handed patients (Figure 3.8). In unusual industrial settings, when the nondominant hand is predominantly stressed, carpal tunnel syndrome may favor the nondominant hand (Falck and Aarnio 1983).

Carpal tunnel syndrome has its highest incidence between 40 and 60 years of age. It is rare before age 20 or after age 80. The age distribution of patients in a typical clinical series is shown in Figure 3.9 (Phalen 1966).

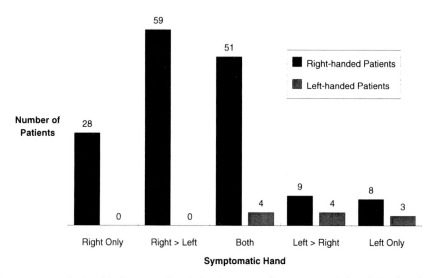

Figure 3.8 Relationship between hand dominance and symptomatic hand(s) of patients with carpal tunnel syndrome. (Data from Reinstein 1981.)

The retrospective epidemiologic study entitled "Carpal Tunnel Syndrome in Rochester, Minnesota, 1961 to 1980" provides a population-based survey of carpal tunnel syndrome with care taken to ascertain cases that came to medical attention and to define the criteria for diagnosis (Stevens et al. 1988). The results match those in the clinical series. Figure 3.10 shows the age distribution of the first episode of carpal tunnel syndrome in this population. Table 3.1 shows the incidence of carpal tunnel syndrome in the population.

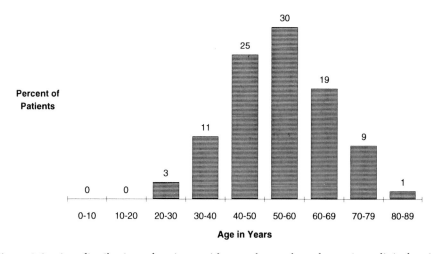

Figure 3.9 Age distribution of patients with carpal tunnel syndrome in a clinical series. (Data from Phalen 1966.)

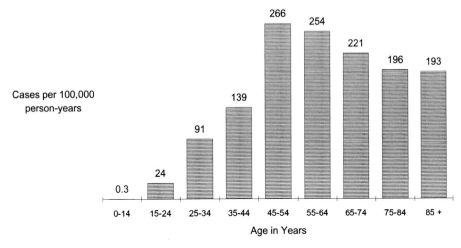

Figure 3.10 Age distribution of incidence of carpal tunnel syndrome in the citizens of Rochester, Minnesota. (Data from Stevens et al. 1988.)

The increasing incidence during the period of the study might be influenced by the increased awareness of the syndrome by patients or the increased diagnostic acumen of physicians. In addition, as discussed in Chapter 7, the sensitivity of nerve conduction tests had improved between 1960 and 1980.

A survey in Santa Clara County, California, suggests that carpal tunnel syndrome may now be more common there than it was in Rochester, Minnesota, earlier ("Occupational Disease Surveillance" 1989). The California survey ascertained patients who came to medical attention during 1988 for carpal tunnel syndrome in a county of 1.4 million people. Results showed that 7,214 cases of carpal tunnel syndrome were reported (515 per 100,000 population), even though only 30% of physicians replied to the query. Unfortunately, the study has been marred by incomplete case finding and poor case definition.

There is little cross-cultural data on the prevalence of carpal tunnel syndrome. A door-to-door survey among the Parsi population of Bombay, India, found that carpal tunnel syndrome, with a prevalence of 557 cases per 100,000 population, was the most common neurologic disorder in this community (Bhar-

Table 3.1 Carpal tunnel syndrome in Rochester, Minnesota: age-adjusted incidence per 100,000 patient years

Years	Women	Men	Total
1961–65	132	33	88
1966–70	151	40	102
1971–65	133	58	100
1976–80	173	68	125
1961–80	149	52	105

(Data from Stevens et al. 1988.)

ucha et al. 1991). In contrast, one report maintains that there is a low incidence of carpal tunnel syndrome in black South Africans, but this study did not undertake thorough case finding and does not provide adequate data for comparison to the more complete studies (Goga 1990).

DEFINITIONS OF CARPAL TUNNEL SYNDROME

The Rochester, Minnesota epidemiologic study used the following criteria for diagnosis of carpal tunnel syndrome (Stevens et al. 1988):

1. Diagnosis of carpal tunnel syndrome in the patient's medical record.
2. History of "transient or persisting numbness or paresthesias of fingers innervated by the median nerve that was typically aggravated by, or occurred during activities such as, driving, reading, or sewing." If paresthesias involved all fingers of one hand, but other factors were typical for carpal tunnel syndrome, the diagnosis was still accepted.
3. Exclusion of alternative diagnoses (but consideration of the possibility of coexisting diagnoses) such as "cervical radiculopathy, thoracic outlet syndrome, peripheral neuropathy, brachial plexus lesions, proximal median nerve entrapment, other upper extremity mononeuropathies, and Raynaud's phenomenon."

Note that these criteria relied on clinical judgment for interpretation of items two and three. No physical examination or electromyographic criteria were considered, but physical and electromyographic data on the patients were available to the reviewers and might have influenced their interpretation of the history and differential diagnosis. Of the 1,016 patients in the series, only 3 lacked confirmatory evidence of the diagnosis by additional characteristic history, physical examination, or electromyography. This work stands out as a lucid attempt at explicit definition of diagnostic criteria.

The National Institute of Occupational Safety and Health (NIOSH) has proposed a surveillance case definition of work-related carpal tunnel syndrome (Matte et al. 1989, 24):

Criteria A, B, and C must be met:

A. Symptoms suggestive of carpal tunnel syndrome: "paresthesia, hypoesthesia, pain or numbness affecting at least part of the median nerve distribution of the hand."

B. Objective findings consistent with carpal tunnel syndrome:
Either, (1) One or more of the following physical findings: Tinel sign, Phalen sign, or "decreased or absent sensation to pin prick in the median nerve distribution of the hand." Or, (2) "Electrodiagnostic findings of median nerve dysfunction across the carpal tunnel."

C. Evidence of work relatedness: One or more of the following: Frequent, repetitive or forceful hand work on affected side; sustained awkward hand position; use of vibrating tools; prolonged pressure over wrist or base of palm; temporal relationship of symptoms to work or association with carpal tunnel syndrome in co-workers.

This definition is more restrictive than the Rochester definition; it requires objective support of the diagnosis either from physical examination or from nerve conduction tests. As noted, the physical findings used are subject to both false-positive and false-negative results.

When the NIOSH criteria were applied to a series of patients, Katz et al. (1991) found that 38% of patients appeared to be classified incorrectly. This conclusion was based on a "gold standard" of nerve conduction studies to make the "correct" classification. Chapter 8 discusses why a nerve conduction standard may inevitably be "fool's gold."

DIAGNOSTIC CRITERIA FOR CARPAL TUNNEL SYNDROME

Explicit definitions of carpal tunnel syndrome are important for epidemiologic studies. Each definition is tailored to the aims of the study: for example, a definition may be used that minimizes either false-positive or false-negative diagnoses. A research definition, however, does not solve the problem of making a correct diagnosis in difficult individual patients.

For many patients with hand symptoms, we have imperfect diagnostic tools to determine whether or not symptoms that might be those of carpal tunnel syndrome are indeed the consequence of focal dysfunction of the median nerve. At times, the most reliable diagnostic criterion is the opinion of an experienced clinician (Katz et al. 1990). Without doubt, in many cases the diagnosis of carpal tunnel syndrome is clear-cut. In other cases, particularly when clinical confirmation of the diagnosis is unavailable or when multiple conditions may be contributing to arm and hand symptoms and signs, the clinical diagnosis is less certain.

Carpal tunnel syndrome is a diagnosis largely based on symptoms. The high incidence of asymptomatic nerve compression, the inaccuracies of diagnostic signs and tests, the possibility of multiple common conditions contributing to hand symptoms, and the natural variations in the ways patients experience and describe symptoms all contribute to diagnostic uncertainty. There will always be patients in whom carpal tunnel syndrome is a possible but unproven diagnosis.

When the diagnosis of carpal tunnel syndrome is uncertain, the clinician should be aware of the uncertainty and be wary of unnecessarily aggressive therapy. An uncertain diagnosis implies that if carpal tunnel syndrome is present, any median nerve injury is likely to be mild. In this setting, observation over time or clinical trials of conservative therapies often provide the best diagnostic and therapeutic strategies.

Table 3.2 offers a classification of types of median neuropathy that may occur at the carpal tunnel. Many patients will be on the border between one class and another. The scheme is proposed to aid clinical decisions by thinking about carpal tunnel syndrome both clinically and pathophysiologically. Detailed discussion of the pathophysiologic concepts is found in subsequent chapters.

Class 0. *Asymptomatic median nerve pathology.* This is present in a large portion of the clinically normal population. Histopathology may be present in

Table 3.2 Classification of median neuropathies at the carpal tunnel

Class	Symptoms	Signs
0 Asymptomatic	None	None
1 Intermittently symptomatic	Intermittent positive symptoms	Provocative tests often positive, but neurologic deficit usually absent
2 Persistently symptomatic	Continual symptoms, positive or negative	Neurologic deficit sometimes present
3 Severe	Usually present	Neurologic deficit with evidence of axonal interruption

over 40% of median nerves studied at autopsy, but the more subtle tests of nerve conduction show abnormalities in about 20% of the population, so even the most sensitive available electrodiagnostic tests may not reveal all instances of mild pathologic change in the nerve.

Some patients remain asymptomatic despite electrodiagnostic evidence of definite dysfunction of median nerve myelinated fibers. These patients may have clearly abnormal sensory or motor nerve conduction but have no symptoms or signs of carpal tunnel syndrome and require no specific treatment. One common example is abnormal nerve conduction in an asymptomatic hand, contralateral to a hand with carpal tunnel syndrome. Another example is persistence of abnormal nerve conduction following carpal tunnel surgery that has successfully relieved all symptoms of the median neuropathy.

Class 1. *Intermittently symptomatic median nerve compression.* These patients typically have intermittent hand paresthesias. Neurologic examination shows no sensory or motor deficit. In some, paresthesias can be reproduced by provocative tests.

The paresthesias result from excessive neuronal firing, which may occur whether or not large myelinated fibers have delayed conduction, so these patients may or may not have abnormalities on nerve conduction tests. There is a wide range of severity within in this class.

Class 1A. *Subclinical median nerve irritability.* At the mildest extreme, excessive neuronal firing occurs only with provocative tests; for example, a person has a positive Tinel's sign over the median nerve at the wrist or a positive Phalen's test. These patients may not have any other symptoms of carpal tunnel syndrome; hence, the positive provocative tests are "false-positives" for the diagnosis of carpal tunnel syndrome.

Many people find that their hands "go to sleep" at one time or another. They have mild median nerve irritability that usually is not brought to the attention of a clinician. They do not have sufficient symptoms to establish a diagnosis of carpal tunnel syndrome.

Class 1B. *Mild carpal tunnel syndrome.* At the next level of severity many patients in class 1 have transient symptoms of carpal tunnel syndrome and return to an asymptomatic state. Examples are most women with carpal tunnel syndrome during pregnancy and some patients who develop carpal tunnel syndrome after a few days or weeks of a particular activity, which they then stop. Symptoms may resolve completely; nerve conduction abnormalities may resolve completely or partially. Some individuals will remain in this class for many years, experiencing symptoms from time to time, without progression to more serious nerve dysfunction. Some require no treatment; others respond well to nonoperative therapies such as change of activities or splinting.

Class 1C. *Moderate intermittent carpal tunnel syndrome.* The most severely affected patients in class 1 have recurrence of hand symptoms many times a week. At this stage they usually have evidence of local slowing of nerve conduction across the carpal tunnel. Neurologic examination will usually show no fixed neurologic deficit. Some benefit from conservative therapy; in others, troublesome symptoms are eventually treated with surgery.

Class 2. *Persistently symptomatic carpal tunnel syndrome.* These patients are much more likely than patients in class 1 to have deficits on neurologic examination and will usually have abnormal median nerve conduction. When sensory loss in the median distribution is present, symptoms and signs of excessive neuronal firing such as paresthesias and Phalen's sign may become less prominent (Phalen 1966). These patients rarely obtain lasting relief with nonsurgical therapy, but symptoms and signs will be completely relieved with surgery in most patients in this class.

Figure 8.1 contrasts patients with intermittent symptoms and patients with persistent symptoms in regard to electrodiagnostic and clinical findings. In an individual case it may be difficult to decide whether to classify a patient in class 1 or class 2. Rarely, a patient with persistent symptoms has normal nerve conduction studies and no deficit on neurologic examination. Before subjecting these patients to surgery, the history and response to provocative tests must be extremely reliable.

Class 3. *Severe carpal tunnel syndrome* with clinical evidence of median nerve axonal interruption. These patients may have thenar atrophy, fibrillations or neuropathic motor units on electromyography, or evidence of small-fiber sensory or sympathetic dysfunction. Most are symptomatic, but an occasional patient is unaware of symptoms until physical signs are discovered. Most of these patients will have some improvement following carpal tunnel surgery, but recovery of neurologic function may be delayed or incomplete.

REFERENCES

Aiache AE, Delagi EF. A pure sign of lumbrical function. Plast Reconstr Surg 1974;54:312–15.

Aratari E, Regesta G, Rebora A. Carpal tunnel syndrome appearing with prominent skin symptoms. Arch Dermatol 1984;120:517–19.

Besson I, Couturier F, De-Giacomini P, Caze MC, Reboux JF. Involvement of the median nerve associated with cutaneous lesions and trophic disorders of the fingers (letter in French). Presse Med 1989;18:1207.

Bharucha NE, Bharucha AE, Bharucha EP. Prevalence of peripheral neuropathy in the Parsi community of Bombay. Neurology 1991;41:1315–17.

Birkbeck MQ, Beer TC. Occupation in relation to the carpal tunnel syndrome. Rheumatol Rehabil 1975;14:218–21.

Borg K, Lindblom U. Increase of vibration threshold during wrist flexion in patients with carpal tunnel syndrome. Pain 1986;26:211–19.

Borg K, Lindblom U. Diagnostic value of quantitative sensory testing (QST) in carpal tunnel syndrome. Acta Neurol Scand 1988;78:537–41.

Braun RM, Davidson K, Doehr S. Provocative testing in the diagnosis of dynamic carpal tunnel syndrome. J Hand Surg 1989;14A:195–97.

Cherington M. Proximal pain in carpal tunnel syndrome. Arch Surg 1974;108:69.

Crymble B. Brachial neuralgia and the carpal tunnel syndrome. Br Med J 1968;3:470–71.

Daras M, Tuchman AJ, Spector S, Zalzal P, Rogoff B. Tinel's sign. A reappraisal of its use (letter in French). Presse Med 1987;16:918.

Dawson DM, Hallett M, Millender LH. Carpal tunnel syndrome. Entrapment neuropathies. 2nd ed. Boston: Little, Brown, 1990;25–92.

Desjacques P, Egloff-Baer S, Roth G. Lumbrical muscles and the carpal tunnel syndrome. Electromyogr Clin Neurophysiol 1980;20:443–49.

Durkan JA. A new diagnostic test for carpal tunnel syndrome. J Bone Joint Surg 1991;73A:535–38.

Falck B, Aarnio P. Left-sided carpal tunnel syndrome in butchers. Scand J Work Environ Health 1983;9:291–97.

Fast A, Parikh S, Ducommun EJ. Dermatitis-sympathetic dysfunction in carpal tunnel syndrome. A case report. Clin Orthop 1989;247:124–26.

Franklin GM, Haug JA, Peck NB, Heyer N, Checkoway H. Occupational carpal tunnel syndrome in Washington state, 1984–1987. Neurology 1990;40:420.

Gainer JV Jr, Nugent GR. Carpal tunnel syndrome: report of 430 operations. South Med J 1977;70:325–28.

Gelberman RH, Szabo RM, Williamson RV, Dimick MP. Sensibility testing in peripheral-nerve compression syndromes. An experimental study in humans. J Bone Joint Surg 1983;65A:632–38.

Gellman H, Gelberman RH, Tan AM, Botte MJ. Carpal tunnel syndrome. An evaluation of the provocative diagnostic tests. J Bone Joint Surg 1986;68A:735–37.

Gelmers HJ. The significance of Tinel's sign in the diagnosis of carpal tunnel syndrome. Acta Neurochir (Wien) 1979;49:255–58.

Gilliatt RW, Wilson TG. A pneumatic-tourniquet test in the carpal-tunnel syndrome. Lancet 1953;2:595–97.

Gilliatt RW, Wilson TG. Ischaemic sensory loss in patients with peripheral nerve lesions. J Neurol Neurosurg Psychiatry 1954;17:104–14.

Goga IE. Carpal tunnel syndrome in black South Africans. J Hand Surg 1990;15B:96–99.

Golding DN, Rose DM, Selvarajah K. Clinical tests for carpal tunnel syndrome: an evaluation. Br J Rheumatol 1986;25:388–90.

Hodgkins ML, Grady D. Carpal tunnel syndrome. West J Med 1988;148:217–20.

Hybbinette CH, Mannerfelt L. The carpal tunnel syndrome. A retrospective study of 400 operated patients. Acta Orthop Scand 1975;46:610–20.

Katz JN, Larson MG, Fossel AH, Liang MH. Validation of a surveillance case definition of carpal tunnel syndrome. Am J Public Health 1991;81:189–93.

Katz JN, Larson MG, Sabra A, Krarup C, Stirrat CR, Sethi R, Eaton HM, Fossel AH, Liang MH. The carpal tunnel syndrome: diagnostic utility of the history and physical examination findings. Ann Intern Med 1990;112:321–27.

Katz JN, Stirrat CR. A self-administered hand diagram for the diagnosis of carpal tunnel syndrome. J Hand Surg 1990;15A:360–63.

Kremer M, Gilliatt RW, Golding JSR, Wilson TG. Acroparaesthesiae in the carpal-tunnel syndrome. Lancet 1953;2:595.

Krendel DA, Jobsis M, Gaskell PC Jr, Sanders DB. The flick sign in carpal tunnel syndrome (letter). J Neurol Neurosurg Psychiatry 1986;49:220–21.

Kummel BM, Zazanis GA. Shoulder pain as the presenting complaint in carpal tunnel syndrome. Clin Orthop 1973;92:227–30.

LaBan MM, Friedman NA, Zemenick GA. "Tethered" median nerve stress test in chronic carpal tunnel syndrome. Arch Phys Med Rehabil 1986;67:803–4.

LaBan MM, MacKenzie JR, Zemenick GA. Anatomic observations in carpal tunnel syndrome as they relate to the tethered median nerve stress test. Arch Phys Med Rehabil 1989;70:44–46.

LaBan MM, Zemenick GA, Meerschaert JR. Neck and shoulder pain. Presenting symptoms of carpal tunnel syndrome. Mich Med 1975;74:549–50.

Logigian EL, Busis NA, Berger AR, Bruyninckx F, Khalil N, Shahani BT, Young RR. Lumbrical sparing in carpal tunnel syndrome: anatomic, physiologic, and diagnostic implications. Neurology 1987;37:1499–1505.

Lundborg G, Gelberman RH, Minteer-Convery M, Lee YF, Hargens AR. Median nerve compression in the carpal tunnel—functional response to experimentally induced controlled pressure. J Hand Surg 1982;7:252–59.

Marchettini P, Cline M, Ochoa JL. Innervation territories for touch and pain afferents of single fascicles of the human ulnar nerve. Brain 1990;113:1491–1500.

Matte TD, Baker EL, Honchar PA. The selection and definition of targeted work-related conditions for surveillance under SENSOR. Am J Public Health 1989;79 Suppl:21–25.

Maxwell JA, Clough CA, Reckling FW, Kelly CR. Carpal tunnel syndrome. A review of cases treated surgically. J Kans Med Soc 1973;74:190–93.

Mossman SS, Blau JN. Tinel's sign and the carpal tunnel syndrome. Br Med J [Clin Res] 1987;294:680.

Ochoa JL. Neuropathic pains, from within: personal experiences experiments, and reflections on mythology. In: Dimitrijevic M, Wall PD, Lindblom U, eds. Recent achievements in restorative neurology 3: altered sensation and pain. Basel: S Karger, 1990; 100–111.

Occupational disease surveillance: carpal tunnel syndrome. MMWR 1989;38:485–89.

Paine KW, Polyzoidis KS. Carpal tunnel syndrome. Decompression using the Paine retinaculotome. J Neurosurg 1983;59:1031–36.

Phalen GS. The carpal-tunnel syndrome. Seventeen years' experience in diagnosis and treatment of six hundred fifty-four hands. J Bone Joint Surg 1966;48A:211–28.

Phalen GS. The carpal-tunnel syndrome. Clinical evaluation of 598 hands. Clin Orthop 1972;83:29–40.

Pryse-Phillips WE. Validation of a diagnostic sign in carpal tunnel syndrome. J Neurol Neurosurg Psychiatry 1984;47:870–72.

Quinlan AG. Carpal tunnel syndrome presenting as a complete median-nerve palsy with trophic changes. Br Med J 1967;1:32.

Reinstein L. Hand dominance in carpal tunnel syndrome. Arch Phys Med Rehabil 1981;62:202–3.

Roquer J, Herraiz J. Validity of Flick sign in CTS diagnosis (letter). Acta Neurol Scand 1988;78:351.

Seror P. Carpal tunnel syndrome. Value of a new diagnostic test (letter in French). Presse Med 1987a;16:914.

Seror P. Tinel's sign in the diagnosis of carpal tunnel syndrome. J Hand Surg 1987b;12B:364–65.

Seror P. Phalen's test in the diagnosis of carpal tunnel syndrome. J Hand Surg 1988;13B:383–85.

Spindler HA, Dellon AL. Nerve conduction studies and sensibility testing in carpal tunnel syndrome. J Hand Surg 1982;7:260–63.

Spinner RJ, Bachman JW, Amadio PC. The many faces of carpal tunnel syndrome. Mayo Clin Proc 1989;64:829–36.

Stevens JC, Sun S, Beard CM, O'Fallon WM, Kurland LT. Carpal tunnel syndrome in Rochester, Minnesota, 1961 to 1980. Neurology 1988;38:134–38.

Szabo RM, Gelberman RH, Dimick MP. Sensibility testing in patients with carpal tunnel syndrome. J Bone Joint Surg 1984;66A:60–64.

Tinel J. Le signe du "fourmillement" dans les lésions des nerfs périphériques. Presse Med 1915;47:388–89.

Torebjörk HE, Ochoa JL, Schady W. Referred pain from intraneural stimulation of muscle fascicles in the median nerve. Pain 1984;18:145–56.

Tountas CP, MacDonald CJ, Meyerhoff JD, Bihrle DM. Carpal tunnel syndrome. A review of 507 patients. Minn Med 1983;66:479–82.

Wilson-MacDonald J, Caughey MA, Myers DB. Diurnal variation in nerve conduction, hand volume, and grip strength in the carpal tunnel syndrome. Br Med J [Clin Res] 1984;289:1042.

Yamaguchi D, Lipscomb P, Soule E. Carpal tunnel syndrome. Minn Med 1965;48:22–31.

Yates SK, Yaworski R, Brown WF. Relative preservation of lumbrical versus thenar motor fibres in neurogenic disorders. J Neurol Neurosurg Psychiatry 1981;44:768–74.

4

Differential Diagnosis of Carpal Tunnel Syndrome

Diagnosis of carpal tunnel syndrome is often considered in patients with hand or arm pains, paresthesias, stiffness, weakness, or muscular atrophy. In patients with symptoms that are typically neuropathic, such as paresthesias, weakness, spasms, and atrophy, the differential diagnosis centers around other disorders of nerve including focal or diffuse diseases of peripheral nerves, brachial plexus, nerve roots, and cervical spinal cord. In patients who present with arm and hand pain or stiffness, disorders of joint, bone, tendon, and soft tissue are often at the forefront of the differential diagnosis. The diagnostic task is often complicated if more than one condition is contributing to limb symptoms and especially if one condition is causing limb symptoms and also contributing to the pathogenesis of carpal tunnel syndrome.

Introductory discussions of diseases of the hand and arm are available elsewhere (Cailliet 1982; Hadler 1984; Lister 1984; American Society for Surgery of the Hand 1990). Choosing the entities to include in this chapter has been a challenge. Is angina pectoris in the differential diagnosis since it can present with arm pain? Is hyperventilation in the differential diagnosis since it can cause acral paresthesias? The problem of proximal arm pain in carpal tunnel syndrome is reviewed in Chapter 3, yet diseases of the shoulder joint will rarely be confused with carpal tunnel syndrome. This chapter will focus only on the diagnosis of those conditions that are most likely to be confused with carpal tunnel syndrome. The following two chapters review the relation of carpal tunnel syndrome to other medical conditions.

NEUROLOGIC DIFFERENTIAL DIAGNOSIS

Hand paresthesias and hand, wrist, or forearm pain may characterize a number of upper extremity neuropathies. Other median neuropathies are discussed in detail in Chapters 17 and 18. Fully developed ulnar or radial neuropathies, brachial plexopathies, and cervical radiculopathies should be easily separable from carpal tunnel syndrome by findings on neurologic examination (Stewart

1987; Dawson et al. 1990). The diagnosis is complicated when multiple neuropathic abnormalities coexist or when symptoms are atypical and unaccompanied by signs of nerve dysfunction.

Among 400 patients operated on for carpal tunnel syndrome, Hybbinette and Mannerfelt (1975) identified 7 patients who obtained no benefit from carpal tunnel surgery and in whom an alternative neurologic diagnosis was made postoperatively:

Cervical radiculopathy	4
Syringomyelia	1
Neurosarcoma of the brachial plexus	1
Postradiation brachial plexopathy	1

Ulnar Neuropathy

Ulnar neuropathies, like carpal tunnel syndrome, can present with hand paresthesias, hand weakness, or upper extremity pain. In the fully developed case with nonanomalous anatomy, the distinction from carpal tunnel syndrome is simple. Sensory loss will usually be limited to the little finger and ulnar half of the ring finger. Motor loss will affect the hand intrinsic muscles except for the opponens pollicis, flexor pollicis brevis, abductor pollicis brevis, and median lumbricals. Flexor carpi ulnaris and the ulnar-innervated finger flexors may be weak with more proximal lesions. Diagnostic complexity increases when evaluating mild cases without objective signs, cases with simultaneous disease of median and ulnar nerves, or cases with anomalous patterns of innervation.

Chapter 1 discusses the anomalies of motor and sensory innervation, such as the "all median hand" or ulnar innervation of thenar muscles (Rowntree 1949). Chapter 7 includes a discussion of use of nerve conduction studies to clarify anomalous innervations.

Many patients with carpal tunnel syndrome report paresthesias or have sensory loss that includes the medial half of the ring finger or even the little finger. Hands with carpal tunnel syndrome, but without clinical evidence of ulnar neuropathy, are more likely than control hands to have abnormal thresholds for vibration perception in the little finger (Imai et al. 1990). In one series, over one fourth of hands with carpal tunnel syndrome had abnormalities by monofilament testing of tactile thresholds or two-point discrimination sensory testing in the little finger (Silver et al. 1985). Most of these abnormalities improved following carpal tunnel release surgery without surgery on Guyon's canal. This observation might be explained by anomalous patterns of innervation or by imprecise sensory mapping, but the incidence exceeds that usually reported for median innervation of the little finger (Stopford 1918). Silver et al. (1985) speculate that ulnar nerve compression at Guyon's canal often coexists with carpal tunnel syndrome and that section of the flexor retinaculum may rearrange wrist anatomy enough to also decrease ulnar nerve compression in Guyon's canal.

Electrodiagnostic testing of patients with carpal tunnel syndrome should include both median and ulnar nerve conduction studies (American Association of Electrodiagnostic Medicine 1992). Interpretation of the results is complicated by conflicting reports on the incidence of ulnar nerve conduction test abnormalities in patients with carpal tunnel syndrome; this is discussed in more detail in Chapter 7.

Radial Neuropathies

A complete radial neuropathy with wristdrop will not be mistaken for carpal tunnel syndrome. Isolated neuropathy of the superficial branch of the radial nerve is also distinctive; patients have no weakness but do have paresthesias, numbness, and sometimes pain or hyperpathia localized to the dorsal lateral aspect of the hand.

Posterior interosseous neuropathy, when fully developed, is easily identified by weakness in the distal extensor muscles innervated by the posterior interosseous branch of the radial nerve. Mild radial tunnel syndrome is a more problematic diagnosis; a number of authors believe that posterior interosseous nerve entrapment at the radial tunnel can cause forearm pain alone, without associated muscular weakness (Stewart 1987). In some of these patients, nocturnal awakening with arm pain is purportedly a prominent symptom (Carfi and Ma 1985). To the extent that this controversial syndrome exists, its presentation with pain and tenderness over the extensor mass of the forearm, distal to the lateral epicondyle, should be distinguishable from the presentation of carpal tunnel syndrome, in which pain will be more ventral when it includes the forearm. Radial tunnel syndrome is much less likely than carpal tunnel syndrome to be accompanied by paresthesias.

Brachial Plexus Lesions

The symptomatic presentation of an abnormality in the brachial plexus will vary both with the portion of the plexus affected and with the cause of the plexopathy. In most cases the extent of neurologic signs will clearly distinguish a brachial plexopathy from carpal tunnel syndrome. The distinction between neuralgic amyotrophy and proximal median neuropathies is discussed in Chapter 17.

The sensory changes of upper brachial plexopathies may overlap the median cutaneous sensory distribution. Patients with these upper plexopathies often have abnormal median distal sensory nerve conduction tests, even though the pathology is much more proximal than the carpal tunnel; an abnormal median distal sensory latency in these cases is not necessarily evidence of coexistent carpal tunnel syndrome.

Patients with lower brachial plexopathies may develop weakness and atrophy in hand intrinsic muscles. These patients should be distinguishable from those with carpal tunnel syndrome by weakness in ulnar-innervated hand intrinsic muscles. They should differ from patients with combined ulnar and median neuropathies by preservation of sensation in the median distribution. In patients with lower brachial plexopathies, nerve conduction studies can also be helpful by showing normal median motor and sensory conduction while ulnar sensory action potentials are abnormal (Gilliatt et al. 1978). If the thenar muscles are severely atrophied, the median thenar compound muscle action potential amplitude will, of course, be decreased, and the median motor nerve conduction velocity may be slowed. Figure 4.1 illustrates the pattern of sensory loss in a patient with a form of brachial plexopathy who was initially thought to have a median neuropathy.

Cervical Radiculopathy

The neurologic signs and symptoms of cervical radiculopathies may overlap those of carpal tunnel syndrome. Forearm and upper arm pain may be a feature of either disorder, but neck pain is more characteristic of cervical radiculopathy. A key historical point of differentiation is timing of symptoms: radiculopathies usually have steady, rather than intermittent, nocturnal or rest-induced paresthesias. The pain of radiculopathies may be persistent even when paresthesias are intermittent. The symptoms of radiculopathy may be increased by neck turning or

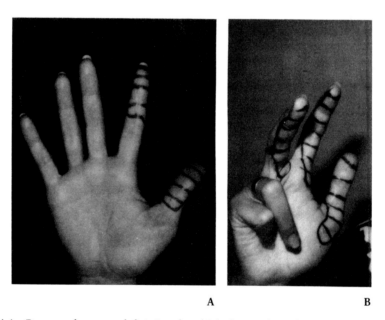

A   B

Figure 4.1 Pattern of sensory deficit in a brachial plexopathy. This 36-year-old woman was initially thought to have a median neuropathy based on progressive sensory loss in the pattern shown (**A, B**). Evolution of her findings over years eventually led to the diagnosis of brachial plexopathy. Brachial plexus exploration confirmed this diagnosis with pathologic evidence of localized hypertrophic demyelination.

occasionally by arm stretching or decreased occasionally by gentle manual neck traction. Spurling's sign (induction of arm pain and paresthesias by turning the head toward the symptomatic side and extending the neck) is indicative of radiculopathy.

C-6 radiculopathy may cause cutaneous sensory symptoms on the lateral hand and pain in the arm or forearm. Sensory findings are typically most noticeable on the dorsum of the hand, particularly on the thumb, index finger, and web space between them. Motor changes, such as deltoid or biceps weakness, and depression of the biceps reflex, when present, clearly indicate a radiculopathy or other proximal abnormality rather than a median neuropathy.

The sensory symptoms of a C-7 radiculopathy center on the middle finger and its neighbors. Prominence of sensory symptoms on the dorsum of the hand is atypical for carpal tunnel syndrome. When weakness is present, forearm muscles innervated by the median nerve, especially the pronators, may be weak, but triceps will also be weak, and thenar muscles will be spared. A depressed triceps jerk clearly favors a radiculopathy.

Radiculopathy is much rarer at C-8 than at C-7 or C-6. Weakness, when present, includes not only median-innervated thenar muscles but also ulnar-innervated hand intrinsic muscles and distal radial-innervated muscles such as the extensor indicis proprius. Sensory changes are in the ulnar, rather than the median, territory.

Patients with radiculopathy alone should have normal nerve conduction studies. Sensory nerve action potential amplitude should be normal in radiculopathy, even from digits with well-established sensory loss (Conrad and Benecke 1979).

Diseases of the Central Nervous System

The neurologist will rarely have trouble separating carpal tunnel syndrome from central nervous system causes of focal arm symptoms. Every patient with suspected carpal tunnel syndrome should have a screening neurologic history and examination without shortsighted limitation of the evaluation to the patient's arm. For example, patients with multiple sclerosis may note focal hand paresthesias. Syringomyelia or tumors of the cervical spinal cord may cause sensory and motor deficits limited to the hand. Transient ischemic attacks or focal sensory seizures can cause intermittent hand symptoms.

Patients with cervical myelopathies may present with hand sensory symptoms and weakness of hand intrinsic muscles. Usually, the extent of neurologic abnormality, often including the legs, will make the diagnosis clear. Lesions of the upper cervical cord at the level of the foramen magnum can be particularly challenging when hand numbness and clumsiness develop insidiously, and hand intrinsic weakness precedes other neurologic signs. In one series of 57 patients with extramedullary foramen magnum tumors, 3 were initially misdiagnosed as having carpal tunnel syndrome (Yasuoka et al. 1978).

Patients with motor neuron disease occasionally have striking weakness and atrophy of thenar muscles, but examination will usually reveal more widespread motor dysfunction and absence of median sensory abnormalities.

Patients using canes or crutches are vulnerable to development of carpal tunnel syndrome. This is well described in paraplegics and has also been noted in patients with residual weakness from polio (Aljure et al. 1985; Gellman et al. 1988a, 1988b; Werner et al. 1989).

Thenar Hypoplasia

Congenital thenar hypoplasia is a rare condition. It may present clinically with bilateral or unilateral "atrophy" (really hypotrophy) localized to thenar muscles without pain or sensory abnormalities. Although presumably present from birth, it may escape recognition until midchildhood or even adulthood. Cavanagh et al. (1979) reported a woman who first became symptomatic in her late forties and was initially misdiagnosed as having carpal tunnel syndrome. The patients have strikingly weak and atrophic thenar muscles. Neurologic examination is otherwise normal. Nerve conduction studies show normal median sensory conduction. Median motor conduction studies show absent or small thenar compound muscle action potentials, but electromyographic needle examination of these muscles shows no evidence of neuropathic changes. Diagnosis is confirmed by the presence on hand and wrist X rays of bony malformations that may include the carpals, first metacarpal, or thumb phalanges.

Su et al. (1972) reported a 33-year-old woman who had unilateral congenital absence of the opponens pollicis, the abductor pollicis brevis, the superficial head of the flexor pollicis brevis, and the recurrent thenar branch of the median nerve. The patient had a normal adductor pollicis and deep head of flexor pollicis brevis and no skeletal deformities of the hand.

NONNEUROLOGIC DIFFERENTIAL DIAGNOSIS
Tenosynovitis

Tenosynovitis, or inflammation of the synovial tendon sheaths, is manifested by pain elicited by tendon movement. There may be accompanying signs of inflammation such as swelling, warmth, redness, and tenderness. Tenosynovitis may be isolated to a single tendon, or it may be more generalized. It may be secondary to a systemic inflammatory process such as rheumatoid arthritis, gout, or infection. Tendon overuse may cause tenosynovitis. Often, tenosynovitis is "idiopathic."

A common form of localized tenosynovitis affects the abductor pollicis longus and extensor pollicis brevis tendons (De Quervain's tenosynovitis). Patients with De Quervain's tenosynovitis have aching discomfort over the radial styloid that increases with wrist and thumb movement. Pain may radiate to the forearm or into the hand. The classic sign is increase in pain when the thumb is held in flexion while the wrist is deviated ulnarly (Finkelstein's sign).

Another common area of tenosynovitis in the forearm involves the extensor muscles that arise from the lateral humeral epicondyle, often called lateral epicondylitis or tennis elbow. The characteristics are focal tenderness near the lateral epicondyle and increase in pain with wrist extension against resistance.

Medial epicondylitis (golfer's elbow) is less common than lateral epicondylitis. As the name implies, pain and tenderness typically involve the ulnar-innervated wrist and finger flexors originating from the medial epicondyle. Pain is increased by wrist flexion against resistance.

Tenosynovitis may be localized to other forearm tendons such as those of the biceps or the extensor carpi radialis (Brooker 1977). Tenosynovitis can affect the flexor digitorum superficialis or flexor digitorum profundus tendons in the palm. Patients with this condition may note pain with finger flexion (Lapedus and Guidotti 1972). The pain may be in the palm or radiate to the dorsum of the hand.

Some patients describe forearm pain induced by forearm use. Many of these patients have nonspecific clinical findings, and terms like *tendinitis* or *chronic muscular strain* are applied loosely for want of a more specific diagnostic term.

Trigger finger refers to the phenomenon of a finger suddenly snapping or catching during flexion so that reextension is blocked. It most commonly occurs in the thumb, middle, or ring fingers. It may arise with or without preceding clinical evidence of tendinitis of the finger flexor tendons. On examination a nodule may be palpable on the affected tendon proximal to the metacarpalphalangeal joint.

These focal tendon problems are usually clearly separable from carpal tunnel syndrome by history and physical examination. Diagnosis may be more difficult, however, when tenosynovitis coexists with carpal tunnel syndrome. For example, Phalen (1972) found De Quervain's tenosynovitis in 4, tennis elbow in 15, and trigger finger or thumb in 32 of 384 patients with carpal tunnel syndrome. It is not clear whether these associations reflect coincident occurrence of common conditions, increased detection of a second condition once symptoms of the first draw attention to the arm, or a pathogenic link between two conditions.

Osteoarthritis

Osteoarthritis of the finger joints most commonly involves the distal interphalangeal joints. It presents with joint stiffness and deformity (Heberden's nodes at the distal or, less commonly, Bouchard's nodes at the proximal interphalangeal joints). Finger pain may be prominent, particularly with finger use, but lack of paresthesias and presence of focal deformities and tenderness should make osteoarthritis hard to confuse with carpal tunnel syndrome.

The basal joints of the thumb, particularly of the metacarpal-trapezial joint, are the most common site of osteoarthritis in the hand. Osteoarthritis of the basal joints of the thumb presents with wrist pain localized to the base of the thumb. The pain increases with wrist use, so that the hand may have a dull ache after use or by the end of the day. The pain may interfere with sleep but will rarely appear anew during sleep or be most troublesome on arising. Physical examination shows tenderness localized to the base of the metacarpal of the thumb. Pain can often be reproduced by rotation and compression of the metacarpal at this joint. Joint crepitus and instability are late findings (Lister 1984).

Osteoarthritis of the metacarpal-trapezial joint, particularly in more advanced cases, is often accompanied by other joint or tendon involvement (Melone et al. 1987). Examples are scaphoid-trapezial arthritis, deformity of the metacarpal-phalangeal joint of the thumb, trigger digits, or tenosynovitis of the wrist. Scaphoid-trapezial arthritis may be marked by tenderness over the thenar eminence distal to the scaphoid tubercle. Patients with either scaphoid-trapezial arthritis or metacarpal-trapezial arthritis may have an increased incidence of carpal tunnel syndrome (Sarkin 1975; Crosby et al. 1978).

Inflammatory Arthropathies

Patients with inflammatory arthropathies in the hand will have focal joint warmth, tenderness, swelling, and redness. In contrast, carpal tunnel syndrome by itself causes no more than occasional, mild diffuse hand swelling without localized signs of inflammation. When parasthesias or signs of median neuropathy accompany inflammatory signs, carpal tunnel syndrome and arthritis may both be present. Rheumatoid arthritis, gout, pseudogout, and other inflammatory arthropathies of the wrist and hand as causes of carpal tunnel syndrome are discussed in Chapter 5.

Hand Infection

An infection in the thenar or deep palmar spaces may present with palm or wrist pain but should be distinguishable from carpal tunnel syndrome by classic local signs of inflammation—warmth, swelling, redness, and tenderness. A deep palmar space infection, when fully developed, presents with swelling that is prominent on the dorsal aspect of the hand with some loss of palmar concavity and fixed finger posture. The tenderness is present day or night, but throbbing, nocturnal pain may become prominent as the pressure of pus develops in the closed space. When these infections have a fulminant course, they are rarely confused with carpal tunnel syndrome; however, as pressure increases in the carpal canal, acute carpal tunnel syndrome may appear as a secondary manifestation of the infection.

When the carpal canal or deep palmar space is infected with indolent organisms such as mycobacteria or fungi, symptoms of carpal tunnel syndrome may precede physical evidence of inflammation by months. A more detailed discussion of carpal tunnel syndrome complicating granulomatous infections appears in Chapter 6.

Hand Stiffness

Patients with carpal tunnel syndrome frequently complain of hand or finger stiffness. On rare occasion, a carpal tunnel syndrome patient describes the stiffness as the most troublesome symptom. When hand stiffness is prominent, differential diagnosis includes the stiffness of rheumatoid or osteoarthritis. Both rheumatoid stiffness and carpal tunnel stiffness may be prominent on awakening. The patient with scleroderma or with eosinophilia myalgia syndrome may describe stiff hands or fingers because of skin tightness.

Patients with Dupuytren's contracture may complain of stiff fingers and are easily identified by presence of contracture on examination. Both Phalen (1966) and Yamaguchi et al. (1965) found that about 2% of their patients with carpal tunnel syndrome also had Dupuytren's contracture.

Diabetics may develop painless limitation of finger joint motion. Diabetic limited finger joint mobility may appear in young insulin-dependent diabetics before development of neuropathy or carpal tunnel syndrome (Rosenbloom 1989). The patient's inability to fully extend the distal and proximal interphalangeal joints is evident when the patient tries unsuccessfully to place the palm flat on a table. Older diabetics with limited finger joint mobility are more likely than other diabetics to have carpal tunnel syndrome or abnormal distal median nerve conduction without typical symptoms of carpal tunnel syndrome (Chaudhuri et al. 1989).

Two neurologic syndromes enter into the differential diagnosis of hand stiffness. Writer's cramp is a focal dystonia characterized by recurring hand or forearm cramping with use. Although the dystonia may be uncomfortable, pain is rarely a prominent feature, and paresthesias are absent. Myotonia can also present with hand cramping and stiffness. In patients with myotonic dystrophy, weakness and atrophy of hand intrinsic muscles might complicate the diagnosis.

Ganglia and Hand Tumors

Ganglion cysts (ganglia) are the most common soft tissue masses in the hand or wrist. They are fibrous cysts filled with clear mucinous fluid that arise from the synovium of joints or tendons. A few are posttraumatic. In most cases they present as painless masses and offer little diagnostic challenge. They may cause chronic wrist pain, and the most common location is the dorsum of the wrist. Dellon and Seif (1978) have proposed that this pain may be caused by compression of the terminal fibers of the posterior interosseous nerve by the ganglion.

On rare occasions, ganglia may occur in the carpal canal. In one series of 89 hand ganglia, 2 were in the carpal canal and associated with carpal tunnel syndrome (Hvid-Hansen 1970). When in the carpal canal, they may be palpable intermittently or not at all.

A large variety of other hand tumors can occur (Johnson et al. 1985). On occasion, hand tumors may compress the median nerve and cause carpal tunnel syndrome as the presenting feature. A list of hand masses that have been reported in patients with carpal tunnel syndrome is presented in Table 6.4. When hand tumors such as osteoid osteoma involve bone, night pain may be a prominent symptom. Chapter 19 discusses tumors of the median nerve.

Raynaud's Phenomenon

Raynaud's phenomenon is blanching or cyanosis of digits precipitated by cold or emotional stress (Blunt and Porter 1981). Blanching is reversible and episodic and is often followed by red fingers from reactive hyperemia. One or more digits of the hands or feet change color and may feel painful, numb, or heavy during an episode of Raynaud's phenomenon. An occasional patient with carpal tunnel syndrome will note finger blanching coincident with occurrence of hand pain and paresthesia (Garland et al. 1957). Nonetheless, it is rarely difficult to distinguish Raynaud's phenomenon from carpal tunnel syndrome based on the patient's description of symptoms.

The conditions may coexist. At the Mayo Clinic about 1% of patients seen with carpal tunnel syndrome also had Raynaud's (Linscheid et al. 1967). In most of these patients with both conditions, an underlying collagen disease was the common cause. A typical example is scleroderma, which is commonly accompanied by Raynaud's and which may also cause carpal tunnel syndrome (Sukenik et al. 1987). Rheumatoid arthritis, systemic lupus erythematosus, or systemic vasculitis may also cause both syndromes. The two syndromes may coexist in chronic renal failure patients on hemodialysis (Schwarz et al. 1984). Other potential causes of both syndromes include myxedema, trauma, and vibration white finger (see discussion of this entity in Chapter 13). Unilateral Raynaud's phenomenon may, on rare occasion, be caused by arterial compression at the thoracic outlet; if the lower brachial plexus is simultaneously compressed, cutaneous parasthesias are more likely to involve the little and ring fingers rather than a classic median nerve distribution.

Loebe and Heidrich (1988) found subtle laboratory evidence of cold-induced digital artery vasospasm in 4 of 40 patients with carpal tunnel syndrome. Their technique showed a similar incidence of arterial abnormalities in patients without carpal tunnel syndrome, supporting their conclusion that carpal tunnel syndrome is not important in the pathogenesis of Raynaud's phenomenon.

In patients with both conditions, release of the flexor retinaculum will usually relieve symptoms of carpal tunnel syndrome without alleviating the symptoms of Raynaud's (Linscheid et al. 1967). However, Waller and Dathan (1985) reported amelioration of Raynaud's after carpal tunnel surgery.

Chronic Wrist Pain

Evaluation of chronic wrist pain is often difficult. Differential diagnosis includes carpal tunnel syndrome, sequelae of wrist trauma, and many of the inflammatory conditions discussed earlier.

Chronic posttraumatic wrist pain may be secondary to chronic intercarpal or carpal-metacarpal sprains. The wrist may seem weak. Examination discloses point tenderness over the wrist (Joseph et al. 1981). Occult fractures, especially of the scaphoid, or avascular necrosis of carpal bones may also present with chronic wrist pain. These may not be evident on plain wrist X rays and may require radionuclide scanning, CT scanning, or tomograms for detection (Gilula et al. 1984).

Avascular lunate necrosis (Kienbock's disease) is particularly important in this regard because it may present with insidious onset of pain without preceding trauma (Gelberman and Szabo 1984). Pain in Kienbock's disease may be prominent at night. Diagnosis in early cases may be concealed by normal wrist X rays. Clues favoring avascular lunate necrosis rather than carpal tunnel syndrome are absence of paresthesias, presence of pain on wrist movement, and compromise of wrist range of motion.

SUMMARY

This chapter reviews some of the conditions that might initially be mistaken for carpal tunnel syndrome or conditions that carpal tunnel syndrome might mimic by presenting with atypical symptoms. Chapter 3 on clinical presentation, Chapters 17 and 18 on median neuropathies outside the carpal tunnel, and Chapters 5 and 6 on carpal tunnel syndrome and other medical conditions cover additional topics on the diagnosis of carpal tunnel syndrome.

REFERENCES

Aljure J, Eltorai I, Bradley WE, Lin JE, Johnson B. Carpal tunnel syndrome in paraplegic patients. Paraplegia 1985;23:182–86.

American Association of Electrodiagnostic Medicine. Guidelines in electrodiagnostic medicine. Muscle Nerve 1992;15:229–253.

American Society for Surgery of the Hand. The hand examination and diagnosis. 3rd ed. New York: Churchill Livingstone, 1990.

Blunt RJ, Porter JM. Raynaud's syndrome. Semin Arthritis Rheum 1981;10:282.

Brooker AF. Extensor carpi radialis tenosynovitis. Orthop Rev 1977;5:99–100.

Cailliet R. Hand pain and impairment. 3rd ed. Philadelphia: FA Davis, 1982.

Carfi J, Ma DM. Posterior interosseous syndrome revisited. Muscle Nerve 1985;8:499–502.

Cavanagh NP, Yates DA, Sutcliffe J. Thenar hypoplasia with associated radiologic abnormalities. Muscle Nerve 1979;2:431–36.

Chaudhuri KR, Davidson AR, Morris IM. Limited joint mobility and carpal tunnel syndrome in insulin-dependent diabetes. Br J Rheumatol 1989;28:191–94.

Conrad B, Benecke R. How valid is the distal sensory nerve action potential for differentiating between radicular and non-radicular nerve lesions? Acta Neurol Scand 1979;60 Supp 73:122.

Crosby EB, Linscheid RL, Dobyns JH. Scaphotrapezial trapezoidal arthrosis. J Hand Surg 1978;3:223–34.

Dawson DM, Hallett M, Millender LH. Entrapment neuropathies. 2nd ed. Boston: Little, Brown, 1990.

Dellon AL, Seif SS. Anatomic dissections relating the posterior interosseous nerve to the carpus, and the etiology of dorsal wrist ganglion pain. J Hand Surg 1978;3:326–32.

Garland H, Bradshaw JP, Clark JM. Compression of the median nerve in the carpal tunnel and its relation to acroparaesthesiae. Br Med J 1957;1:730.

Gelberman RH, Szabo RM. Kienbock's disease. Orthop Clin North Am 1984;15:355–67.

Gellman H, Chandler DR, Petrasek J, Sie I, Adkins R, Waters RL. Carpal tunnel syndrome in paraplegic patients. J Bone Joint Surg 1988A;70:517–19.

Gellman H, Sie I, Waters RL. Late complications of the weight-bearing upper extremity in the paraplegic patient. Clin Orthop 1988b;233:132–35.

Gilliatt RW, Willison RG, Dietz V, Williams IR. Peripheral nerve conduction in patients with a cervical rib and band. Ann Neurol 1978;4:124–29.

Gilula LA, Destouet JM, Weeks PM, Young LV, Wray RC. Roentgenographic diagnosis of the painful wrist. Clin Orthop 1984;187:52–63.

Hadler NM. Medical management of the regional musculoskeletal diseases. Orlando, FL: Grune & Stratton, 1984.

Hvid-Hansen O. On the treatment of ganglia. Acta Chir Scand 1970;136:471–76.

Hybbinette CH, Mannerfelt L. The carpal tunnel syndrome. A retrospective study of 400 operated patients. Acta Orthop Scand 1975;46:610–20.

Imai T, Matsumoto H, Minami R. Asymptomatic ulnar neuropathy in carpal tunnel syndrome. Arch Phys Med Rehabil 1990;71:992–94.

Johnson J, Kilgore E, Newmeyer W. Tumorous lesions of the hand. J Hand Surg 1985;10A:284–86.

Joseph RB, Linscheid RL, Dobyns JH, Bryan RS. Chronic sprains of the carpometacarpal joints. J Hand Surg 1981;6:172–80.

Lapedus PW, Guidotti FP. Stenosing tenovaginitis of the wrist and fingers. Clin Orthop 1972;83:87–90.

Linscheid RL, Peterson LF, Juergens JL. Carpal-tunnel syndrome associated with vasospasm. J Bone Joint Surg 1967;49A:1141–46.

Lister G. The hand: diagnosis and indications. 2nd ed. New York: Churchill Livingstone, 1984.

Loebe M, Heidrich H. The carpal tunnel syndrome—a disease underlying Raynaud's phenomenon? Angiology 1988;39:891–901.

Melone CP Jr, Beavers B, Isani A. The basal joint pain syndrome. Clin Orthop 1987;220:58–67.

Phalen GS. The carpal-tunnel syndrome. Seventeen years' experience in diagnosis and treatment of six hundred fifty-four hands. J Bone Joint Surg 1966;48A:211–28.

Phalen GS. The carpal-tunnel syndrome. Clinical evaluation of 598 hands. Clin Orthop 1972;83:29–40.

Rosenbloom AL. Limitation of finger joint mobility in diabetes mellitus. J Diabetic Complications 1989;3:77–87.

Rowntree T. Anomalous innervation of the hand muscles. J Bone Joint Surg 1949;31B:505–10.

Sarkin TL. Osteo-arthritis of the trapeziometacarpal joint. S Afr Med J 1975;49:392–94.

Schwarz A, Keller F, Seyfert S, Poll W, Molzahn M, Distler A. Carpal tunnel syndrome: a major complication in long-term hemodialysis patients. Clin Nephrol 1984;22:133–37.

Silver MA, Gelberman RH, Gellman H, Rhoades CE. Carpal tunnel syndrome: associated abnormalities in ulnar nerve function and the effect of carpal tunnel release on these abnormalities. J Hand Surg 1985;10A:710–13.

Stewart JD. Focal peripheral neuropathies. New York: Elsevier, 1987.

Stopford JSB. The variation in distribution of the cutaneous nerves of the hand and digits. J Anat 1918;53:14–25.

Su CT, Hoopes JE, Daniel R. Congenital absence of the thenar muscles innervated by the median nerve. Report of a case. J Bone Joint Surg 1972;54A:1087–90.

Sukenik S, Abarbanel JM, Buskila D, Potashnik G, Horowitz J. Impotence, carpal tunnel syndrome and peripheral neuropathy as presenting symptoms in progressive systemic sclerosis (letter). J Rheumatol 1987;14:641–43.

Waller DG, Dathan JR. Raynaud's syndrome and carpal tunnel syndrome. Postgrad Med J 1985;61:161–62.

Werner R, Waring W, Davidoff G. Risk factors for median mononeuropathy of the wrist in postpoliomyelitis patients. Arch Phys Med Rehabil 1989;70:464–67.

Yamaguchi D, Lipscomb P, Soule E. Carpal tunnel syndrome. Minn Med 1965;48:22–31.

Yasuoka S, Okazaki H, Daube JR, MacCarty CS. Foramen magnum tumors. Analysis of 57 cases of benign extramedullary tumors. J Neurosurg 1978;49:828–38.

5

Carpal Tunnel Syndrome with Other Medical Conditions: Part I

Compression of the median nerve in the carpal canal is the primary pathologic process underlying carpal tunnel syndrome. For a given wrist position, the capacity of the canal is fixed; any expansion of a portion of its contents will increase pressure in the canal and compress the median nerve. Pressure in the carpal canal varies with wrist position. Chapter 12 discusses changes of canal pressure with wrist motion and the relation between canal pressure and median nerve compression. Chapter 13 reviews the role of wrist motion and use in the development of carpal tunnel syndrome.

Anomalous canal contents can decrease the space available for normal structures. The contents of the carpal canal might expand from edema, inflammation, hemorrhage, abnormal deposits such as calcium or uric acid, or infiltrative diseases such as amyloidosis. A canal smaller than average—whether from congenital variation or acquired deformity—will develop a proportionately larger increase in pressure for a given expansion of canal contents. A pre-existing abnormality of the median nerve, such as a diffuse peripheral neuropathy or a more proximal nerve injury or compression, can increase the likelihood that focal entrapment of the median nerve in the carpal tunnel will become symptomatic.

Most cases of carpal tunnel syndrome are unrelated to a causal anomaly or systemic illness. The most commonly associated systemic illnesses are diabetes mellitus, rheumatoid arthritis, and hypothyroidism. Carpal tunnel syndrome may complicate pregnancy or occur with other hormonal changes. Collagen diseases and acromegaly are rarer causes. Some patients have a history of prior wrist fracture or blunt trauma. Patients may have other coincident musculoskeletal conditions including De Quervain's tenosynovitis, trigger finger or thumb, Raynaud's phenomenon, lateral humeral epicondylitis (tennis elbow), or disease of the shoulder.

Table 5.1 and Figure 5.1 provide estimates of the incidence of various diseases associated with carpal tunnel syndrome based on the combined results of some of the larger clinical series (Yamaguchi et al. 1965; Phalen 1966; Maxwell et al. 1973; Hybbinette and Mannerfelt 1975; Gainer and Nugent 1977; Loong

Table 5.1 Diagnoses found in 2,705 carpal tunnel syndrome patients

Diagnosis	Number	Diagnosis	Number
Amyloidosis	12	Leukemia	1
Anomalous muscles	3	Median artery thrombosis	1
Asthma	2	Mononeuropathy multiplex	3
Brain tumor	2	Multiple myeloma	4
Carcinoma	2	Multiple sclerosis	1
Carpal tunnel lipoma	1	Mycosis fungoides	1
Collagen disease	12	Neurofibromatosis	1
Dyschondroplasia	2	Peripheral neuropathy	14
Emphysema	2	Pernicious anemia	1
Epilepsy	1	Plantar fasciitis	2
Ganglion	9	Polycythemia	1
Gout	10	Psoriasis	3
Herpes zoster at T-1	1	Raynaud's phenomenon	12
Hodgkin's disease	1	Sarcoidosis	3
Hurler's syndrome	3	Tietze's syndrome	2
Hypertension	7	Tuberculosis	6

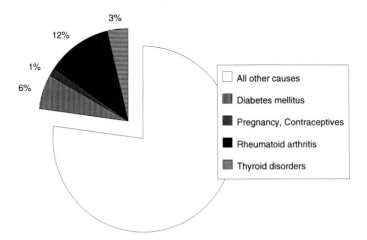

Figure 5.1 The four most common diagnostic associations among 2,705 patients with carpal tunnel syndrome were rheumatoid arthritis, diabetes mellitus, thyroid disorders, and pregnancy or use of oral contraceptives.

1977). The diagnostic criteria for carpal tunnel syndrome and for associated conditions, the rigor with which associated conditions were sought, and the referral patterns vary from series to series, so these incidences are first approximations at best. Figure 5.1 shows the frequency of the most common associations found in these series. Table 5.1 lists some of the rarer associations. The list does not discriminate between chance and pathogenic associations.

In each series the sum of patients with an identified associated disease represents only a fraction of the patients in the series. With follow-up, most cases of carpal tunnel syndrome remain idiopathic. Phillips (1967) followed 41 patients with idiopathic carpal tunnel syndrome for seven years; during the follow-up period, no systemic diseases were recognized that may have contributed to the development of carpal tunnel syndrome.

Lists such as those in Table 5.1 and Figure 5.1 are relatively easy to produce but leave a number of questions unanswered:

1. If a patient has disease X, what is his or her risk of developing carpal tunnel syndrome?
2. Should a patient with carpal tunnel syndrome be tested for previously undiagnosed disease Y?
3. If a patient has carpal tunnel syndrome and disease Z, is treatment of disease Z likely to lead to improvement in carpal tunnel syndrome?

Wherever possible, the discussion that follows tries to address these issues.

CARPAL CANAL STENOSIS

Note that small canal size is not listed in Table 5.1 or Figure 5.1, yet a mismatch between canal size and size of canal contents is invariably part of the compressive process. Newer imaging techniques provide additional data on canal size.

The cross-sectional area of the carpal canal can be estimated from plain radiographs, computed tomography (CT) scans, or magnetic resonance imaging (MRI) scans. More detail is provided in Chapter 11. Some authors have suggested that small canal size, or carpal canal stenosis, explains the vulnerability of some patients to development of carpal tunnel syndrome (Dekel et al. 1980; Gelmers 1981; Bleecker et al. 1985). While this hypothesis is intuitively attractive, other studies of carpal canal size have not confirmed it (Winn and Habes 1990).

Deformities of the Carpal Canal

Bony anomalies or deformities can reduce the cross-sectional area of the canal. Carpal tunnel syndrome can develop as a late sequel of deformities caused by carpal or radial fractures or other wrist trauma (Lewis and Miller 1922; Abbott and Saunders 1933; Cannon and Love 1946). Congenital anomalies causing carpal tunnel syndrome include a hypoplastic scaphoid with dysplastic radius, anomalous distal radius projecting into the canal, or anterior subluxation of carpal bones *(Madelung's deformity)* (Izhar-ul-Haque 1982; Radford and Matthewson 1987; Luchetti et al. 1988). A patient with carpal osteopetrosis presented with carpal tunnel syndrome (Rakic et al. 1986).

CONNECTIVE TISSUE DISEASES

Inflammation in the carpal canal, particularly in the synovium of the flexor tendons, can cause or contribute to median nerve compression. When collagen disease causes flexor tenosynovitis or infection inflames the carpal canal, the mechanism of carpal tunnel syndrome is clear. In contrast, some cases of systemic inflammatory disease are reported with concomitant carpal tunnel syndrome but without evidence that the two diagnoses are pathogenically linked.

Tenosynovitis

Tenosynovitis is frequently listed as a cause of carpal tunnel syndrome. For example, Hybbinette and Mannerfelt (1975) list "tenosynovitis, non-specific chronic or fibrosis" as the condition producing carpal tunnel syndrome in 43% of their 400 patients. Interpreting the literature on tenosynovitis is difficult because of the variety of meanings given to the term in different reports. Hybbinette and Mannerfelt make the diagnosis based on synovial thickening or edema of flexor tendons in the carpal canal identified by the surgeon at time of carpal tunnel release. Phalen (1966) found similar pathology. He reported macroscopic flexor synovial thickening or edema in 203 of 212 carpal tunnel operations. However, Phalen refrained from calling this thickening and edema *synovitis*. Histologic examination showed fibrosis and thickening in about one half the cases, chronic inflammation suggestive of rheumatoid arthritis in about one third, and no pathologic change in nearly one sixth. Other studies of flexor synovium from patients undergoing carpal tunnel surgery have confirmed that the most common synovial histologic changes are fibrosis and edema rather than inflammation (Faithfull et al. 1986; Neal et al. 1987; Fuchs et al. 1991).

There is an association between carpal tunnel syndrome and other tenosynovial diseases, including trigger finger, De Quervain's tenosynovitis, Dupuytren's contracture, lateral epicondylitis, olecranon bursitis, and shoulder periarthritis (subdeltoid bursitis, bicipital tendinitis, calcific tendinitis, adhesive capsulitis) (Murray-Leslie and Wright 1976). Rarely, however, is there direct evidence that synovial inflammation is the cause of carpal tunnel syndrome, even when it is coincident with these other conditions. A number of hypotheses might explain these associations:

1. Both conditions might be caused by some unknown tenosynovial diathesis.
2. Both conditions might be caused by the patient's pattern of arm use. The role of arm use in causing carpal tunnel syndrome is discussed in Chapter 13.
3. Carpal tunnel syndrome symptoms might be caused by a change in

pattern of arm use secondary to another arm condition. For example, if the patient used his or her arm less because of shoulder periarthritis, edema might increase in the carpal canal.
4. Carpal tunnel syndrome might be detected more often once other arm conditions focus attention on the arm.

Some clinicians use the term *tenosynovitis* loosely as a diagnosis for arm pain, particularly when no physical findings are present or if the patient has areas of arm or forearm tenderness. Often, there is little pathologic justification for this usage. Recently, other ill-defined terms such as *cumulative trauma disorder* or *repetitive strain disorder* are replacing *tenosynovitis* in this context; unfortunately, these terms replace unproven pathologic implications with unproven pathogenic implications.

There is evidence on electron micrographs that some patients with carpal tunnel syndrome have abnormal collagen in their flexor retinacula (Staubesand and Fischer 1980; Stransky et al. 1989). The relationship between these findings, "tenosynovitis," and the pathogenesis of carpal tunnel syndrome is undefined.

Rheumatoid Arthritis

Rheumatoid arthritis is the systemic inflammatory illness most commonly associated with carpal tunnel syndrome. In the combined series of carpal tunnel patients, 321 of 2,705 had rheumatoid arthritis (12%). The prevalence of rheumatoid arthritis was 9% in another carpal tunnel syndrome series (Crow 1960).

The prevalence of carpal tunnel syndrome in rheumatoid patients varies from series to series. The prevalence was 24% in a series from Philadelphia, 22% in an Australian series, but only 2% in a Chinese series (McCormack et al. 1970; Moran et al. 1986). Carpal tunnel syndrome may be present prior to evident arthropathy (Richards 1984). Fleming et al. (1976), looking carefully for early extraarticular symptoms in rheumatoid patients, found median nerve sensory symptoms in over one half of patients within one year of onset of rheumatoid arthritis. Patients with rheumatoid arthritis who were over 40 years old had a 42% incidence of carpal tunnel symptoms compared with an incidence of 13% in age-matched nonrheumatoid controls (Herbison et al. 1973).

Patients with rheumatoid arthritis frequently have signs of flexor tenosynovitis, such as tenderness localized to the flexor tendon or triggering or limitation of digital flexion or extension. Gray and Gottlieb (1977) divided their rheumatoid patients on the basis of presence or absence of signs of hand flexor tenosynovitis. The incidence of carpal tunnel syndrome was 47% in the former group and 13% in the latter.

In advanced rheumatoid disease, carpal deformities can contribute to median nerve compression. For example, in a case of dorsal carpal dislocation with flexor tendon rupture, the distal ulna was displaced into the carpal canal and compressed the median nerve (Craig and House 1984).

Early in the course of rheumatoid arthritis, many patients who have symptoms suggestive of carpal tunnel syndrome have normal median distal motor and sensory latencies (Chamberlain and Corbett 1970). Conversely, occasional patients with rheumatoid arthritis have abnormal median nerve conduction studies but no symptoms of carpal tunnel syndrome. Table 5.2 shows the correlation of nerve conduction tests and symptoms in one series of rheumatoid patients (Barnes and Currey 1967).

The incidence of abnormal tests is undoubtedly low by current standards: This series used a median distal motor latency greater than 5.0 msec or a distal sensory latency of greater than 4.0 msec as the indication of abnormality.

Successful medical treatment of rheumatoid arthritis will often relieve the symptoms of carpal tunnel syndrome. With treatment, reduced symptoms of median nerve irritation parallel reduction of the inflammatory disease in hand tendons and joints. Nerve conduction studies may also show improvement (Vemireddi et al. 1979). When symptoms persist despite medical therapy, carpal tunnel surgery is often successful. In some cases, flexor synovectomy is performed in addition to division of the flexor retinaculum (Nalebuff 1969; Ranawat and Straub 1970; Hooper 1972).

Carpal tunnel syndrome may occur as a complication of wrist arthroplasty performed for rheumatoid carpal disease (Lamberta et al. 1980).

Sclerodermatous Disorders

Scleroderma accounts for only a small number of carpal tunnel syndrome patients, both because scleroderma is much rarer than rheumatoid arthritis and because carpal tunnel syndrome is an infrequent complication of scleroderma. Of 125 scleroderma patients questioned yearly for neurologic symptoms, 4 were found to have carpal tunnel syndrome (Lee et al. 1984). Average follow-up was for two and one half years, although some patients were followed much longer. An additional patient had a mononeuritis multiplex with separate episodes of right ulnar neuropathy, a possible lateral cutaneous neuropathy of the calf, and a distal right median sensory neuropathy. In some cases, carpal tunnel syndrome accompanied active hand flexor tenosynovitis, but other cases had no evidence of joint or connective tissue disease as a local cause of median nerve compression. When carpal tunnel syndrome precedes clinical evidence of scleroderma, it is impossible to tell whether the occurrence of the two conditions in the same

Table 5.2 Carpal tunnel syndrome and median nerve conduction in 45 patients with rheumatoid arthritis

	Median Nerve Conduction	
	Abnormal	Normal
Patients with signs or symptoms of carpal tunnel syndrome	15	9
Patients without signs or symptoms of carpal tunnel syndrome	7	14

(Data from Barnes and Currey 1967.)

patient is by chance or by a pathogenic link (Sukenik et al. 1987; Barr and Blair 1988; Berth-Jones et al. 1990).

Toxic oil syndrome, an inflammatory illness caused by ingesting adulterated rapeseed oil, has clinical features overlapping those of scleroderma (Alonso-Ruiz et al. 1986). Among 214 patients with toxic oil syndrome, 31 had symptoms suggestive of carpal tunnel syndrome. Symptoms evolved from 1 to 17 months after onset of the toxic oil syndrome. Abnormal nerve conduction studies in 11 cases supported the diagnosis of carpal tunnel syndrome (Olmedo Garzón et al. 1983).

Carpal tunnel syndrome is a common complication of eosinophilic fasciitis, a rare inflammatory condition of subcutaneous fascia. Superficially, eosinophilic fasciitis resembles scleroderma since both cause stiffening and thickening of soft tissue of the extremities. Unlike scleroderma, it predominantly inflames subcutaneous fascia and spares dermis and viscera. The wrist and forearms are often sites of this inflammation. Physical findings include focal induration and loss of joint range of motion. Hand involvement and Raynaud's phenomenon, both common features of scleroderma, are not typical of eosinophilic fasciitis. In small series of patients with eosinophilic fasciitis, between one fourth and three fourths of patients had carpal tunnel syndrome (Barnes et al. 1979; Jones et al. 1986; Lakhanpal et al. 1988).

Both carpal tunnel syndrome and mononeuropathy multiplex with median nerve involvement have been reported in patients with eosinophilia-myalgia syndrome (Selwa et al. 1990; Shulman 1990).

Polymyalgia Rheumatica

Carpal tunnel syndrome may precede or accompany the muscular symptoms of polymyalgia rheumatica (Miller and Stevens 1978; Richards 1980; Chan and Kaye 1982). Patients with polymyalgia may have a multifocal synovitis. Radionuclide bone scanning suggested a wrist synovitis in 11 of 25 polymyalgic patients. Two of these patients had clinical carpal tunnel syndrome (O'Duffy et al. 1980). The symptoms of carpal tunnel syndrome may improve with steroid therapy of the polymyalgia (Ahmed and Braun 1978).

There is a report of coexistent polymyalgia rheumatica, carpal tunnel syndrome, and wrist chondrocalcinosis in three patients (Richards 1981). Another unusual case is that of a 48-year-old man who developed wrist pain and tenderness with median distribution hypoesthesia (Merianos et al. 1983). Median nerve conduction studies were normal. Erythrocyte sedimentation rate was 25 mm per hour. At carpal tunnel surgery, biopsy of a persistent median artery showed giant cell arteritis.

Systemic Lupus Erythematosus

Carpal tunnel syndrome may occur in patients with lupus. At times, carpal tunnel syndrome precedes any systemic symptoms, and the association may be fortuitous (Sidiq et al. 1972). However, in a survey of lupus patients for neuromuscular complications, 10 of 30 patients with definite lupus by American Rheumatism Association criteria had symptoms of carpal tunnel syndrome, and 7 of the 10 had abnormal median nerve conduction studies (Omdal et al. 1988).

Gout

Gout may cause either acute or chronic carpal tunnel syndrome (Champion 1969). Of 2,705 patients with carpal tunnel syndrome, 3 patients had gout. Conversely, of 10 patients with gout of the hand, 4 had carpal tunnel syndrome (Moore and Weiland 1985). The typical gouty patient with carpal tunnel syndrome has tophi on the flexor tendon synovium in the carpal canal (Akizuki and Matsui 1984; Janssen and Rayan 1987). The combination of tophi and carpal tunnel syndrome may be bilateral (Pledger et al. 1976; Green et al. 1977). Patients usually get symptomatic relief with carpal tunnel release. In one case, tophi oozing from the wound delayed healing (Lianga et al. 1986).

Chondrocalcinosis

Patients with chondrocalcinosis of the wrists may have either symptoms of carpal tunnel syndrome or asymptomatic slowing of median distal nerve conduction (Gerster et al. 1980; Lagier et al. 1984; Binder et al. 1989). Among 22 patients with evidence of chondrocalcinosis on wrist X rays, 14 had prolonged median distal motor latencies, and 8 of these had clinical carpal tunnel syndrome. The calcification was not grossly evident at surgery. At times chondrocalcinosis may present with acute wrist inflammation, or "pseudogout," confirmed by wrist X ray or by demonstration of calcium pyrophosphate crystals in the carpal canal. Acute carpal tunnel syndrome may accompany the pseudogout (Spiegel et al. 1976; Lewis and Fiddian 1982; Goodwin and Arbel 1985).

Miscellaneous Connective Tissue Diseases

Any illness that causes carpal synovial inflammation, infiltration, or edema may lead to median nerve compression. Small series or case reports link other rheumatic conditions and carpal tunnel syndrome. Some 3% to 6% of patients with primary Sjögren's syndrome have carpal tunnel syndrome (Binder et al. 1988; Andonopoulos et al. 1990).

Winkelmann et al. (1982) reported five patients with carpal tunnel syndrome accompanying cutaneous connective tissue diseases, such as morphia, fasciitis, discoid lupus, or lupus panniculitis. In two patients synovial biopsy showed lymphoproliferative changes. Both the carpal tunnel syndrome and skin disease may improve with chloroquine therapy.

Of six patients with palmar fasciitis and polyarthritis, two had carpal tunnel syndrome (Medsger et al. 1982). This syndrome may be a harbinger of carcinoma of the ovary.

A patient with mixed connective tissue syndrome had bilateral carpal tunnel syndrome and bilateral trigeminal sensory neuropathies (Vincent and Van-

Houzen 1980). Prednisone therapy gave symptomatic improvement of both the carpal tunnel syndrome and the systemic inflammatory disease.

Benign joint hypermobility is manifested by increased joint range of motion. Often, patients with this condition can hyperflex at the wrists and hyperabduct at the thumbs to touch the thumbs to their ipsilateral forearm. March et al. (1988) described four patients with benign joint hypermobility who developed symptoms of carpal tunnel syndrome from sleeping with their wrists habitually hyperflexed; symptoms resolved with change of sleep postures.

Other case reports link carpal tunnel syndrome to dermatomyositis/polymyositis, multicentric reticulohistiocytosis, or lymphoma (Quinones et al. 1966; Miller 1967; Flam et al. 1972).

ENDOCRINOPATHIES
Diabetes Mellitus

Diabetes mellitus is one of the most common systemic illnesses found in association with carpal tunnel syndrome. In the combined series of 2,705 patients with carpal tunnel syndrome, 166 were diabetic. Dieck and Kelsey (1985) examined 40 women with carpal tunnel syndrome, aged 45 to 74 years, in a hospital-based case-control study. Patients with carpal tunnel syndrome had a history of diabetes nearly three times more frequently than controls did. The 95% confidence interval was 1.3 to 6.5 times.

Nerve entrapment in the carpal tunnel is only one of many peripheral neuropathic complications of diabetes (Brown and Asbury 1984). By the time they develop symptoms of carpal tunnel syndrome, patients with diabetes usually have some evidence of a generalized peripheral neuropathy by examination or by nerve conduction studies (Leffert 1969). Diabetic carpal tunnel syndrome is very rare in diabetic children (Rosenbloom 1984).

Nerve conduction studies in diabetics without symptoms of carpal tunnel syndrome often show focal abnormalities of motor and sensory conduction across the carpal tunnel in excess of the abnormalities noted in the ipsilateral ulnar nerve (Ozaki et al. 1988). In diabetics, abnormal conduction across the carpal tunnel is more common in women than in men and increases in frequency with increasing age. Conduction may be abnormal across the carpal tunnel when other nerve conduction studies do not give evidence of a more diffuse neuropathy (Comi et al. 1985).

In patients who present with carpal tunnel syndrome and are not known to be diabetic, the chance of detecting diabetes by routine screening is very low. Pal et al. (1986) screened 42 patients with idiopathic carpal tunnel syndrome and found only a single patient with an abnormal glucose tolerance test. Chaplin and Kasdan (1985) found that 2 of 100 carpal tunnel syndrome patients had high fasting blood sugars; both of these patients had absent Achilles tendon reflexes. Isselin and Gariot (1989) found a fasting plasma glucose greater than 140 mg/dl in 3% of patients with carpal tunnel syndrome or other nerve entrapment in the arm.

There is an interesting case report linking the symptoms of carpal tunnel syndrome to the site of insulin injection (Bell and Clements 1983):

> A 27 year old woman with a 14 year history of insulin-dependent diabetes presented with bilateral hand pain, thenar atrophy, median distribution sensory loss, and abnormal median nerve conduction. She switched her insulin injection sites from her arms to elsewhere on her body with resultant improvement in hand symptoms and in median sensory finger-to-wrist nerve conduction studies. Arm symptoms recurred temporarily when insulin injection in the arms was briefly resumed.

Unfortunately, treatment of diabetic carpal tunnel syndrome is rarely this simple. There is little available data on surgery for diabetic carpal tunnel syndrome. Brown and Asbury (1984, 9) state: "When of short duration, these entrapment neuropathies appear to respond to accepted treatment in a manner similar to that found in patients without polyneuropathy." However, if the diabetic carpal tunnel syndrome has progressed to the stage of objective motor or sensory deficit, postoperative neurologic recovery will be less likely than in idiopathic carpal tunnel syndrome of similar severity.

Thyroid Disease

Either hypothyroidism or hyperthyroidism can cause carpal tunnel syndrome. In the combined series of 2,705 carpal tunnel syndrome patients, there were 94 cases of thyroid disease. Hypothyroidism was more frequent than hyperthyroidism. After doing thyroid function tests in 100 patients with carpal tunnel syndrome, Chaplin and Kasdan (1985) found only one thyroid abnormality, which was not confirmed on repeat testing.

In hypothyroid patients, swelling of the contents of the carpal tunnel can cause median nerve compression with typical carpal tunnel syndrome symptoms. At times, in addition to synovial swelling, hypothyroid patients have a more generalized arthropathy that may affect multiple joints and cause arthralgia, joint swelling, and stiffness (Frymoyer and Bland 1973). Carpal tunnel syndrome can be the initial clinical manifestation of hypothyroidism (Golding 1970; Olive and Hennessey 1988). A mild elevation of thyroid-stimulating hormone (TSH) may be the earliest laboratory confirmation of the thyroid deficiency.

Estimates of the incidence of carpal tunnel syndrome in hypothyroid patients vary. In 1958, Murray and Simpson (1958) reported that 26 of 35 myxedematous patients had acroparesthesias. Among 20 patients with hypothyroidism, Rao et al. (1980) found 3 patients with clinical symptoms of carpal tunnel syndrome and 6 patients with asymptomatic prolongation of median distal sensory latency. Among 24 patients with central nervous system effects of hypothyroidism, 6 had carpal tunnel syndrome, and 4 others had evidence of peripheral neuropathy (Cremer et al. 1969). Hypothyroidism rarely causes a diffuse peripheral neuropathy (Fincham and Cape 1968). Most hypothyroid patients with carpal tunnel syndrome do not have clinical or electrical evidence of more diffuse neuropathy. Thyroid replacement therapy can lead to complete symptomatic relief of carpal tunnel syndrome (Frymoyer and Bland 1973).

Carpal tunnel syndrome has been reported in patients receiving lithium for manic-depressive illness (Wood and Jacoby 1986; Deahl 1988). In these cases, the mechanism appeared to be lithium-induced hypothyroidism, and symptoms of carpal tunnel syndrome resolved with thyroid replacement therapy despite continuation of lithium treatment.

Carpal tunnel syndrome rarely accompanies hyperthyroidism. Both the symptoms and electrical abnormalities of carpal tunnel syndrome may improve following radioactive iodine treatment of Graves' disease (Beard et al. 1985).

Estrogens, Progesterone, Gonadotrophins

Carpal tunnel syndrome is a frequent complication of pregnancy (Tobin 1967). Symptoms typically increase in frequency and severity in the third trimester and usually resolve rapidly postpartum or even toward the end of pregnancy (Gould and Wissinger 1978; Massey 1978; Wand 1990). Over 20% of pregnant women may have symptoms of carpal tunnel syndrome; symptoms are bilateral in about one half of the women. However, the incidence of physical signs of carpal tunnel syndrome (positive Phalen's test, abnormal sensory signs or opponens weakness) is much lower—2% in one series (Ekman-Ordeberg et al. 1987).

Gestational carpal tunnel syndrome is usually uncomplicated by other arm conditions, but cases have been reported of carpal tunnel syndrome with eosinophilic fasciitis, De Quervain's tenosynovitis, or "reflex sympathetic dystrophy" in pregnancy (Schumacher et al. 1985; Simon et al. 1988; Amdur and Levin 1989).

Gestational carpal tunnel syndrome may be more common in primiparae (Ekman-Ordeberg et al. 1987). Recurrence with subsequent pregnancies is not inevitable (Tobin 1967).

Median nerve conduction studies are normal, more often than not, in gestational carpal tunnel syndrome (Melvin et al. 1969; Nicholas et al. 1971). Distal sensory latency is more likely to be abnormal than distal motor latency. When latencies are abnormal, they typically improve postpartum and rarely remain mildly abnormal after symptoms have resolved (Gould and Wissinger 1978).

Symptoms usually can be controlled during pregnancy with use of nocturnal wrist splints (Ekman-Ordeberg et al. 1987). Other reported therapies include local steroid injection in the carpal canal (Godfrey 1983). Vitamin B_6 therapy, 100 to 200 mg daily, has also been proposed (Ellis 1987). (The controversy about vitamin B_6 therapy for carpal tunnel syndrome is discussed in Chapter 14.) An occasional patient with gestational carpal tunnel syndrome requires surgical release of the flexor retinaculum.

The high incidence of carpal tunnel syndrome during pregnancy is commonly attributed to fluid retention with an increase in carpal canal pressure secondary to edema. A recent study suggests that the median nerves of pregnant women have an increased susceptibility to local anesthetics (Butterworth et al. 1990). Whether this susceptibility is evidence of median nerve compression in the carpal tunnel or of hormonally-induced changes in nerve physiology is unknown.

Occurrence of symptoms of carpal tunnel syndrome during breast-feeding is rarer than occurrence of symptoms during pregnancy (Snell et al. 1980; Yagnik 1987). Wand (1989, 1990) described 24 women who developed symptoms of carpal tunnel syndrome during lactation. They typically became symptomatic a few weeks postpartum, had persistent symptoms during the months of lactation, and improved within a few weeks of weaning. Compared with women with gestational carpal tunnel syndrome, women with lactational carpal tunnel syndrome are older, more likely to be primiparous, and less likely to have peripheral edema. It is unclear whether carpal tunnel syndrome with lactation has a hormonal cause or whether it is related to wrist positioning during breast-feeding.

Kotowicz et al. (1988) reported an unusual case of carpal tunnel syndrome accompanying galactorrhea and amenorrhea secondary to a prolactin-secreting pituitary adenoma. This case, lactation-associated carpal tunnel syndrome, and the observation that prolactin levels may be increased in acromegaly and hypothyroidism have led to speculation about the role of prolactin in the pathogenesis of carpal tunnel syndrome. Rossi et al. (1984) measured prolactin levels in patients with idiopathic carpal tunnel syndrome and did not find evidence for an association.

Use of oral contraceptives can be followed by development of carpal tunnel syndrome. Sabour and Fadel (1970) reported 62 women who developed carpal tunnel syndrome symptoms while on oral contraceptives and had resolution of symptoms within one month of stopping the medication. They suggest that the risk is higher when the estrogen content of the oral contraceptive is higher. Fluid retention may be a pathogenic mechanism.

The relationship between carpal tunnel syndrome and menopause or postmenopausal estrogen use is unclear. Two case-control studies have suggested that postmenopausal estrogen use might be a risk factor for carpal tunnel syndrome with an odds ratio in both studies of 2.4 (Cannon et al. 1981; Dieck and Kelsey 1985). In one of these, the results fell slightly short of statistical significance, and neither study controlled for patient age as a confounding variable. Interpretation of these studies is complicated by case reports of postmenopausal women with symptoms of carpal tunnel syndrome who experienced relief of hand symptoms when placed on estrogen and progesterone replacement therapy (Confino-Cohen et al. 1991).

Another conflicting observation is that there may be an increased occurrence of carpal tunnel syndrome following oophorectomy. Björkqvist et al. (1977) studied 20 women before and after oophorectomy; 3 of the 20 developed symptoms consistent with carpal tunnel syndrome within four months of surgery; 2 of these women, who had normal median distal latencies documented prior to oophorectomy, developed prolonged median distal latencies when they were symptomatic. In a case-control study, hysterectomy with bilateral oophorectomy was a risk factor for development of carpal tunnel syndrome (Cannon et al. 1981).

A 31-year-old woman developed symptoms of carpal tunnel syndrome after taking danazol for treatment of endometriosis (Gray 1978). She also developed a knee effusion. Carpal tunnel syndrome symptoms and the knee effusion resolved one week after stopping danazol.

Growth Hormone

Carpal tunnel syndrome is a common complication of acromegaly. Sternberg (1891), as cited in Pickett et al. (1975), reportedly identified nocturnal hand paresthesias as an early manifestation of acromegaly. Woltman (1941) reported that 10 of 213 acromegalic patients complained of periodic hand pain and documented that, in at least some cases, this was associated with an isolated median neuropathy. In series of acromegalic patients, the incidence of carpal tunnel syndrome may range from 35% to 64% (Bluestone et al. 1971; Pickett et al. 1975; Baum et al. 1986; Podgorski et al. 1988). Carpal tunnel syndrome symptoms are a predictor of growth hormone levels and activity of the acromegaly: 34 of the 63 patients whose acromegaly was active had carpal tunnel syndrome symptoms; only 1 patient without active symptoms had carpal tunnel syndrome symptoms (O'Duffy et al. 1973).

Symptoms of carpal tunnel syndrome may be one of the earliest clinical indications of acromegaly. Patients may also have an arthropathy involving multiple joints that complicates interpretation of their extremity symptoms (Bluestone et al. 1971; Podgorski et al. 1988). Development of carpal tunnel syndrome is independent of glucose intolerance, abnormalities of thyroid function, or development of more diffuse peripheral neuropathy (Jamal et al. 1987). The pathogenic import of raised growth hormone levels is further supported by development of carpal tunnel syndrome in patients receiving growth hormone as experimental treatment for osteoporosis (Aloia et al. 1976).

In unselected patients with carpal tunnel syndrome, the incidence of acromegaly is very low. The cost-effectiveness of screening for acromegaly in carpal tunnel syndrome patients is unknown. A reasonable approach is to be clinically alert for acromegaly but not to undertake laboratory screening for it unless prompted by clinical clues.

In most acromegalic patients, treatment of the acromegaly will relieve the symptoms of carpal tunnel syndrome (Nabarro 1987). Symptoms of carpal tunnel syndrome may regress within two weeks after fall of growth hormone levels (O'Duffy et al. 1973). Median distal motor latency may improve within one week of surgical removal of a pituitary adenoma (Baum et al. 1986). Carpal tunnel syndrome may also improve following suppression of growth hormone secretion with bromocriptine or lergotrile (Kleinberg et al. 1978; Luboshitzky and Barzilai 1980).

Calcium Abnormalities

Carpal tunnel syndrome is rarely associated with disorders of calcium metabolism. Some case reports deserve mention:

- A 78-year-old man presented with years of carpal tunnel syndrome symptoms. At surgery, pseudogout was diagnosed with pyrophosphate crystals in the carpal canal. The pseudogout was caused by hypercalcemia secondary to hyperparathyroidism (Weinstein et al. 1968).
- A patient with carpal tunnel syndrome had hypocalcemia, chronic renal failure, and secondary hyperparathyroidism. Wrist X rays revealed ectopic calcification in the carpal canal (Firooznia et al. 1981).
- A 57-year-old woman presented with bilateral nocturnal hand paresthesias and pain. Serum calcium was elevated to 11.8 mg/dl, and serum parathormone levels were over twice the upper limit of normal. Bilateral median distal motor latencies were markedly prolonged (6.5 and 7.2 msec). Two weeks after surgical removal of a parathyroid adenoma, hand symptoms were absent and median distal motor latencies had improved to 3.8 and 3.7 msec (Palma 1983).
- A 55-year-old woman acutely developed symptoms of carpal tunnel syndrome after carpopedal spasm caused by hypocalcemic tetany (Massey et al. 1978). Symptoms slowly resolved after episodes of spasm were stopped by correction of serum calcium.

REFERENCES

Abbott LC, Saunders JBdeCM. Injuries of the median nerve in fractures of the lower end of the radius. Surg Gynecol Obstet 1933;57:507–16.

Ahmed T, Braun AI. Carpal tunnel syndrome with polymyalgia rheumatica. Arthritis Rheum 1978;21:221–23.

Akizuki S, Matsui T. Entrapment neuropathy caused by tophaceous gout. J Hand Surg 1984;9B:331–32.

Aloia JF, Zanzi I, Ellis K, Jowsey J, Roginsky M, Wallach S, Cohn SH. Effects of growth hormone in osteoporosis. J Clin Endocrinol Metab 1976;43:992–99.

Alonso-Ruiz A, Zea-Mendoza AC, Salazar-Vallinas JM, Rocamora-Ripoll A, Beltrán-Gutíerrez J. Toxic oil syndrome: a syndrome with features overlapping those of various forms of scleroderma. Semin Arthritis Rheum 1986;15:200–212.

Amdur HS, Levin RE. Eosinophilic fasciitis during pregnancy. Obstet Gynecol 1989;73:843–47.

Andonopoulos AP, Lagos G, Drosos AA, Moutsopoulos HM. The spectrum of neurological involvement in Sjögren's syndrome. Br J Rheumatol 1990;29:21–23.

Barnes CG, Currey HL. Carpal tunnel syndrome in rheumatoid arthritis. A clinical and electrodiagnostic survey. Ann Rheum Dis 1967;26:226–33.

Barnes L, Rodnan GP, Medsger TA, Short D. Eosinophilic fasciitis. A pathologic study of twenty cases. Am J Pathol 1979;96:493–517.

Barr WG, Blair SJ. Carpal tunnel syndrome as the initial manifestation of scleroderma. J Hand Surg [Am] 1988;13:366–68.

Baum H, Ludecke DK, Herrmann HD. Carpal tunnel syndrome and acromegaly. Acta Neurochir (Wien) 1986;83:54–55.

Beard L, Kumar A, Estep HL. Bilateral carpal tunnel syndrome caused by Graves' disease. Arch Intern Med 1985;145:345–46.

Bell DS, Clements RS Jr. Reversal of the carpal tunnel syndrome after change of insulin injection sites (letter). Diabetes Care 1983;6:211–12.

Berth-Jones J, Coates PA, Graham-Brown RA, Burns DA. Neurological complications of systemic sclerosis—a report of three cases and review of the literature. Clin Exp Dermatol 1990;15:91–94.

Binder A, Snaith ML, Isenberg D. Sjögren's syndrome: a study of its neurological complications. Br J Rheumatol 1988;27:275–80.

Binder AI, Sheppard MN, Paice E. Extensor tendon rupture related to calcium pyrophosphate crystal deposition disease. Br J Rheumatol 1989;28:251–53.

Björkqvist SE, Lang AH, Punnonen R, Rauramo L. Carpal tunnel syndrome in ovariectomized women. Acta Obstet Gynecol Scand 1977;56:127–30.

Bleecker ML, Bohlman M, Moreland R, Tipton A. Carpal tunnel syndrome: role of carpal canal size. Neurology 1985;35:1599–1604.

Bluestone R, Bywaters EG, Hartog M, Holt PJ, Hyde S. Acromegalic arthropathy. Ann Rheum Dis 1971;30:243–58.

Brown MJ, Asbury AK. Diabetic neuropathy. Ann Neurol 1984;15:2–12.

Butterworth IV JF, Walker FO, Lysak SZ. Pregnancy increases median nerve susceptibility to lidocaine. Anesthesiology 1990;72:962–65.

Cannon BW, Love JG. Tardy median palsy; median neuritis; median thenar neuritis amenable to surgery. Surgery 1946;20:210–16.

Cannon LJ, Bernacki EJ, Walter SD. Personal and occupational factors associated with carpal tunnel syndrome. JOM 1981;23:255–58.

Chamberlain MA, Corbett M. Carpal tunnel syndrome in early rheumatoid arthritis. Ann Rheum Dis 1970;29:149–52.

Champion D. Gouty tenosynovitis and the carpal tunnel syndrome. Med J Aust 1969;1:1030–32.

Chan MK, Kaye RL. Carpal tunnel syndrome as a precursor of polymyalgia rheumatica. Ariz Med 1982;39:517–19.

Chaplin E, Kasdan ML. Carpal tunnel syndrome and routine blood chemistries. Plast Reconstr Surg 1985;75:722–24.

Comi G, Lozza L, Galardi G, Ghilardi MF, Medaglini S, Canal N. Presence of carpal tunnel syndrome in diabetics: effect of age, sex, diabetes duration and polyneuropathy. Acta Diabetol Lat 1985;22:259–62.

Confino-Cohen R, Lishner M, Savin H, Lang R, Ravid M. Response of carpal tunnel syndrome to hormone replacement therapy. Br Med J 1991;303:1514.

Craig EV, House JH. Dorsal carpal dislocation and flexor tendon rupture in rheumatoid arthritis: a case report. J Hand Surg 1984;9A:261–64.

Cremer GM, Goldstein NP, Paris J. Myxedema and ataxia. Neurology 1969;19:37–46.

Crow RS. Treatment of the carpal-tunnel syndrome. Br Med J 1960;1:1611–15.

Deahl MP. Lithium-induced carpal tunnel syndrome. Br J Psychiatry 1988;153:250–51.

Dekel S, Papaioannou T, Rushworth G, Coates R. Idiopathic carpal tunnel syndrome caused by carpal stenosis. Br Med J 1980;280:1297–99.

Dieck GS, Kelsey JL. An epidemiologic study of the carpal tunnel syndrome in an adult female population. Prev Med 1985;14:63–69.

Ekman-Ordeberg G, Salgeback S, Ordeberg G. Carpal tunnel syndrome in pregnancy. A prospective study. Acta Obstet Gynecol Scand 1987;66:233–35.

Ellis JM. Treatment of carpal tunnel syndrome with vitamin B_6. South Med J 1987;80:882–84.

Faithfull DK, Moir DH, Ireland J. The micropathology of the typical carpal tunnel syndrome. J Hand Surg 1986;11B:131–32.

Fincham RW, Cape CA. Neuropathy in myxedema. A study of sensory nerve conduction in the upper extremities. Arch Neurol 1968;19:464–66.

Firooznia H, Golimbu C, Rafii M. Carpal tunnel syndrome as a manifestation of secondary hyperparathyroidism (letter). Arch Intern Med 1981;141:959.

Flam M, Ryan SC, Mah-Poy GL, Jacobs KF, Neldner KH. Multicentric reticulohistiocytosis. Report of a case, with atypical features and electron microscopic study of skin lesions. Am J Med 1972;52:841–48.

Fleming A, Dodman S, Crown JM, Corbett M. Extra-articular features in early rheumatoid disease. Br Med J 1976;1:1241–43.

Frymoyer JW, Bland J. Carpal-tunnel syndrome in patients with myxedematous arthropathy. J Bone Joint Surg 1973;55A:78–82.

Fuchs PC, Nathan PA, Myers LD. Synovial histology in carpal tunnel syndrome. J Hand Surg 1991;16A:753–58.

Gainer JV Jr, Nugent GR. Carpal tunnel syndrome: report of 430 operations. South Med J 1977;70:325–28.

Gelmers HJ. Primary carpal tunnel stenosis as a cause of entrapment of the median nerve. Acta Neurochir (Wien) 1981;55:317–20.

Gerster JC, Lagier R, Boivin G, Schneider C. Carpal tunnel syndrome in chondrocalcinosis of the wrist. Clinical and histologic study. Arthritis Rheum 1980;23:926–31.

Godfrey CM. Carpal tunnel syndrome in pregnancy (letter). Can Med Assoc J 1983;129:928.

Golding DN. Hypothyroidism presenting with musculoskeletal symptoms. Ann Rheum Dis 1970;29:10–14.

Goodwin DR, Arbel R. Pseudogout of the wrist presenting as acute median nerve compression. J Hand Surg 1985;10B:261–62.

Gould JS, Wissinger HA. Carpal tunnel syndrome in pregnancy. South Med J 1978;71:144–45,154.

Gray RG. Bilateral carpal tunnel syndrome and arthritis associated with danazol administration (letter). Arthritis Rheum 1978;21:493–94.

Gray RG, Gottlieb NL. Hand flexor tenosynovitis in rheumatoid arthritis. Prevalence, distribution, and associated rheumatic features. Arthritis Rheum 1977;20:1003–8.

Green EJ, Dilworth JH, Levitin PM. Tophaceous gout. An unusual cause of bilateral carpal tunnel syndrome. JAMA 1977;237:2747–48.

Herbison GJ, Teng C, Martin JH, Ditunno JF Jr. Carpal tunnel syndrome in rheumatoid arthritis. Am J Phys Med 1973;52:68–74.

Hooper J. The surgery of the wrist in rheumatoid arthritis. Aust NZ J Surg 1972;42:135–40.

Hybbinette CH, Mannerfelt L. The carpal tunnel syndrome. A retrospective study of 400 operated patients. Acta Orthop Scand 1975;46:610–20.

Isselin J, Gariot P. Tunnel syndromes and blood glucose anomalies (in French). Ann Chir Main 1989;8:344–46.

Izhar-ul-Haque. Carpal tunnel syndrome due to an anomalous distal end of the radius. A case report. J Bone Joint Surg 1982;64A:943–44.

Jamal GA, Kerr DJ, McLellan AR, Weir AI, Davies DL. Generalised peripheral nerve dysfunction in acromegaly: a study by conventional and novel neurophysiological techniques. J Neurol Neurosurg Psychiatry 1987;50:886–94.

Janssen T, Rayan GM. Gouty tenosynovitis and compression neuropathy of the median nerve. Clin Orthop 1987;216:203–6.

Jones HR Jr, Beetham WP Jr, Silverman ML, Margles SW. Eosinophilic fasciitis and the carpal tunnel syndrome. J Neurol Neurosurg Psychiatry 1986;49:324–27.

Kleinberg DL, Schaaf M, Frantz AG. Studies with lergotrile mesylate in acromegaly. Fed Proc 1978;37:2198–2201.

Kotowicz MA, Turtle JR, Crouch R. Bilateral carpal tunnel syndrome and galactorrhea. Med J Aust 1988;148:252–55.

Lagier R, Boivin G, Gerster JC. Carpal tunnel syndrome associated with mixed calcium pyrophosphate dihydrate and apatite crystal deposition in tendon synovial sheath. Arthritis Rheum 1984;27:1190–95.

Lakhanpal S, Ginsburg WW, Michet CJ, Doyle JA, Moore SB. Eosinophilic fasciitis: clinical spectrum and therapeutic response in 52 cases. Semin Arthritis Rheum 1988;17:221–31.

Lamberta FJ, Ferlic DC, Clayton ML. Volz total wrist arthroplasty in rheumatoid arthritis: a preliminary report. J Hand Surg 1980;5:245–52.

Lee P, Bruni J, Sukenik S. Neurological manifestations in systemic sclerosis (scleroderma). J Rheumatol 1984;11:480–83.

Leffert RD. Diabetes mellitus initially presenting as peripheral neuropathy in the upper limb. J Bone Joint Surg 1969;51A:1004–10.

Lewis D, Miller EM. Peripheral nerve injuries associated with fractures. Trans Am Surg Assoc 1922;40:489–580.

Lewis SL, Fiddian NJ. Acute carpal tunnel syndrome a rare complication of chondrocalcinosis. Hand 1982;14:164–67.

Lianga J, Waslen GD, Penney CJ. Tophaceous gout presenting with bilateral hand contractures and carpal tunnel syndrome (letter). J Rheumatol 1986;13:230–31.

Loong SC. The carpal tunnel syndrome: a clinical and electrophysiological study of 250 patients. Proc Aust Assoc Neurol 1977;14:51–65.

Luboshitzky R, Barzilai D. Bromocriptine for an acromegalic patient. Improvement in cardiac function and carpal tunnel syndrome. JAMA 1980;244:1825–27.

Luchetti R, Mingione A, Monteleone M, Cristiani G. Carpal tunnel syndrome in Madelung's deformity. J Hand Surg 1988;13B:19–22.

March LM, Francis H, Webb J. Benign joint hypermobility with neuropathies: documentation and mechanism of median, sciatic, and common peroneal nerve compression. Clin Rheumatol 1988;7:35–40.

Massey EW. Acroparesthesias in pregnancy (letter). South Med J 1978;71:880.

Massey EW, O'Brian JT, Georges LP. Carpal tunnel syndrome secondary to carpopedal spasm. Ann Intern Med 1978;88:804–5.

Maxwell JA, Clough CA, Reckling FW, Kelly CR. Carpal tunnel syndrome. A review of cases treated surgically. J Kans Med Soc 1973;74:190–93.

McCormack LJ, Cauldwell EW, Anson BJ. Brachial and antebrachial arterial patterns. Surg Gynecol Obstet 1970;96:43–54.

Medsger TA, Dixon JA, Garwood VF. Palmar fasciitis and polyarthritis associated with ovarian carcinoma. Ann Intern Med 1982;96:424–31.

Melvin JL, Burnett CN, Johnson EW. Median nerve conduction in pregnancy. Arch Phys Med Rehabil 1969;50:75–80.

Merianos P, Smyrnis P, Tsomy K, Hager J. Giant cell arteritis of the median nerve simulating carpal tunnel syndrome. Hand 1983;15:249–51.

Miller DG. The association of immune disease and malignant lymphoma. Ann Intern Med 1967;66:507–21.

Miller LD, Stevens MB. Skeletal manifestations of polymyalgia rheumatica. JAMA 1978;240:27–29.

Moore JR, Weiland AJ. Gouty tenosynovitis in the hand. J Hand Surg 1985;10A:291–95.

Moran H, Chen SL, Muirden KD, Jiang SJ, Gu YY, Hopper J, Jiang PL, Lawler G, Chen RB. A comparison of rheumatoid arthritis in Australia and China. Ann Rheum Dis 1986;45:572–78.

Murray IPC, Simpson JA. Acroparaesthesia in myxoedema—a clinical and electromyographic study. Lancet 1958;1:1360–63.

Murray-Leslie CF, Wright V. Carpal tunnel syndrome, humeral epicondylitis, and the cervical spine: a study of clinical and dimensional relations. Br Med J 1976;1:1439–42.

Nabarro JD. Acromegaly. Clin Endocrinol (Oxf) 1987;26:481–512.

Nalebuff EA. Surgical treatment of rheumatoid tenosynovitis in the hand. Surg Clin North Am 1969;49:799–809.

Neal NC, McManners J, Stirling GA. Pathology of the flexor tendon sheath in the spontaneous carpal tunnel syndrome. J Hand Surg 1987;12B:229–32.

Nicholas GG, Noone RB, Graham WP. Carpal tunnel syndrome in pregnancy. Hand 1971;3:80–83.

O'Duffy JD, Hunder GG, Wahner HW. A follow-up study of polymyalgia rheumatica: evidence of chronic axial synovitis. J Rheumatol 1980;7:685–93.

O'Duffy JD, Randall RV, MacCarty CS. Median neuropathy (carpal-tunnel syndrome) in acromegaly. A sign of endocrine overactivity. Ann Intern Med 1973;78:379–83.

Olive KE, Hennessey JV. Marked hyperprolactinemia in subclinical hypothyroidism. Arch Intern Med 1988;148:2278–79.

Olmedo Garzón FJ, Leiva Santana C, Alonso Ruiz A, Riva Meana C. The toxic-oil syndrome: a new cause of the carpal-tunnel syndrome (letter). N Engl J Med 1983;309:1455.

Omdal R, Mellgren SI, Husby G. Clinical neuropsychiatric and neuromuscular manifestations in systemic lupus erythematosus. Scand J Rheumatol 1988;17:113–17.

Ozaki I, Baba M, Matsunaga M, Takebe K. Deleterious effect of the carpal tunnel on nerve conduction in diabetic polyneuropathy. Electromyogr Clin Neurophysiol 1988;28:301–6.

Pal B, Mangion P, Hossain MA. An assessment of glucose tolerance in patients with idiopathic carpal tunnel syndrome (letter). Br J Rheumatol 1986;25:412–13.

Palma G. Carpal tunnel syndrome and hyperparathyroidism (letter). Ann Neurol 1983;14:592.

Phalen GS. The carpal-tunnel syndrome. Seventeen years' experience in diagnosis and treatment of six hundred fifty-four hands. J Bone Joint Surg 1966;48A:211–28.

Phillips RS. Carpal tunnel syndrome as a manifestation of systemic disease. Ann Rheum Dis 1967;26:59–63.

Pickett JB, Layzer RB, Levin SR, Scheider V, Campbell MJ, Sumner AJ. Neuromuscular complications of acromegaly. Neurology 1975;25:638–45.

Pledger SR, Hirsch B, Freiberg RA. Bilateral carpal tunnel syndrome secondary to gouty tenosynovitis: a case report. Clin Orthop 1976;118:188–89.

Podgorski M, Robinson B, Weissberger A, Stiel J, Wang S, Brooks PM. Articular manifestations of acromegaly. Aust NZ J Med 1988;18:28–35.

Quinones CA, Perry HO, Rushton JG. Carpal tunnel syndrome in dermatomyositis and scleroderma. Arch Dermatol 1966;94:20–25.

Radford PJ, Matthewson MH. Hypoplastic scaphoid—an unusual cause of carpal tunnel syndrome. J Hand Surg 1987;12B:236–38.

Rakic M, Elhosseiny A, Ramadan F, Iyer R, Howard RG, Gross L. Adult-type osteopetrosis presenting as carpal tunnel syndrome. Arthritis Rheum 1986;29:926–28.

Ranawat C, Straub LR. Volar tenosynovitis of wrist in rheumatoid arthritis. Arthritis Rheum 1970;13:112–17.

Rao SN, Katiyar BC, Nair KR, Misra S. Neuromuscular status in hypothyroidism. Acta Neurol Scand 1980;61:167–77.

Richards AJ. Carpal tunnel syndrome in polymyalgia rheumatica. Rheumatol Rehabil 1980;19:100–102.

Richards AJ. Chondrocalcinosis and polymyalgia rheumatica in carpal tunnel syndrome (letter). Arthritis Rheum 1981;24:640.

Richards AJ. Carpal tunnel syndrome and subsequent rheumatoid arthritis in the "fibrositis" syndrome. Ann Rheum Dis 1984;43:232–34.

Rosenbloom AL. Skeletal and joint manifestations of childhood diabetes. Pediatr Clin North Am 1984;31:569–89.

Rossi E, Sighinolfi E, Bortolotti P, De-Santis G, Schoenhuber R, Grandi M, Landi A. Nocturnal prolactin secretion in carpal tunnel syndrome. Ital J Neurol Sci 1984;5:405–8.

Sabour MS, Fadel HE. The carpal tunnel syndrome—a new complication ascribed to the "pill." Am J Obstet Gynecol 1970;107:1265–67.

Schumacher HR Jr, Dorwart BB, Korzeniowski OM. Occurrence of De Quervain's tendinitis during pregnancy. Arch Intern Med 1985;145:2083–84.

Selwa JF, Feldman EL, Blaivas M. Mononeuropathy multiplex in tryptophan-associated eosinophilia-myalgia syndrome. Neurology 1990;40:1632–33.

Shulman LE. The eosinophilia-myalgia syndrome associated with ingestion of L-tryptophan. Arthritis Rheum 1990;33:913–17.

Sidiq M, Kirsner AB, Sheon RP. Carpal tunnel syndrome. First manifestation of systemic lupus erythematosus. JAMA 1972;222:1416–17.

Simon JN, Mokriski BK, Malinow AM, Martz DG Jr. Reflex sympathetic dystrophy syndrome in pregnancy. Anesthesiology 1988;69:100–102.

Snell NJ, Coysh HL, Snell BJ. Carpal tunnel syndrome presenting in the puerperium. Practitioner 1980;224:191–93.

Spiegel PG, Ginsberg M, Skosey JL, Kwong P. Acute carpal tunnel syndrome secondary to pseudogout: case report. Clin Orthop 1976;120:185–87.

Staubesand J, Fischer N. The ultrastructural characteristics of abnormal collagen fibrils in various organs. Connect Tissue Res 1980;7:213–17.

Stransky G, Wenger E, Dimitrov L, Weis S. Collagen dysplasia in idiopathic carpal tunnel syndrome. Pathol Res Pract 1989;185:795–98.

Sukenik S, Abarbanel JM, Buskila D, Potashnik G, Horowitz J. Impotence, carpal tunnel syndrome and peripheral neuropathy as presenting symptoms in progressive systemic sclerosis (letter). J Rheumatol 1987;14:641–43.

Tobin SM. Carpal tunnel syndrome in pregnancy. Am J Obstet Gynecol 1967;97:493–98.

Vemireddi NK, Redford JB, PombeJara CN. Serial nerve conduction studies in carpal tunnel syndrome secondary to rheumatoid arthritis: preliminary study. Arch Phys Med Rehabil 1979;60:393–96.

Vincent FM, Van-Houzen RN. Trigeminal sensory neuropathy and bilateral carpal tunnel syndrome: the initial manifestation of mixed connective tissue disease. J Neurol Neurosurg Psychiatry 1980;43:458–60.

Wand JS. The natural history of carpal tunnel syndrome in lactation. J R Soc Med 1989;82:349–50.

Wand JS. Carpal tunnel syndrome in pregnancy and lactation. J Hand Surg 1990;15B:93–95.

Weinstein JD, Dick HM, Grantham SA. Pseudogout, hyperparathyroidism, and carpal-tunnel syndrome. A case report. J Bone Joint Surg 1968;50A:1669–74.

Winkelmann RK, Connolly SM, Doyle JA. Carpal tunnel syndrome in cutaneous connective tissue disease: generalized morphea, lichen sclerosus, fasciitis, discoid lupus erythematosus, and lupus panniculitis. J Am Acad Dermatol 1982;7:94–99.

Winn FJ Jr, Habes DJ. Carpal tunnel area as a risk factor for carpal tunnel syndrome. Muscle Nerve 1990;13:254–58.

Woltman HW. Neuritis associated with acromegaly. Arch Neurol Psychiatry 1941;45:680–82.

Wood KA, Jacoby RJ. Lithium induced hyperthyroidism presenting with carpal tunnel syndrome (letter). Br J Psychiatry 1986;149:386–87.

Yagnik PM. Carpal tunnel syndrome in nursing mothers (letter). South Med J 1987;80:1468.

Yamaguchi D, Lipscomb P, Soule E. Carpal tunnel syndrome. Minn Med 1965;48:22–31.

6

Carpal Tunnel Syndrome with Other Medical Conditions: Part II

AMYLOIDOSIS

The amyloids are a group of proteins that have specific staining properties including birefringence when viewed with polarized light after staining with Congo red. Amyloidosis is a rare cause of nerve compression, but amyloid deposition in the tissues of the carpal tunnel can cause carpal tunnel syndrome. Amyloidosis is not evident by gross inspection of canal contents at surgery; its reported incidence will increase if the surgeon and pathologist search explicitly for it. Many surgeons do not submit tissue from carpal surgery for histologic evaluation. In one report of 345 carpal tunnel releases, only 87 pathologic specimens were available for review (Bastian 1974); 2 of the 87 stained positive for amyloid. In the Mayo Clinic series of 2,784 patients operated on for carpal tunnel syndrome, 1,500 specimens were reviewed for amyloid deposits (Kyle et al. 1989). Some 57 of these specimens were initially reported positive for amyloid, but reexamination of the specimens with Congo red staining and careful searching for amyloid yielded 95 additional cases of carpal tunnel amyloidosis.

Carpal tunnel amyloidosis can be subdivided into localized carpal tunnel amyloidosis, primary systemic amyloidosis, familial amyloidosis, and beta-2-microglobulin amyloidosis associated with hemodialysis and renal failure. In the Mayo Clinic series, which did not include hemodialysis cases, the distribution is shown in Figure 6.1. Regardless of the type or cause of amyloid in the carpal tunnnel, carpal tunnel surgery is usually successful in relieving the symptoms of carpal tunnel syndrome.

Primary Systemic Amyloidosis

Primary systemic amyloidosis is also known as light chain amyloidosis (AL) because of the derivation of the amyloid protein from immunoglobulin light chains. Carpal tunnel syndrome is a prominent or initial manifestation of primary

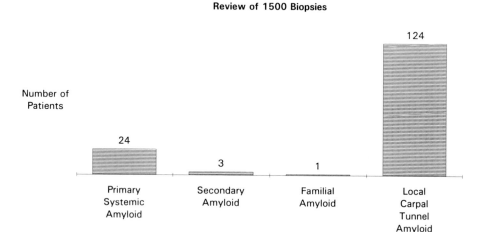

Figure 6.1 Types of amyloid found at the time of carpal tunnel surgery on careful review of 1,500 biopsies by Kyle et al. (1989). None of the patients with amyloid were on hemodialysis. (Data from Kyle et al. 1989.)

systemic amyloidosis in one quarter of the cases (Kyle and Greipp 1983). Systemic manifestations may result from infiltration in other organs, especially heart, kidney, tongue, and gastrointestinal tract. If serum and urine of these patients are screened with immunoprotein electrophoresis, nearly 90% will have abnormalities, most commonly a monoclonal paraprotein (Kelly et al. 1979).

Patients who present with a peripheral neuropathy and serum evidence of a monoclonal gammopathy introduce a differential diagnosis that includes primary systemic amyloidosis, multiple myeloma, osteoclastic myeloma, or "monoclonal gammopathy of undetermined significance." (Kelly 1983). In these patients, nerve conduction evidence of focal slowing across the carpal tunnel should prompt a search for primary systemic amyloidosis or multiple myeloma with amyloidosis (Kelly et al. 1979, 1981). In a series of 19 patients with peripheral neuropathy and monoclonal gammopathy of undetermined significance, only 1 had evidence of carpal tunnel syndrome (Krol-v-Straaten et al. 1985).

Secondary amyloidosis (AA) may result from chronic inflammatory or infectious diseases. In secondary amyloidosis, the amyloid is usually not deposited in the carpal tunnel (Benson et al. 1975). When carpal tunnel syndrome accompanies secondary amyloidosis, the underlying disease, such as rheumatoid arthritis or leprosy, is more likely than amyloidosis to be the cause of the median neuropathy.

Foci of amyloid deposition can be located by scintigraphy with ^{123}I-labeled serum amyloid P protein. In a small series of patients, scanning showed amyloid in the carpal region in primary, but not in secondary, amyloidosis patients (Hawkins et al. 1990).

Local Carpal Tunnel Amyloid Deposits

Many patients who present with carpal tunnel syndrome and local deposition of amyloid in the carpal tunnel will have no evidence of systemic disease or amyloid elsewhere in their bodies. In the Mayo Clinic series, Kyle et al. (1989) followed 124 such patients. Only four of these patients had systemic manifestations of amyloidosis at follow-up. In these four patients, the systemic amyloidosis became apparent 4 to 15 years after the carpal tunnel syndrome was first symptomatic and 4 to 10 years after the amyloid was demonstrated in the carpal tunnel. Nine of the patients had serum evidence of monoclonal gammopathy but did not develop known systemic amyloidosis or multiple myeloma.

Hereditary Neuropathic Amyloidosis, Type II

There are a number of different familial amyloid syndromes, some of which affect the peripheral nervous system (Thomas 1975). Among these, hereditary neuropathic amyloidosis, type II (Indiana or Rukavina type), is distinctive for its presentation with carpal tunnel syndrome as the initial symptom (Mahloudji et al. 1969). The amyloid derives from abnormal transthyretin caused by a single amino acid substitution (Wallace et al. 1988). The carpal tunnel syndrome matches idiopathic carpal tunnel syndrome in its symptoms, distribution of age of onset, varied clinical manifestations, and findings on nerve conduction studies. Amyloid infiltration of the flexor retinaculum can be demonstrated at surgery or by biopsy elsewhere (Lambird and Hartmann 1969).

Hereditary neuropathic amyloidosis, type II may slowly progress to a more generalized peripheral neuropathy. Occasionally, cardiac infiltration may become symptomatic late in the illness. The patients may have vitreous amyloid opacities. Abnormalities of the autonomic nervous system are absent or appear late.

Typically, patients survive for many years after onset of symptoms. Inheritance is autosomal dominant. In the United States, large kindreds have been reported from Maryland and Indiana (Rukavina et al. 1956).

Beta-2-Microglobulin Amyloid and Renal Disease

Renal dialysis patients, particularly hemodialysis patients, have an increased incidence of carpal tunnel syndrome. Symptoms often worsen following a dialysis session and improve before the next session (Jain et al. 1979). The carpal tunnel syndrome occasionally becomes symptomatic within months of institution of dialysis (Mancusi-Ungaro et al. 1976). The typical pattern, however, is for carpal tunnel syndrome symptoms to appear after years of dialysis. Over one half of patients who have been on dialysis for five years develop carpal tunnel syndrome (Scardapane et al. 1979; Halter et al. 1981).

Early papers noted that symptoms of carpal tunnel syndrome were more common in the arm that had a functioning arteriovenous access fistula (Kumar et al. 1975; Warren and Otieno 1975). The shunt, in some patients, may steal radial arterial blood flow from the hand (Gilbert et al. 1988). However, the carpal tunnel syndrome is often bilateral or may affect an arm that has never been used for a shunt (Jain et al. 1979; Halter et al. 1981; Bicknell et al. 1991).

Nerve conduction studies in hemodialysis patients with carpal tunnel syndrome will often give bilateral evidence of median nerve conduction slowing across the carpal tunnel and show electrical evidence of a more diffuse neuropathy (Halter et al. 1981). Bicknell et al. (1991) performed nerve conduction studies on 46 patients on chronic dialysis. Their results are summarized in Figure 6.2. Abnormal median nerve conduction and carpal tunnel syndrome were found in both hemodialysis and peritoneal dialysis patients. All patients who had been on dialysis for seven or more years had abnormal median nerve conduction across the carpal tunnel.

Hemodialysis patients with carpal tunnel syndrome usually report symptomatic relief from carpal tunnel surgery (Teitz et al. 1985). Often, synovial tissue biopsied at the time of surgery will show amyloid deposition (Kachel et al. 1983; Schwarz et al. 1984).

Gejyo et al. (1985) reported that dialysis-associated amyloid was derived from beta-2-microglobulin. The clinical manifestations of beta-2-microglobulin amyloidosis are now known to include carpal tunnel syndrome, juxtaarticular radiolucent bone lesions, and arthropathy with a predilection for large joints (Bardin et al. 1987; Kleinman and Coburn 1989; Sargent et al. 1989; Stone and Hakim 1989; Ullian et al. 1989). Shoulder pain is a common feature (Chattopadhyay et al. 1987). Amyloid deposits can be found in joints, bone, tongue,

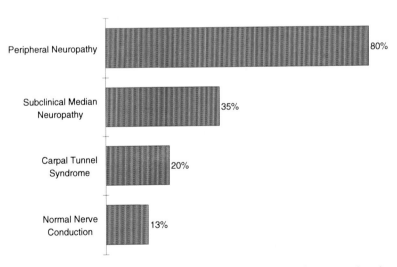

Figure 6.2 Nerve conduction results in 46 patients on chronic dialysis. Peripheral neuropathy and subclinical median neuropathy were diagnosed on the basis of nerve conduction studies. Carpal tunnel syndrome was diagnosed on the basis of typical symptoms and signs and was always accompanied by abnormal median nerve conduction. (Data from Bicknell et al. 1991.)

peritoneal fat, or a variety of other organs (Campistol et al. 1987; Fuchs et al. 1987; Muñoz-Gómez et al. 1987). However, a negative amyloid stain on a peritoneal fat aspiration does not exclude amyloid deposition in the carpal tunnel or elsewhere (Orfila et al. 1988).

Beta-2-microglobulin amyloid is most common with hemodialysis using cuprophane membranes but may also occur with other dialysis techniques including continuous ambulatory peritoneal dialysis (Vandenbroucke et al. 1986; Gagnon et al. 1988).

Even with a careful search, amyloid is not found in all hemodialysis patients with carpal tunnel syndrome (Cornelis et al. 1989). In individual cases, contributory mechanisms of median nerve compression may include local edema, deposition of other substances such as iron in synovial tissue, coexistent peripheral neuropathy, vascular effects of the dialysis shunt, or other coexisting disease (Cary et al. 1986).

DISORDERS OF THE PERIPHERAL NERVE
Generalized Peripheral Neuropathy

Common clinical lore is that patients with peripheral neuropathies are susceptible to carpal tunnel syndrome and other forms of local nerve entrapment (Potts et al. 1980). Susceptibility varies depending on the pathophysiology of the neuropathy. For example, diabetic peripheral neuropathy, as discussed earlier, has a clear association with carpal tunnel syndrome, but for peripheral neuropathy of other causes, the association is less well documented.

Patients with demyelinating neuropathies may be particularly susceptible to developing abnormalities at sites of focal nerve compression. Lambert and Mulder (1964) reported that in some patients with Guillain-Barré syndrome there is preferential slowing of nerve conduction at common sites of nerve compression. This preferential slowing is most evident on sensory nerve conduction studies. Albers et al. (1985) found that in 42% of their patients' median sensory conduction was abnormal, but sural nerve conduction was normal. Symptoms of carpal tunnel syndrome are usually not a clinical feature of Guillain-Barré syndrome.

Diphtheritic neuropathy provides an experimental model of an acute demyelinating neuropathy. Guinea pigs with experimentally induced diphtheritic neuropathy are more vulnerable than guinea pigs without neuropathy to developing focal conduction delay in the plantar nerve (Hopkins and Morgan-Hughes 1969). This local pressure effect is prevented if the guinea pigs are not allowed to put pressure on their hind legs.

Hereditary liability to pressure palsies is another example of a neuropathy that affects myelin and predisposes patients to develop acute or chronic pathology from focal nerve compression. Patients with this condition develop recurrent mononeuropathies at common nerve compression sites including at the carpal tunnel (Earl et al. 1964; Staal et al. 1965; Roos and Thygesen 1972; Debruyne et al. 1980; Dyck 1984). For example, Cruz Martinez et al. (1977) found six cases of clinically evident median neuropathy among 25 patients with this syndrome.

The median neuropathy may be accompanied by radial or ulnar neuropathies. The mononeuropathies may develop suddenly following relatively minor trauma or without obvious cause. Patients with the syndrome often have evidence on nerve conduction studies of diffuse peripheral neuropathy or additional mononeuropathies that are not clinically evident. Only 2 of the 25 patients reported by Cruz Martinez et al. had completely normal median nerve conduction studies. Additional evidence that these patients have a generalized underlying diathesis of peripheral nerve is that they often eventually develop a more symmetric diffuse peripheral neuropathy and that their sural nerve biopsies often show structural abnormalities, even if no symptoms of neuropathy are present in the biopsied limb (Figure 6.3) (Behse et al. 1972).

Despite the prevalence of alcoholic peripheral neuropathy, there is little literature on carpal tunnel syndrome in alcoholics. Is this because diabetics are studied more closely than alcoholics for variations in their peripheral neuropathy? Or is the predominantly axonal neuropathy of alcoholics less vulnerable than diabetic neuropathy to focal nerve compression? Alcoholic peripheral neuropathy regularly involves the feet before it affects the hands, and when it affects the hands, sensory loss follows a "glove" distribution rather than a median cutaneous pattern (Victor 1984). Patients with alcoholic neuropathy are more likely to show abnormal nerve conduction in sural or peroneal nerves than in the median nerve (Behse and Buchthal 1977).

Casey and Le Quesne (1972b) studied median sensory nerve conduction in 16 alcoholics. They compared digital conduction from the tip to the base of the middle finger to more proximal conduction from the tip of the finger to the wrist. The characteristic abnormality in these alcoholic subjects was loss of amplitude of the digital nerve action potential. None of the alcoholics had slowed sensory conduction across the carpal tunnel; in contrast, sensory conduction velocity

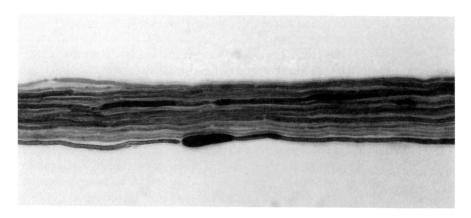

Figure 6.3   Nerve pathology in hereditary liability to pressure palsies. This microdissected bundle of nerve fibers shows several myelin tomaculae ("sausages").

across the carpal tunnel was reduced in patients with carpal tunnel syndrome and in some patients with diabetic neuropathy (Casey and Le Quesne 1972a).

The "Double Crush" Syndrome

Upton and McComas (1973) offered the hypothesis that many patients with carpal tunnel syndrome presented atypical features because nerve fibers were being compressed both at the carpal tunnel and more proximally, often at the level of the cervical nerve roots. They proposed that constriction of axonal flow at a proximal site along the axon made the median nerve unusually sensitive to compression in the carpal canal.

Upton and McComas estimated that over three quarters of their patients with carpal tunnel syndrome had evidence of cervical pathology. In some of their patients, there was dermatomal sensory loss beyond the territory of the median nerve, or there was electromyographic evidence of denervation in a myotomal pattern in arm muscles not supplied by the median nerve; however, in many instances, their evidence of cervical radiculopathy was as sparse as radiologic demonstration of cervical spondylosis, complaints of neck pain or stiffness, or remote history of "whiplash" injury.

Despite lack of any control data by Upton and McComas on the incidence of these common neck abnormalities in the general population, their hypothesis was intuitively appealing; the catch phrase "double crush" is often used in discussions of occurrence of radiculopathies, brachial plexopathies, or proximal median neuropathies in patients with carpal tunnel syndrome. For example, a report of 19 patients with well-documented coexistence of carpal tunnel syndrome and cervical radiculopathy, usually at the level of the sixth or seventh cervical root, describes the patients as having "double crush syndrome" but does not establish whether or not this represents a fortuitous combination of common conditions (Massey et al. 1981). Other cases suggest that carpal tunnel syndrome can occur coincident with more proximal median compression or with brachial plexus compression (Reddy 1984; Zamora et al. 1986).

Hurst et al. (1985) examined 888 patients with carpal tunnel syndrome severe enough to be treated surgically, of whom 271 had the syndrome bilaterally; 112 patients had bilateral surgery. The incidence of "cervical arthritis" was 14% among patients with bilateral carpal tunnel syndrome and only 9% among those with unilateral disease. The authors gratuitously view this as support of the double crush hypothesis without considering such factors as effect of patient age, order of appearance of each syndrome, or impact of unilateral cervical radiculopathy on the results.

Osterman (1988) found that patients with both carpal tunnel syndrome and cervical radiculopathy differed from patients with only carpal tunnel syndrome by having a higher mean age, more prominent proximal arm symptoms, more paresthesias (but less numbness), weaker grip, fewer nerve conduction abnormalities, and a worse response to carpal tunnel surgery. Again, the data does not distinguish whether the conditions coexist by chance or because of a pathogenic link.

Frith and Litchy (1985) reported on nerve conduction findings in 104 "surgically proven" cases of radiculopathy; 18 (17%) of the patients had nerve conduction abnormalities in the median nerve across the carpal tunnel; in 10 of these 18, the radiculopathy was unilateral, but the median nerve abnormalities were bilateral. This data does not establish that the radiculopathy significantly increased the risk of developing a median neuropathy. However, these findings do emphasize the need to consider that a patient might have more than one affliction causing converging neurologic symptoms. The abstract does not specify which of the median nerve abnormalities were symptomatic. The abnormal nerve conduction results alone do not prove a coexistent carpal tunnel syndrome. This diagnosis must be based on clinical findings as well. Wilbourn and Breuer (1986) found only 37 confirmed cases of cervical radiculopathy among 1,183 patients with carpal tunnel syndrome diagnosed in an electromyographic laboratory.

In summary, a small percentage of patients with carpal tunnel syndrome haver another neuropathic condition contributing to arm symptoms. In these patients, thorough neurologic examination and careful electrodiagnostic studies will usually yield the correct diagnoses. The concept of double crush syndrome rarely needs to be invoked to explain the clinical profile of these patients.

INFECTIOUS DISEASES
Rubella Arthritis

Carpal tunnel syndrome may occur as a complication of the polyarthritis that is an occasional sequela of rubella infection or of live rubella immunization (Blennow et al. 1982; Tingle et al. 1985). Adults are more commonly affected than children (Cooper et al. 1969). The syndrome is usually self-limited or improves with antiinflammatory medication (Hale and Ruderman 1973). In one postrubella case that came to carpal tunnel surgery, synovial pathology showed infiltration with polymorphonuclear leukocytes (Ellis 1973).

Out of 23,000 children immunized, 9 developed carpal tunnel syndrome symptoms (Kilroy et al. 1970). In another series, the incidence of postimmunization arthralgia was 3%. In a limited sample, when the arthralgic population was questioned closely, over three quarters had carpal tunnel syndrome symptoms (Thompson et al. 1971). Symptoms appear 10 days to two months following immunization and resolve in one month or less. Median nerve conduction studies may be normal or show transient mild abnormalities.

Lyme Borreliosis

Of 76 patients with symptoms of Lyme disease of greater than four weeks' duration and of sufficient severity to require referral to a Lyme disease clinic, over one quarter had symptoms of carpal tunnel syndrome (Halperin et al. 1989). Only two of these patients had clinical evidence of active wrist tenosynovitis.

Median nerve conduction studies were abnormal in nearly three quarters of the patients with carpal tunnel symptoms. In addition, 3 of 68 patients studied had asymptomatic median nerve conduction abnormalities. Patients often had clinical improvement in carpal tunnel symptoms and sometimes had median nerve conduction improvement, following antibiotic treatment of the Lyme disease. Patients with carpal tunnel syndrome may or may not have other peripheral nervous system manifestations of Lyme disease.

Granulomatous Infections of the Hand

Carpal tunnel syndrome may occur as a complication of granulomatous infection in the carpal canal with a variety of different organisms. Table 6.1 provides examples.

These patients often present with insidious onset of carpal tunnel syndrome symptoms, and the syndrome may evolve gradually over months or years. Local wrist swelling and other signs of focal inflammation may or may not be present (Klofkorn and Steigerwald 1976; Bush and Schneider 1984). Sporotrichosis may also cause cutaneous nodules on the hand or in a lymphangitic pattern on the arm (Hagemann 1968).

Some cases have been treated with local steroid injections before coming to carpal tunnel surgery; however, the effect of steroids on the natural history of the infection is unknown (Langa et al. 1986). In a patient with bilateral tuberculous infection of the carpal canal, one side had previously been treated with steroid injection without evidence that this treatment retarded or promoted the course of infection (Gouet et al. 1984).

Table 6.1 Granulomatous infection of the carpal tunnel

Organism	Reference
Mycobacterium tuberculosis	Suso et al. 1988
	Langa et al. 1986
	Lee 1985
	Gouet et al. 1984
	Bush and Schneider 1984
	Klofkorn and Steigerwald 1976
Atypical mycobacteria	Prince et al. 1988
	Randall et al. 1982
	Stratton et al. 1978
	Gunther et al. 1977
	Cheatum et al. 1976
	Kaplan and Clayton 1969
	Kelly et al. 1967
Histoplasma capsulatum	Randall et al. 1982
	Strayer et al. 1981
Sporothrix schenckii	Stratton et al. 1981
	Hagemann 1968

Carpal tunnel syndrome may be the first evidence of a systemic granulomatous infection. The classical gross surgical finding of granulomatous infection is "rice bodies" (Stratton et al. 1978). These are fibrinous masses, shaped like rice grains, 2 to 20 mm long, visible in the carpal canal. They may also be seen with noninfectious inflammatory diseases. At times, granulomatous tenosynovitis may not be recognized until a second or third exploration of the carpal tunnel is undertaken when the initial surgery has given no more than transient relief of symptoms (Kelly et al. 1967; Langa et al. 1986).

Leprosy

Patients with leprosy can develop a progressive median neuropathy, although ulnar neuropathy is more common in these patients (Baccaredda-Boy et al. 1963; Callaway et al. 1965). Initially, symptoms may be intermittent and mimic those of carpal tunnel syndrome. Later in the disease, motor and sensory loss become irreversible. Brand (1956) examined over 2,000 affected hands and found the following patterns:

Isolated ulnar neuropathy	46%
Median and ulnar neuropathy	52%
Median, ulnar, and radial neuropathy	1.5%
Isolated median neuropathy	0.5%

In addition, patients often have cutaneous sensory neuropathies from disease of intradermal nerve branches (Callaway et al. 1965).

At carpal tunnel surgery, the median nerve may be thickened and edematous and show necrosis, giant cells, and occasionally acid-fast organisms on biopsy (Callaway et al. 1965; Selby 1974). The median nerve may also be infected more proximally, in the forearm (Antia et al. 1970).

Miscellaneous Infections

Carpal tunnel syndrome may accompany toxic shock syndrome (Sahs et al. 1983). In some patients with toxic shock syndrome, carpal tunnel syndrome develops acutely secondary to hand swelling.

A case report details carpal tunnel syndrome in a 47-year-old woman whose symptoms began three weeks after receiving the swine flu/Victoria A influenza vaccine (Hasselbacher 1977). A causal relationship between the vaccination and development of carpal tunnel syndrome is unproven.

References to cases of acute median nerve compression by gonococcal or pyogenic infections of the wrist are given in Table 6.5.

ANOMALOUS CANAL ANATOMY OR MASSES

At the time of carpal tunnel surgery, the surgeon sometimes discovers anomalous structures within the canal. Examples include ectopic or accessory muscles, bony anomalies, a persistent median artery, or a variety of tumors. On occasion, physical examination findings such as a palpable palmar mass or swelling, triggering of a flexor tendon, or clicking with wrist movement are clues to these structures (Neviaser 1974; Aghasi et al. 1980; Asai et al. 1986; Desai et al. 1986). The palmar mass may be present for years prior to development of symptoms of carpal tunnel syndrome (Hayes 1974). Carpal tunnel X rays at times reveal a deformity or unexpected calcification (Sutro 1969; Louis and Dick 1973; Pritsch et al. 1980; Firooznia et al. 1981; Edwards et al. 1984; Weiber and Linell 1987). Soft tissue anomalies or tumors may be detected preoperatively by computed tomography (CT) or magnetic resonance imaging (MRI) scanning (Mesgarzadeh et al. 1989; Feyerabend et al. 1990; Reicher and Kellerhouse 1990). These anomalies are rare, and knowledge of their existence preoperatively will rarely be important for patient management. Some surgeons routinely X-ray the wrist before carpal tunnel surgery; however, extensive preoperative imaging to study canal contents is seldom justified.

Anomalous contents of the canal are rare in patients with carpal tunnel syndrome. Table 6.2 lists anomalous canal contents reported in the combined series of 2,705 patients that is shown in Table 5.1. Phalen (1966) qualified his estimation of the incidence of anomalies, stating that he might overlook some because of his operative approach through a transverse incision without careful exploration of the contents of the canal.

Congenital Muscular Anomalies

Table 6.3 lists anomalous muscles that may compress the median nerve in the carpal tunnel or distal forearm. Occasionally, children with anomalous muscles have symptoms of carpal tunnel syndrome, but most patients with anomalous muscles do not develop carpal tunnel syndrome until adulthood.

At times, anomalous muscles become symptomatic following trauma or in association with other pathology within the canal; an example is accessory lumbricals discovered in conjunction with a fibroma or a degenerative synovial cyst (Butler and Bigley 1971; Nather and Pho 1981; Asai et al. 1986; Desai et al. 1986). The anomalous muscle within the canal may not cause nerve compression until it hypertrophies with use (Abbott and Saunders 1933). The anomaly may be present unilaterally in patients with bilateral carpal tunnel syndrome (Gleason and Abraham 1982). In many instances, the muscle anomaly is an incidental

Table 6.2 Anomalous carpal canal contents in 2,705 patients with carpal tunnel syndrome

Ganglion	12
Tumor	3
Anomalous muscle belly	7
Thrombosed median artery	2

Table 6.3 Anomalous muscles in carpal tunnel syndrome

Anomalous Muscle	Reference
Palmaris longus	Bang et al. 1988
	Schlafly and Lister 1987
	Meyer and Pflaum 1987
	Crandall and Hamel 1979
	Brones and Wilgis 1978
	Backhouse and Churchill-Davidson 1975
Ectopic lumbrical	Robinson et al. 1989
	Desai et al. 1986
	Asai et al. 1986
	Nather and Pho 1981
	Jabaley 1978
	Schultz et al. 1973
	Eriksen 1973
	Butler and Bigley 1971
	Touborg-Jensen 1970
Flexor digitorum profundus	Winkelman 1983
Flexor digitorum superficialis	Ametewee et al. 1985
	Gleason and Abraham 1982
	Hutton et al. 1981
	Aghasi et al. 1980
	Probst and Hunter 1975
	Neviaser 1974
	Hayes 1974
	Smith 1971
Abductor digiti quinti	Jackson and Harkins 1972
Palmaris profundus	Floyd et al. 1990
	Fatah 1984
	Carstam 1984
	Walton and Cutler 1971

finding at surgery and seems no more important in the pathogenesis of the nerve compression than any of the contents of the canal.

The palmaris profundus appears in about 1 in 1,600 hands (Carstam 1984). It originates deep in the forearm, becomes superficial above the wrist, and passes through the carpal canal to insert in the deep palmar fascia. The muscle may be attached to the median nerve with connective tissue (Walton and Cutler 1971; Floyd et al. 1990). It may be an incidental finding at carpal tunnel surgery; it has been noted in patients presenting with carpal tunnel syndrome at ages 62, 72, and 85 years (Carstam 1984; Fatah 1984).

The palmaris longus typically originates in the forearm. Its tendon usually passes volar to the flexor retinaculum to insert on the palmar fascia or thenar muscles. The muscle is subject to numerous variations (Reimann et al. 1944). The tendon of palmaris longus has been found under the flexor retinaculum or between the ligament and the median nerve in cases of carpal tunnel syndrome (Brones and Wilgis 1978). In another variant, the body of the palmaris longus may compress the median nerve just proximal to the carpal canal (Backhouse and Churchill-Davidson 1975; Dorin and Mann 1984; Meyer and Pflaum 1987; Schlafly and Lister 1987).

Median Artery

A persistent median artery accompanies the median nerve in the carpal canal in 1% to 16% of arms (Coleman and Anson 1961; Pecket et al. 1973). The median nerve at times is bifid with branches on either side of the artery. The anomalous artery may be unilateral or bilateral. At times the pulse of the median artery may be palpable in the proximal palm.

The pathogenic import of a patent median artery is not always clear. Individuals may have palpable median arteries without evidence of carpal tunnel syndrome or bilateral carpal tunnel syndrome with a unilateral median artery (Chalmers 1978; Barfred et al. 1985). Chalmers found a persistent median artery in 6% of his patients with carpal tunnel syndrome, and Barfred et al. found a persistent median artery in 2% of their patients, not clearly more than would be found in an asymptomatic population. However, both Chalmers and Barfred et al. argue that carpal tunnel syndrome patients with a persistent median artery are more likely than other carpal tunnel syndrome patients to have symptoms occurring during hand use and less likely to experience nocturnal hand paresthesia. There was a lower mean age and a higher percentage of males among the patients with patent median arteries.

Barfred et al. recommend median artery resection at the time of carpal tunnel surgery if normal digital blood supply can be proven while the median artery is clamped. In contrast, Chalmers recommends flexor retinaculum release without resection of the artery.

The median artery may thrombose, spontaneously or posttraumatically, causing subacute presentation of symptoms of carpal tunnel syndrome, sudden onset of hand pain and paresthesia, or sudden deterioration of chronic carpal tunnel syndrome (Jackson and Campbell 1970; Maxwell et al. 1973b; Levy and Pauker 1978). Treatment includes carpal tunnel exploration and resection of the thrombosed artery.

Dickinson and Kleinert (1991) reported a patient on hemodialysis who developed carpal tunnel syndrome secondary to an enlarged median artery with ectopic calcification.

A patient with an arteriovenous malformation in the palm presented with chronic symptoms of carpal tunnel syndrome (Chopra et al. 1979). On physical examination, the hand was warm and swollen. Symptoms were relieved with release of the flexor retinaculum.

Median Nerve Anomalies

Brachial hypertrophy is a very rare condition characterized by progressive unilateral limb hypertrophy with onset in childhood (Figure 6.4). When patients with brachial hypertrophy develop carpal tunnel syndrome, the nerve may be thickened with proliferation of perineural collagen (Shenoy et al. 1980). In the angioosteohypertrophy syndrome (Klippel-Trenaunay-Weber syndrome), other anomalies may accompany brachial hypertrophy and carpal tunnel syndrome (Owens et al. 1973).

Schweitzer and Miller (1973) described a bifid median nerve with unexplained thickening of epineurium and perineurium in a patient with carpal tunnel syndrome. However, a bifid median nerve is a rare variation not usually associated with nerve pathology (Lanz 1977). In other patients with carpal tunnel syndrome and a bifid median nerve, the anomalous nerve division is not necessarily the cause of the carpal tunnel syndrome (Baruch and Hass 1977; Moneim 1982; Amadio 1987).

Space-Occupying Lesions

Masses of varied histology are discovered, in rare instances, at the time of carpal tunnel surgery. The most common are ganglion cysts (Trevaskis et al. 1967; Hvid-Hansen 1970; Harvey and Bosanquet 1981; McMinn 1985; Lewis et al. 1986; Kerrigan et al. 1988). Table 6.4 lists other hand tumors and masses that have been found in the carpal canal.

A lipoma may also develop in the deep palmar space, distal to the carpal tunnel, and cause median nerve compression (Oster et al. 1989).

Other Unusual Canal Contents

The ulnar nerve has been found beside the median nerve in the carpal canal (Eskesen et al. 1981; Galzio et al. 1987). Both nerves may be compressed so that the patient presents with evidence of both median and ulnar neuropathy at the wrist.

Iatrogenic objects that may be found in the canal and compress the median nerve include a tendon graft prosthesis or a prosthetic carpal bone (DeLuca and Cowen 1975; Lichtman et al. 1982; Björnsson et al. 1984). In one patient, the broken tip of an acupuncture needle was found embedded in the median nerve at the time of surgery (Southworth and Hartwig 1990).

OBESITY

Obesity is sometimes listed among the causes of carpal tunnel syndrome. For example, Maxwell et al. (1973a) classified 14% of their carpal tunnel syndrome patients as obese but provided no data on incidence of obesity in a control population. A case control study found obesity in 27% of carpal tunnel syndrome patients and in 12% of controls, but the risk ratio was not statistically

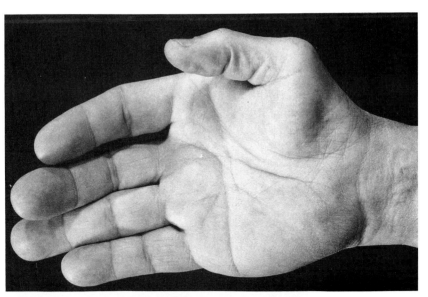

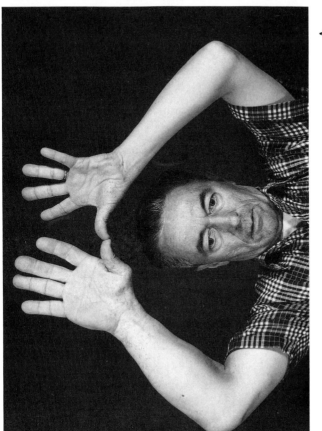

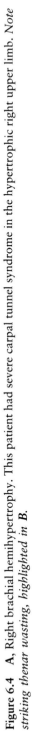

Figure 6.4 A, Right brachial hemihypertrophy. This patient had severe carpal tunnel syndrome in the hypertrophic right upper limb. *Note striking thenar wasting, highlighted in* **B**.

Table 6.4 Tumors and masses in the carpal tunnel

Tumor or Mass	Reference
Carpal osteophyte	Engel et al. 1978
Chondroma, osteochondroma	Nather and Chong 1986 Gahhos and Cuono 1984 Tompkins 1967
Degenerative or detritus cyst	Pritsch et al. 1980
Distended ulnar bursa	Linscheid 1979
Epithelioid sarcoma	Patel et al. 1986
Lipoma	Kremchek and Kremchek 1988 Brand and Gelberman 1988 Hybbinette and Mannerfelt 1975 Paarlberg et al. 1972
Median nerve tumors	See Chapter 19
Mesodermal tumor	Ernst and Konermann 1982
Osteoid osteoma	Herndon et al. 1974
Pigmented villonodular synovitis	Chidgey et al. 1988
Squamous cell carcinoma	Mackay and Barua 1990 Dandy and Munro 1973
Tendon fibrous histiocytoma	Iqbal 1982
Tendon fibroma	Sarma et al. 1986 Brown and Coulson 1974

significant (Cannon et al. 1981). Neither study defined obesity. A case control study in adult women with carpal tunnel syndrome found that a weight gain of 4 kg or more in the previous five years was a possible risk factor for development of carpal tunnel syndrome (Dieck and Kelsey 1985). An association between carpal tunnel syndrome and obesity is possible but unproven.

HAND EDEMA

Hand swelling of diverse causes can trigger carpal tunnel syndrome. Reported cases are as varied as congestive heart failure, hand swelling after an insect sting, vibration-induced angioedema, or postmastectomy lymphedema (Lazaro 1972; Arnold 1977; Ganel et al. 1979; Wener et al. 1983; Mandawat 1985; Barker et al 1986).

ACUTE CARPAL TUNNEL SYNDROME

Prominent carpal tunnel syndrome may develop suddenly in rare circumstances. Acute trauma is the most common of these. Colles' fracture of the distal radius is the prototypic injury. While most patients do not develop median neuropathy after Colles' fracture, some do report mild paresthesias in the median cutaneous distribution that resolve spontaneously as focal swelling recedes. In one series, 19 of 300 Colles' fracture patients had more severe acute median neuropathy (Sponsel and Palm 1965). Sometimes median nerve function improves after readjusting the patient's splint to neutral rather than wrist-flexed posture. When severe median neuropathy is present with dense anesthesia and impaired two-point discrimination, the flexor retinaculum should be released acutely (Bauman et al. 1981). In these cases, a hematoma or swelling is often found in the canal at surgery; if the canal appears normal, nerve compression in the distal forearm by hematoma or bone displacement should be considered (Lewis 1978). When the neuropathy is milder, the patient can be kept under observation. Sponsel and Palm found that 8 of their 19 patients required delayed carpal tunnel surgery. The risk of median nerve compression increases with volar displacement of a fragment of the distal radius (Paley and McMurtry 1987).

Acute carpal tunnel syndrome can also occur with other wrist and hand fractures, such as fractures of the scaphoid and metacarpals, or with carpal-metacarpal fracture dislocations (McClain and Wissinger 1976; Weiland et al. 1976; Olerud and Lonnquist 1984). Acute carpal tunnel syndrome may also occur with blunt palm trauma without fracture (Ametewee 1983).

When hand trauma is severe—for example, after wringer or roller hand-crushing injuries—acute median nerve compression is very common, and many surgeons prophylactically section the flexor retinaculum (Primiano and Reef 1974; Askins et al. 1986). In the most severe cases, a forearm fasciotomy may be required to prevent development of a forearm compartment syndrome.

Carpal tunnel syndrome may develop following hand or forearm surgery. For example, a case developed following placement of a compression plate for nonunion of an ulnar fracture, and another occurred after tendon graft prosthesis placement (DeLuca and Cowen 1975; Bauman et al. 1981).

Foreign bodies that penetrate the wrist can cause acute carpal tunnel syndrome. Examples include thorns or glass fragments (Sterling et al. 1972; Goldberg and Levy 1977).

Hemorrhage in the carpal canal can cause acute nerve compression. Hemorrhage may occur after minor trauma with pigmented villonodular synovitis of the flexor synovium, with anticoagulation, in acute or chronic leukemia, in hemophilia, or spontaneously (Hartwell and Kurtay 1966; Case 1967; McClain and Wissinger 1976; Khunadorn et al. 1977; Howie and Buxton 1984; Moneim and Gribble 1984; Kilpatrick et al. 1985; Nkele 1986; Chidgey et al. 1988; Copeland et al. 1989). One patient on heparin developed an antecubital hematoma after venipuncture. Carpal tunnel symptoms were prominent after the acute antecubital hematoma resolved. At carpal tunnel surgery, a small hematoma was found in the carpal canal (Kohn et al. 1976).

Table 6.5 lists some other uncommon causes of acute carpal tunnel syndrome. Often the patient will give a history of chronic mild acroparesthesias preceding a sudden symptomatic crescendo (Weiber and Linell 1987). If a long-

Table 6.5 Unusual causes of acute carpal tunnel syndrome

Cause	Reference
Hand burns	Adamson et al. 1971
Gonococcal tenosynovitis	DeHertogh et al. 1988
Gout	Morgan 1985
Insect sting	Barker et al. 1986
	Lazaro 1972
Intense wrist use	Jones and Scheker 1988
Median artery thrombosis	de Graad and Rodseth 1989
	Maxwell et al. 1973b
Pregnancy	Adamson et al. 1971
Prolonged wrist flexion	Belsole and Greeley 1988
Pseudogout	Goodwin and Arbel 1985
	Lewis and Fiddian 1982
	Spiegel et al. 1976
Pyogenic hand infection	Gerardi et al. 1989
	Oates 1960
Pyogenic forearm infection	Swift and McDonald 1976
Ruptured palmaris longus tendon	Lourie et al. 1990
Snake bite	Schweitzer and Lewis 1981
Tight handcuffs*	Stone and Laureno 1991
	Levin and Felsenthal 1984
	Dorfman and Jayaram 1978

*Usually accompanied by superficial radial neuropathy.

standing anomaly or mass is present, the cause of the sudden deterioration may not be evident (Ametewee et al. 1985).

DELAYED EFFECTS OF TRAUMA

Chronic carpal tunnel syndrome may persist as a residual symptom following Colles' fracture and other wrist or hand injuries (Chapman et al. 1982). Paget's (1865) original cases of distal median nerve compression were posttraumatic. The incidence of chronic carpal tunnel syndrome was 31% in one group of patients followed after Colles' fractures (Altissimi et al. 1986). In some patients, symptoms will resolve slowly in the months following the fracture: In a group of patients with displaced fractures, 17% had symptoms of median neuropathy three months after injury, but only 12% had symptoms six months after injury (Stewart et al. 1985).

Carpal tunnel syndrome is reported as a delayed effect of arm crush injuries, hook of the hamate fractures, or posttraumatic ulna-minus (Manske 1978; Murray et al. 1979; Askins et al. 1986; Nathan and Meadows 1987; Bishop and Beckenbaugh 1988). When an episode of very heavy lifting causes wrist trauma and synovial edema, carpal tunnel syndrome may be a delayed complication (Elliott and Elliott 1979).

Hand burns, even if superficial, may predispose to delayed appearance of carpal tunnel syndrome (Fissette et al. 1981). Electrical burns of the hand, in particular, can cause distal median nerve injury (DiVincenti et al. 1969; Solem et al. 1977; Rosenberg 1989). The mechanism of injury can include tenosynovial edema, nerve compression in the forearm by damaged tissue such as necrotic muscle, or direct electrical injury to the nerve.

Carpal tunnel syndrome may occur following distal hand tendon injuries (Browne and Snyder 1975). The injuries need not be severe enough to disrupt the tendons. In an extreme case, a 23-year-old man had resection in the distal palm of an injured flexor digitorum superficialis tendon. Four weeks later he developed median distribution hypoesthesia. At carpal tunnel surgery, the proximal portion of the divided tendon and adherent scar tissue were compressing the median nerve (Sturim and Edmond 1980). A similar sequence of events can follow digital avulsion injuries (Milroy et al. 1984).

The tendon of flexor digitorum profundus may rupture without evident trauma. Hypertrophic synovial reaction may develop around the ruptured tendon in the carpal tunnel and contribute to median nerve compression (Jackson 1990).

Symptoms of median neuropathy may appear as a late effect following partial median nerve laceration in the forearm. Exploration may reveal a neuroma in continuity in the forearm, with the nerve distal to the neuroma swollen and compressed as it enters the carpal tunnel. Symptoms may resolve after section of the flexor retinaculum, while the neuroma is left undisturbed (McGrath and Polayes 1979; Martinelli et al. 1985).

Distal median neuropathy can occur following motor vehicle accidents (Guyon and Honet 1977). Typically, the driver is gripping the steering wheel tightly at the time of impact. Symptoms of median neuropathy develop immediately or within two weeks of the accident (Haas et al. 1981). Among 21 patients with carpal tunnel syndrome resulting from steering wheel impact, Label (1991) found that 71% recovered within five months when treated with splinting; the remaining 29% underwent carpal tunnel surgery.

GENETIC CONSIDERATIONS

Although most cases of carpal tunnel syndrome are sporadic, a number of familial instances of the syndrome are known. Reports usually suggest autosomal dominant transmission (Danta 1975; Gray et al. 1979; Mochizuki et al. 1981; Braddom 1985; McDonnell et al. 1987; Golik et al. 1988; Michaud et al. 1990). Symptoms may begin in childhood or adulthood. The flexor retinaculum is abnormally thickened in some of these families (Michaud et al. 1990). Associations with other hand conditions include an increased incidence of trigger finger or susceptibility to mallet finger (Gray et al. 1979; Jones and Peterson 1988). In some families, patients may develop other entrapment neuropathies (Fowler et al. 1986). On occasion, carpal tunnel syndrome may be the first symptomatic manifestation of hereditary sensory motor neuropathy (Folkers et al. 1978). Hereditary liability to pressure palsies is discussed with other peripheral neuropathies. Familial amyloidosis, type II, as discussed earlier, may cause carpal tunnel syndrome, but in many familial aggregations of carpal tunnel syndrome, amyloid stains have been negative.

A genetic linkage analysis in one family found no link to varied blood markers (Sparkes et al. 1985). In cases of sporadic carpal tunnel syndrome, there was no association with HLA type (Vanwijck and Bouillenne 1986).

Carpal tunnel syndrome can be a manifestation of mucopolysaccharidoses and mucolipidoses. These storage diseases present in childhood with coarse features, stiff joints, dwarfism, and other anomalies. Inheritance is usually recessive. Carpal tunnel syndrome may be severe and is often accompanied by marked thickening of the flexor retinaculum. Patients may have trigger finger and other evidence of flexor tenosynovitis. Table 6.6 provides references linking carpal tunnel syndrome to these disorders. Despite the severity of the nerve compression, many patients will improve following carpal tunnel surgery, but tendon release and postoperative hand therapy may be necessary (Pronicka et al. 1988).

Watson-Jones (1949) gave one of the earliest descriptions of carpal tunnel syndrome in a connective tissue disorder, describing bilateral carpal tunnel syndrome in a 20-year-old man with Léri's pleonosteosis. Yeoman (1961) reported a

Table 6.6 Carpal tunnel syndrome in mucopolysaccharidoses and mucolipidoses

Syndrome	Reference
Hurler's (MPS-IH)	MacDougal et al. 1977
Scheie's (MPS-IS)	Vinals-Torras et al. 1985 Miner and Schimke 1975 Fisher et al. 1974 McKusick 1972
Hunter's (MPS-II)	Miner and Schimke 1975
Maroteaux-Lamy (MPS-VI)	Peterson et al. 1975 McKusick 1972
pseudo-Hurler's (ML-III)	MacDougal et al. 1977 Starreveld and Ashenhurst 1975 Gellis et al. 1975
I-cell disease (ML-II)	MacDougal et al. 1977
Unknown metabolic defect	Bundey et al. 1974 Karpati et al. 1973

MPS = Mucopolysaccharidosis.
ML = Mucolipidosis.

Table 6.7 Carpal tunnel syndrome and inherited connective tissue disorders

Disorder	Reference
Weill-Marchesani syndrome	Dellon et al. 1984 McKusick 1972
Schwartz-Jampel syndrome	Cruz Martinez et al. 1984
Lipoid proteinosis	Gordon et al. 1971
Osteochondritis dissecans	Auld and Chesney 1979

similar case. It is likely that these cases are also examples of mucopolysaccharidosis (McKusick 1972).

Table 6.7 lists examples of carpal tunnel syndrome occurring in other inherited connective tissue disorders.

CARPAL TUNNEL SYNDROME IN CHILDREN

Carpal tunnel syndrome is rare in children. In addition to the familial and metabolic causes mentioned in the preceding section, some additional causes are listed in Table 6.8.

There are a few case reports of carpal tunnel syndrome in children or adolescents without a clear cause (Lettin 1965; Feingold et al. 1980; Sainio et al. 1987). In some teenagers, symptoms were temporally related to increasing arm

Table 6.8 Causes of childhood carpal tunnel syndrome

Cause	Reference
Aberrant lumbricals with cystic degeneration of the synovium	Asai et al. 1986
Bleeding diathesis (e.g., hemophilia)	Khunadorn et al. 1977 Case 1967
Brachial hypertrophy	Shenoy et al. 1980
Angioosteohypertrophy (Klippel-Trenaunay-Weber)	Poilvache et al. 1989
Lipoblastomatosis	Paarlberg et al. 1972
Median nerve tumors	See Chapter 19
Melorheostosis	Bostman and Bakalim 1985 Barfred and Ipsen 1985
Rubella infection or immunization	Blennow et al. 1982 Thompson et al. 1971 Kilroy et al. 1970 Cooper et al. 1969
Skeletal anomalies	Radford and Matthewson 1987

use in athletics (Gibson and Manske 1987). In a five-year-old boy, symptoms improved after steroid injection in the wrist and after he stopped the habit of sleeping with his wrists flexed (Lagos 1971). A nine-year-old boy developed carpal tunnel syndrome from a hypertrophic flexor retinaculum seven years after partial laceration of the ligament (Poilvache et al. 1989). Some children have a combination of carpal tunnel syndrome and trigger finger (McArthur et al. 1969; Maurer et al. 1980; Poilvache et al. 1989).

Two newborns had long median distal motor latencies on nerve conduction studies, one after a radial wrist hematoma developed following radial artery puncture for blood gas sampling and the other after a radial artery cutdown (Koenigsberger and Moessinger 1977).

Table 6.9 Carpal tunnel syndrome as a drug side effect

Drug	Note
Danazol Sikka et al. 1983	See "Estrogens" in Chapter 5
Diazepam Hines and Hughes 1974	Wrist phlebitis at site of intravenous injection
Disulfiram Howard 1982	Associated with wrist arthritis
Fluoxetine Barnhart 1991	Associated with allergic rash
Lithium Deahl 1988 Wood and Jacoby 1986	Secondary to hypothyroidism
Nonsteroidal antiinflammatories	Occasional patients report worsening when these are used to treat carpal tunnel syndrome
Oral contraceptives	See "Estrogens" in Chapter 5
Propanolol, metoprolol Emara and Saadah 1988	
Quinidine Sukenik et al. 1987	Might also occur with drug-induced lupus from other drugs
Thalidomide Clemmensen et al. 1984	Three patients reported
Tranylcypromine Harrison et al. 1983	Possible role of B_6 deficiency
Warfarin Copeland et al. 1989 Nkele 1986 Hartwell and Kurtay 1966	Hemorrhage in carpal tunnel

MEDICATION SIDE EFFECTS

Carpal tunnel syndrome has been reported as a side effect of some drugs (Table 6.9). These are all very rare occurrences, documented only with case reports.

SCREENING

If no clues to the cause of carpal tunnel syndrome are evident on a general history and physical examination, laboratory screening for causes of carpal tunnel syndrome is rarely worthwhile. In 100 patients with carpal tunnel syndrome who underwent laboratory screening, the abnormalities found were two high fasting blood sugars, one abnormal thyroid function test, and two high sedimentation rates (Chaplin and Kasdan 1985). The thyroid function was normal when rechecked. Both patients with high blood sugars had absent Achilles tendon reflexes.

SUMMARY

Most cases of carpal tunnel syndrome are idiopathic, but carpal tunnel syndrome may be seen as a manifestation of a wide variety of medical conditions. At times, it may be the first clinical evidence of a systemic disease. Every patient with carpal tunnel syndrome deserves a general history and physical examination to avoid overlooking one of these medical conditions.

REFERENCES

Abbott LC, Saunders JBdeCM. Injuries of the median nerve in fractures of the lower end of the radius. Surg Gynecol Obstet 1933;57:507–16.

Adamson JE, Srouji SJ, Horton CE, Mladick RA. The acute carpal tunnel syndrome. Plast Reconstr Surg 1971;47:332–36.

Aghasi MK, Rzetelny V, Axer A. The flexor digitorum superficialis as a cause of bilateral carpal-tunnel syndrome and trigger wrist. A case report. J Bone Joint Surg 1980;62A: 134–35.

Albers JW, Donofrio PD, McGonagle TK. Sequential electrodiagnostic abnormalities in acute inflammatory demyelinating polyradiculoneuropathy. Muscle Nerve 1985;8:528–39.

Altissimi M, Antenucci R, Fiacca C, Mancini GB. Long-term results of conservative treatment of fractures of the distal radius. Clin Orthop 1986;206:202–10.

Amadio PC. Bifid median nerve with a double compartment within the transverse carpal canal. J Hand Surg 1987;12A:366–68.

Ametewee K. Carpal tunnel syndrome produced by a post traumatic calcific mass. Hand 1983;15:212–15.

Ametewee K, Harris A, Samuel M. Acute carpal tunnel syndrome produced by anomalous flexor digitorum superficialis indicis muscle. J Hand Surg 1985;10B:83–84.

Antia NH, Pandya SS, Dastur DK. Nerves in the arm in leprosy: I. Clinical electrodiagnostic and operative aspects. Int J Lepr 1970;38:12–29.

Arnold AG. The carpal tunnel syndrome in congestive cardiac failure. Postgrad Med J 1977;53:623–24.

Asai M, Wong AC, Matsunaga T, Akahoshi Y. Carpal tunnel syndrome caused by aberrant lumbrical muscles associated with cystic degeneration of the tenosynovium: a case report. J Hand Surg 1986;11A:218–21.

Askins G, Finley R, Parenti J, Bush D, Brotman S. High-energy roller injuries to the upper extremity. J Trauma 1986;26:1127–31.

Auld CD, Chesney RB. Familial osteochondritis dissecans and carpal tunnel syndrome. Acta Orthop Scand 1979;50:727–30.

Baccaredda-Boy A, Mastropaoli C, Pastorino P, Sacco G, Farris G. Electromyographic findings in leprosy. Int J Lepr 1963;31:531–32.

Backhouse KM, Churchill-Davidson D. Anomalous palmaris longus muscle producing carpal tunnel-like compression. Hand 1975;7:22–24.

Bang H, Kojima T, Tsuchida Y. A case of carpal tunnel syndrome caused by accessory palmaris longus muscle. Handchir Mikrochir Plast Chir 1988;20:141–43.

Bardin T, Zingraff J, Shirahama T, Noel LH, Droz D, Voisin MC, Drueke T, Dryll A, Skinner M, Cohen AS, et al. Hemodialysis-associated amyloidosis and beta-2 microglobulin. Clinical and immunohistochemical study. Am J Med 1987;83:419–24.

Barfred T, Hjlund AP, Bertheussen K. Median artery in carpal tunnel syndrome. J Hand Surg 1985;10A:864–67.

Barfred T, Ipsen T. Congenital carpal tunnel syndrome. J Hand Surg 1985;10A:246–48.

Barker B, Bloch T, Vakili ST, Waller BF. One pathologist went to mow, went to mow a meadow. (letter). JAMA 1986;255:200.

Barnhart ER, ed. Physicians' desk reference. 45th ed. Oradell, NJ: Medical Economics Data, 1991.

Baruch A, Hass A. Anomaly of the median nerve (letter). J Hand Surg 1977;2:331–32.

Bastian FO. Amyloidosis and the carpal tunnel syndrome. Am J Clin Pathol 1974;61:711–17.

Bauman TD, Gelberman RH, Mubarak SJ, Garfin SR. The acute carpal tunnel syndrome. Clin Orthop 1981;156:151–56.

Behse F, Buchthal F. Alcoholic neuropathy: clinical, electophysiological, and biopsy findings. Ann Neurol 1977;2:95–110.

Behse F, Buchthal F, Carlsen F, Knappeis GG. Hereditary neuropathy with liability to pressure palsies. Brain 1972;95:777–94.

Belsole RJ, Greeley JM. Surgeon's acute carpal tunnel syndrome: an occupational hazard? J Fla Med Assoc 1988;75:369–70.

Benson MD, Brandt KD, Cohen AS, Cathcart ES. Neuropathy, M components, and amyloid. Lancet 1975;1:10–12.

Bicknell JM, Lim AC, Raroque HG, Tzamaloukas AH. Carpal tunnel syndrome, subclinical median mononeuropathy, and peripheral polyneuropathy: common early chronic complications of chronic peritoneal dialysis and hemodialysis. Arch Phys Med Rehabil 1991;72:378–81.

Bishop AT, Beckenbaugh RD. Fracture of the hamate hook. J Hand Surg 1988;13A:135–39.

Björnsson HA, Gestsson J, Ekelund L, Haffajee D. Silastic scaphoid implants in osteoarthritis of the radioscaphoid joint. J Hand Surg 1984;9B:177–80.

Blennow G, Bekassy AN, Eriksson M, Rosendahl R. Transient carpal tunnel syndrome accompanying rubella infection. Acta Paediatr Scand 1982;71:1025–28.

Bostman OM, Bakalim GE. Carpal tunnel syndrome in a melorheostotic limb. J Hand Surg 1985;10B:101–2.

Braddom RL. Familial carpal tunnel syndrome in three generations of a black family. Am J Phys Med 1985;64:227–34.

Brand MG, Gelberman RH. Lipoma of the flexor digitorum superficialis causing triggering at the carpal canal and median nerve compression. J Hand Surg 1988;13A:342–44.

Brand PW. Treatment of leprosy: II. The role of surgery. N Engl J Med 1956;254:64–67.

Brones MF, Wilgis EF. Anatomical variations of the palmaris longus, causing carpal tunnel syndrome: case reports. Plast Reconstr Surg 1978;62:798–800.

Brown LP, Coulson DB. Triggering at the carpal tunnel with incipient carpal-tunnel syndrome. Report of an unusual case. J Bone Joint Surg 1974;56A:623–24.

Browne EZ Jr, Snyder CC. Carpal tunnel syndrome caused by hand injuries. Plast Reconstr Surg 1975;56:41–43.

Bundey SE, Ashenhurst EM, Dorst JP. Mucolipidosis, probably a new variant with joint deformity and peripheral nerve dysfunction. Birth Defects 1974;10:484–90.

Bush DC, Schneider LH. Tuberculosis of the hand and wrist. J Hand Surg 1984;9A:391–98.

Butler B Jr, Bigley EC Jr. Aberrant index (first) lumbrical tendinous origin associated with carpal-tunnel syndrome. A case report. J Bone Joint Surg 1971;53A:160–62.

Callaway JC, Fite GL, Riordan DC. Ulnar and median neuritis due to leprosy. Int J Lepr 1965;32:285–91.

Campistol JM, Cases A, Torras A, Soler M, Muñoz-Gómez J, Montoliu J, López-Pedret J, Revert L. Visceral involvement of dialysis amyloidosis. Am J Nephrol 1987;7:390–93.

Cannon LJ, Bernacki EJ, Walter SD. Personal and occupational factors associated with carpal tunnel syndrome. JOM 1981;23:255–58.

Carstam N. A rare anomalous muscle, palmaris profundus, found when operating at the wrist for neurological symptoms. A report of two cases. Bull Hosp Joint Dis 1984;44:163–67.

Cary NR, Sethi D, Brown EA, Erhardt CC, Woodrow DF, Gower PE. Dialysis arthropathy: amyloid or iron? Br Med J [Clin Res] 1986;293:1392–94.

Case DB. An acute carpal tunnel syndrome in a haemophiliac. Br J Clin Pract 1967;21:254–55.

Casey EB, Le Quesne PM. Digital nerve action potentials in healthy subjects, and in carpal tunnel and diabetic patients. J Neurol Neurosurg Psychiatry 1972a;35:612–23.

Casey EB, Le Quesne PM. Electrophysiological evidence for a distal lesion in alcoholic neuropathy. J Neurol Neurosurg Psychiatry 1972b;35:624–30.

Chalmers J. Unusual causes of peripheral nerve compression. Hand 1978;10:168–75.

Chaplin E, Kasdan ML. Carpal tunnel syndrome and routine blood chemistries. Plast Reconstr Surg 1985;75:722–24.

Chapman DR, Bennett JB, Bryan WJ, Tullos HS. Complications of distal radial fractures: pins and plaster treatment. J Hand Surg 1982;7:509–12.

Chattopadhyay C, Ackrill P, Clague RB. The shoulder pain syndrome and soft-tissue abnormalities in patients on long-term haemodialysis. Br J Rheumatol 1987;26:181–87.

Cheatum DE, Hudman V, Jones SR. Chronic arthritis due to *Mycobacterium intracellulare*. Sacroiliac, knee, and carpal tunnel involvement in a young man and response to chemotherapy. Arthritis Rheum 1976;19:777–81.

Chidgey LK, Szabo RM, Wiese DA. Acute carpal tunnel syndrome caused by pigmented villonodular synovitis of the wrist. Clin Orthop 1988;228:254–57.

Chopra JS, Khanna SK, Murthy JM. Congenital arteriovenous fistula producing carpal tunnel syndrome. J Neurol Neurosurg Psychiatry 1979;42:815–17.

Clemmensen OJ, Olsen PZ, Andersen KE. Thalidomide neurotoxicity. Arch Dermatol 1984;120:338–41.

Coleman SS, Anson BJ. Arterial patterns in the hand based upon a study of 650 specimens. Surg Gynecol Obstet 1961;113:409–24.

Cooper LZ, Ziring PR, Weiss HJ, Matters BA, Krugman S. Transient arthritis after rubella vaccination. Am J Dis Child 1969;118:218–25.

Copeland J, Wells HG Jr, Puckett CL. Acute carpal tunnel syndrome in a patient taking Coumadin. J Trauma 1989;29:131–32.

Cornelis F, Bardin T, Faller B, Verger C, Allouache M, Raymond P, Rottembourg J, Tourliere D, Benhamou C, Noel LH, et al. Rheumatic syndromes and beta 2–

microglobulin amyloidosis in patients receiving long-term peritoneal dialysis. Arthritis Rheum 1989;32:785–88.

Crandall RC, Hamel AL. Bipartite median nerve at the wrist. Report of a case. J Bone Joint Surg 1979;61A:311.

Cruz Martinez A, Arpa J, Perez-Conde MC, Ferrer MT. Bilateral carpal tunnel in childhood associated with Schwartz-Jampel syndrome. Muscle Nerve 1984;7:66–72.

Cruz Martinez A, Perez Conde MC, Ramon Y Cajal S, Martinez A. Recurrent familiar polyneuropathy with liability to pressure palsies. Electromyogr Clin Neurophysiol 1977;17:101–24.

Dandy DJ, Munro DD. Squamous cell carcinoma of skin involving the median nerve. Br J Dermatol 1973;89:527–31.

Danta G. Familial carpal tunnel syndrome with onset in childhood. J Neurol Neurosurg Psychiatry 1975;38:350–55.

Deahl MP. Lithium-induced carpal tunnel syndrome. Br J Psychiatry 1988;153:250–51.

Debruyne J, Dehaene I, Martin JJ. Hereditary pressure-sensitive neuropathy. J Neurol Sci 1980;47:385–94.

de Graad M, Rodseth DJ. Median artery thrombosis as a cause of carpal tunnel syndrome (letter). S Afr Med J 1989;76:78–79.

DeHertogh D, Ritland D, Green R. Carpal tunnel syndrome due to gonococcal tenosynovitis. Orthopedics 1988;11:199–200.

Dellon AL, Trojak JE, Rochman GM. Median nerve compression in Weill-Marchesani syndrome. Plast Reconstr Surg 1984;74:127–30.

DeLuca FN, Cowen NJ. Median-nerve compression complicating a tendon graft prosthesis. J Bone Joint Surg 1975;57A:553.

Desai SS, Pearlman HS, Patel MR. Clicking at the wrist due to fibroma in an anomalous lumbrical muscle: a case report and review of literature. J Hand Surg 1986;11A:512–14.

Dickinson JC, Kleinert JM. Acute carpal-tunnel syndrome casued by a calcified median artery. J Bone Joint Surg 1991;73A:610–11.

Dieck GS, Kelsey JL. An epidemiologic study of the carpal tunnel syndrome in an adult female population. Prev Med 1985;14:63–69.

DiVincenti FC, Moncrief JA, Pruitt BA Jr. Electrical injuries: a review of 65 cases. J Trauma 1969;9:497–507.

Dorfman LJ, Jayaram AR. Handcuff neuropathy. JAMA 1978;239:957.

Dorin D, Mann RJ. Carpal tunnel syndrome associated with abnormal palmaris longus muscle. South Med J 1984;77:1210–11.

Dyck PJ. Inherited neuronal degeneration and atrophy affecting peripheral motor, sensory, and autonomic neurons. In: Dyck PJ, Thomas PK, Lambert EH, Bunge R, eds. Peripheral neuropathy. 2nd ed. Philadelphia: WB Saunders, 1984;1600–79.

Earl CJ, Fullerton PM, Wakefield GS, Schutta HS. Hereditary neuropathy, with liability to pressure palsies. Q J Med 1964;33:481–98.

Edwards AJ, Sill BJ, Macfarlane I. Carpal tunnel syndrome due to dystrophic calcification. Aust NZ J Surg 1984;54:491–92.

Elliott GB, Elliott KA. The torture or stretch arthritis syndrome (a modern counterpart of the medieval "manacles" and "rack"). Clin Radiol 1979;30:313–15.

Ellis W. Rubella arthritis (letter). Br Med J 1973;4:549.

Emara MK, Saadah AM. The carpal tunnel syndrome in hypertensive patients treated with beta-blockers. Postgrad Med J 1988;64:191–92.

Engel J, Zinneman H, Tsur H, Farin I. Carpal tunnel syndrome due to carpal osteophyte. Hand 1978;10:283–84.

Eriksen J. A case of carpal tunnel syndrome on the basis of an abnormally long lumbrical muscle. Acta Orthop Scand 1973;44:275–77.

Ernst HU, Konermann H. Mesodermal tumor as a cause of carpal tunnel syndrome. Handchir Mikrochir Plast Chir 1982;14:220–22.

Eskesen V, Rosenørn J, Osgaard O. Atypical carpal tunnel syndrome with compression of the ulnar and median nerves. Case report. J Neurosurg 1981;54:668–69.

Fatah MF. Palmaris profundus of Frohse and Fränkel in association with carpal tunnel syndrome. J Hand Surg 1984;9B:142–44.

Feingold MH, Hidvegi E, Horwitz SJ. Bilateral carpal tunnel syndrome in an adolescent. Am J Dis Child 1980;134:394–95.

Feyerabend T, Schmitt R, Lanz U, Warmuth-Metz M. CT morphology of benign median nerve tumors. Report of three cases and a review. Acta Radiol 1990;31:23–25.

Firooznia H, Golimbu C, Rafii M. Carpal tunnel syndrome as a manifestation of secondary hyperparathyroidism (letter). Arch Intern Med 1981;141:959.

Fisher RC, Horner RL, Wood VE. The hand in mucopolysaccharide disorders. Clin Orthop 1974;104:191–99.

Fissette J, Onkelinx A, Fandi N. Carpal and Guyon tunnel syndrome in burns at the wrist. J Hand Surg 1981;6:13–15.

Floyd T, Burger RS, Sciaroni CA. Bilateral palmaris profundus causing bilateral carpal tunnel syndrome. J Hand Surg 1990;15A:364–66.

Folkers K, Ellis J, Watanabe T, Saji S, Kaji M. Biochemical evidence for a deficiency of vitamin B_6 in the carpal tunnel syndrome based on a crossover clinical study. Proc Natl Acad Sci USA 1978;75:3410–12.

Fowler CP, Harrison MJ, Snaith ML. Familial carpal and tarsal tunnel syndrome (letter). J Neurol Neurosurg Psychiatry 1986;49:717–18.

Frith RW, Litchy WJ. Electrophysiologic abnormalities of peripheral nerves in patients with cervical radiculopathy. Muscle Nerve 1985;8:613.

Fuchs A, Jagirdar J, Schwartz IS. Beta 2–microglobulin amyloidosis (AB2M) in patients undergoing long-term hemodialysis. A new type of amyloid. Am J Clin Pathol 1987;88:302–7.

Gagnon RF, Lough JO, Bourgouin PA. Carpal tunnel syndrome and amyloidosis associated with continuous ambulatory peritoneal dialysis. Can Med Assoc J 1988;139:753–55.

Gahhos F, Cuono CB. Periosteal chondroma: another cause of carpal tunnel syndrome. Ann Plast Surg 1984;12:275–78.

Galzio RJ, Magliani V, Lucantoni D, D'Arrigo C. Bilateral anomalous course of the ulnar nerve at the wrist causing ulnar and median nerve compression syndromes. J Neurosurg 1987;67:754–56.

Ganel A, Engel J, Sela M, Brooks M. Nerve entrapments associated with postmastectomy lymphedema. Cancer 1979;44:2254–59.

Gejyo F, Yamada T, Odani S, Nakagawa Y, Arakawa M, Kunitomo T, Kataoka H, Suzuki M, Hirasawa Y, Shirahama T, et al. A new form of amyloid protein associated with chronic hemodialysis was identified as beta 2–microglobulin. Biochem Biophys Res Commun 1985;129:701–6.

Gellis SS, Feingold M, Kelly TE. Picture of the month. Am J Dis Child 1975;129:1059–60.

Gerardi JA, Mack GR, Lutz RB. Acute carpal tunnel syndrome secondary to septic arthritis of the wrist. J Am Osteopath Assoc 1989;89:933–34.

Gibson CT, Manske PR. Carpal tunnel syndrome in the adolescent. J Hand Surg 1987;12A:279–81.

Gilbert MS, Robinson A, Baez A, Gupta S, Glabman S, Haimov M. Carpal tunnel syndrome in patients who are receiving long-term renal hemodialysis. J Bone Joint Surg 1988;70A:1145–53.

Gleason TF, Abraham E. Bilateral carpal tunnel syndrome associated with unilateral duplication of the flexor digitorum superficialis muscle: a case report. Hand 1982;14:48–50.

Goldberg A, Levy M. Carpal tunnel syndrome and artificial tenodesis of index tendon due to "nailing" of the tendon by a palm tree thorn (in Hebrew). Harefuah 1977;92:514.

Golik A, Modai D, Pervin R, Marcus EL, Fried K. Autosomal dominant carpal tunnel syndrome in a Karaite family. Isr J Med Sci 1988;24:295–97.

Goodwin DR, Arbel R. Pseudogout of the wrist presenting as acute median nerve compression. J Hand Surg 1985;10B:261–62.

Gordon H, Gordon W, Botha V, Edelstein I. Lipoid proteinosis. Birth Defects 1971;7:164–77.

Gouet P, Castets M, Touchard G, Payen J, Alcalay M. Bilateral carpal tunnel syndrome due to tuberculosis tenosynovitis: a case report (letter). J Rheumatol 1984;11:721–22.

Gray RG, Poppo MJ, Gottlieb NL. Primary familial bilateral carpal tunnel syndrome. Ann Intern Med 1979;91:37–40.

Gunther SF, Elliott RC, Brand RL, Adams JP. Experience with atypical mycobacterial infection in the deep structures of the hand. J Hand Surg 1977;2:90–96.

Guyon MA, Honet JC. Carpal tunnel syndrome or trigger finger associated with neck injury in automobile accidents. Arch Phys Med Rehabil 1977;58:325–27.

Haas DC, Nord SG, Bome MP. Carpal tunnel syndrome following automobile collisions. Arch Phys Med Rehabil 1981;62:204–6.

Hagemann PO. Sporotrichosis tendonitis and tenosynovitis. Trans Am Clin Climatol Assoc 1968;79:193–98.

Hale MS, Ruderman JE. Carpal tunnel syndrome associated with rubella immunization. Am J Phys Med 1973;52:189–94.

Halperin JJ, Volkman DJ, Luft BJ, Dattwyler RJ. Carpal tunnel syndrome in Lyme borreliosis. Muscle Nerve 1989;12:397–400.

Halter SK, DeLisa JA, Stolov WC, Scardapane D, Sherrard DJ. Carpal tunnel syndrome in chronic renal dialysis patients. Arch Phys Med Rehabil 1981;62:197–201.

Harrison W, Stewart J, Lovelace R, Quitkin F. Case report of carpal tunnel syndrome associated with tranylcypromine. Am J Psychiatry 1983;140:1229–30.

Hartwell SW Jr, Kurtay M. Carpal tunnel compression caused by hematoma associated with anticoagulant therapy. Report of a case. Cleve Clin Q 1966;33:127–29.

Harvey FJ, Bosanquet JS. Carpal tunnel syndrome caused by a simple ganglion. Hand 1981;13:164–66.

Hasselbacher P. Neuropathy after influenza vaccination (letter). Lancet 1977;1:551–52.

Hawkins PN, Lavender JP, Pepys MB. Evaluation of systemic amyloidosis by scintigraphy with I[123]-labeled serum amyloid P component. N Engl J Med 1990;323:508–13.

Hayes CW Jr. Anomalous flexor sublimis muscle with incipient carpal tunnel syndrome. Case report. Plast Reconstr Surg 1974;53:479–83.

Herndon JH, Eaton RG, Littler JW. Carpal-tunnel syndrome. An unusual presentation of osteoid-osteoma of the capitate. J Bone Joint Surg 1974;56A:1715–18.

Hines RA, Hughes CV. Carpal tunnel syndrome and diazepam (intravenously) (letter). JAMA 1974;228:697.

Hopkins AP, Morgan-Hughes JA. The effect of local pressure in diphtheritic neuropathy. J Neurol Neurosurg Psychiatry 1969;32:614–23.

Howard JF. Arthritis and carpal tunnel syndrome associated with disulfiram (antabuse) therapy. Arthritis Rheum 1982;25:1494–96.

Howie CR, Buxton R. Acute carpal tunnel syndrome due to spontaneous haemorrhage. J Hand Surg 1984;9B:137–38.

Hurst LC, Weissberg D, Carroll RE. The relationship of the double crush to carpal tunnel syndrome (an analysis of 1,000 cases of carpal tunnel syndrome). J Hand Surg 1985;10B:202–4.

Hutton P, Kernohan J, Birch R. An anomalous flexor digitorum superficialis indicis muscle presenting as carpal tunnel syndrome. Hand 1981;13:85–86.

Hvid-Hansen O. On the treatment of ganglia. Acta Chir Scand 1970;136:471–76.

Hybbinette CH, Mannerfelt L. The carpal tunnel syndrome. A retrospective study of 400 operated patients. Acta Orthop Scand 1975;46:610–20.

Iqbal QM. Triggering of the finger at the flexor retinaculum. Hand 1982;14:53–55.

Jabaley ME. Personal observations on the role of the lumbrical muscles in carpal tunnel syndrome. J Hand Surg 1978;3:82–84.

Jackson DW, Harkins PD. An aberrant muscle belly of the abductor digiti quinti associated with median nerve paresthesias. Bull Hosp Joint Dis 1972;33:111–15.

Jackson IT, Campbell JC. An unusual cause of carpal tunnel syndrome. A case of thrombosis of the median artery. J Bone Joint Surg 1970;52B:330–33.

Jackson SH. Profundus tendon disruption resulting in carpal tunnel syndrome. Orthopedics 1990;13:887–89.

Jain VK, Cestero RV, Baum J. Carpal tunnel syndrome in patients undergoing maintenance hemodialysis. JAMA 1979;242:2868–69.

Jones NF, Peterson J. Epidemiologic study of the mallet finger deformity. J Hand Surg 1988;13A:334–38.

Jones WA, Scheker LR. Acute carpal tunnel syndrome: a case report. J Hand Surg 1988;13B:400–401.

Kachel HG, Altmeyer P, Baldamus CA, Koch KM. Deposition of an amyloid-like substance as a possible complication of regular dialysis treatment. Contrib Nephrol 1983;36:127–32.

Kaplan H, Clayton M. Carpal tunnel syndrome secondary to *Mycobacterium kansasii* infection. JAMA 1969;208:1186–88.

Karpati G, Carpenter S, Eisen AA, Feindel W. Familial multiple peripheral nerve entrapments—an unusual manifestation of a peripheral neuropathy. Trans Am Neurol Assoc 1973;98:267–69.

Kelly JJ Jr. The electrodiagnostic findings in peripheral neuropathy associated with monoclonal gammopathy. Muscle Nerve 1983;6:504–9.

Kelly JJ Jr, Kyle RA, Miles JM, O'Brien PC, Dyck PJ. The spectrum of peripheral neuropathy in myeloma. Neurology 1981;31:24–31.

Kelly JJ Jr, Kyle RA, O'Brien PC, Dyck PJ. The natural history of peripheral neuropathy in primary systemic amyloidosis. Ann Neurol 1979;6:1–7.

Kelly PJ, Karlson AG, Weed LA, Lipscomb PR. Infection of synovial tissues by mycobacteria other than *Mycobacterium tuberculosis*. J Bone Joint Surg 1967;49A:1521–30.

Kerrigan JJ, Bertoni JM, Jaeger SH. Ganglion cysts and carpal tunnel syndrome. J Hand Surg 1988;13A:763–65.

Khunadorn N, Schlagenhauff RE, Tourbaf K, Papademetriou T. Carpal tunnel syndrome in hemophilia. NY State J Med 1977;77:1314–15.

Kilpatrick T, Leyden M, Sullivan J, Lawler G, Grossman H. Acute median nerve compression by haemorrhage from acute myelomonocytic leukaemia. Med J Aust 1985;142:51–52.

Kilroy AW, Schaffner W, Fleet WF Jr, Lefkowitz LB Jr, Karzon DT, Fenichel GM. Two syndromes following rubella immunization. Clinical observations and epidemiological studies. JAMA 1970;214:2287–92.

Kleinman KS, Coburn JW. Amyloid syndromes associated with hemodialysis. Kidney Int 1989;35:567–75.

Klofkorn RW, Steigerwald JC. Carpal tunnel syndrome as the initial manifestation of tuberculosis. Am J Med 1976;60:583–86.

Koenigsberger MR, Moessinger AC. Iatrogenic carpal tunnel syndrome in the newborn infant. J Pediatr 1977;91:443–45.

Kohn D, Bush A, Kessler I. Risk of venepuncture (letter). Br Med J 1976;2:1133.

Kremchek TE, Kremchek EJ. Carpal tunnel syndrome caused by flexor tendon sheath lipoma. Orthop Rev 1988;17:1083–85.

Krol-v-Straaten MJ, Ackerstaff RG, De-Maat CE. Peripheral polyneuropathy and monoclonal gammopathy of undetermined significance. J Neurol Neurosurg Psychiatry 1985;48:706–8.

Kumar S, Trivedi HL, Smith EK. Carpal tunnel syndrome: a complication of arteriovenous fistula in hemodialysis patients. Can Med Assoc J 1975;113:1070–72.

Kyle RA, Eilers SG, Linscheid RL, Gaffey TA. Amyloid localized to tenosynovium at carpal tunnel release. Natural history of 124 cases. Am J Clin Pathol 1989;91:393–97.

Kyle RA, Greipp PR. Amyloidosis (AL). Clinical and laboratory features in 229 cases. Mayo Clin Proc 1983;58:665–83.

Label LS. Carpal tunnel syndrome resulting from steering wheel impact. Muscle Nerve 1991;14:904.

Lagos JC. Compression neuropathy in childhood. Dev Med Child Neurol 1971;13:531–32.

Lambert EH, Mulder DW. Nerve conduction in the Guillain-Barré syndrome. Electroencephalogr Clin Neurophysiol 1964;17:86.

Lambird PA, Hartmann WH. Hereditary amyloidosis, the flexor retinaculum, and the carpal tunnel syndrome. Am J Clin Pathol 1969;52:714–19.

Langa V, Posner MA, Hoffman S, Steiner GC. Carpal tunnel syndrome secondary to tuberculous tenosynovitis. Bull Hosp Joint Dis 1986;46:137–42.

Lanz U. Anatomical variations of the median nerve in the carpal tunnel. J Hand Surg 1977;2:44–53.

Lazaro III L. Carpal-tunnel syndrome from an insect sting. A case report. J Bone Joint Surg 1972;54A:1095–96.

Lee KE. Tuberculosis presenting as carpal tunnel syndrome. J Hand Surg 1985;10:242–45.

Lettin AWF. Carpal tunnel syndrome in a girl aged 11. Proc R Soc Med 1965;58:183.

Levin RA, Felsenthal G. Handcuff neuropathy: two unusual cases. Arch Phys Med Rehabil 1984;65:41–43.

Levy M, Pauker M. Carpal tunnel syndrome due to thrombosed persisting median artery. A case report. Hand 1978;10:65–68.

Lewis MH. Median nerve decompression after Colles's fracture. J Bone Joint Surg 1978;60B:195–96.

Lewis RC Jr, Nordyke MD, Foreman KA. Median nerve compression caused by a synovial cyst. Bull Hosp Joint Dis 1986;46:68–71.

Lewis SL, Fiddian NJ. Acute carpal tunnel syndrome a rare complication of chondrocalcinosis. Hand 1982;14:164–67.

Lichtman DM, Alexander AH, Mack GR, Gunther SF. Kienbock's disease—update on silicone replacement arthroplasty. J Hand Surg 1982;7:343–47.

Linscheid RL. Carpal tunnel syndrome secondary to ulnar bursa distension from the intercarpal joint: report of a case. J Hand Surg 1979;4:191–92.

Louis DS, Dick HM. Ossifying lipofibroma of the median nerve. J Bone Joint Surg 1973;55A:1082–84.

Lourie GM, Levin LS, Toby B, Urbaniak J. Distal rupture of the palmaris longus tendon and fascia as a cause of acute carpal tunnel syndrome. J Hand Surg 1990;15A:367–69.

MacDougal B, Weeks PM, Wray RC Jr. Median nerve compression and trigger finger in the mucopolysaccharidoses and related diseases. Plast Reconstr Surg 1977;59:260–63.

Mackay IR, Barua JM. Perineural tumour spread: an unusual cause of carpal tunnel syndrome. J Hand Surg 1990;15B:104–5.

Mahloudji M, Teasdall RD, Adamkiewicz JJ, Hartmann WH, Lambird PA, McKusick VA. The genetic amyloidoses with particular reference to hereditary neuropathic amyloidosis, type II (Indiana or Rukavina type). Medicine (Baltimore) 1969;48:1–37.

Mancusi-Ungaro A, Corres JJ, Di-Spaltro F. Median carpal tunnel syndrome following a vascular shunt procedure in the forearm. Case report. Plast Reconstr Surg 1976;57:96–97.

Mandawat MK. Congestive heart failure and carpal tunnel syndrome: a rare association. J Indian Med Assoc 1985;83:287.

Manske PR. Fracture of the hook of the hamate presenting as carpal tunnel syndrome. Hand 1978;10:181–83.

Martinelli P, Poppi M, Gaist G, Padovani R, Pozzati E. Posttraumatic neuroma of the median nerve: a cause of carpal tunnel syndrome. Eur Neurol 1985;24:13–15.

Massey EW, Riley TL, Pleet AB. Coexistent carpal tunnel syndrome and cervical radiculopathy (double crush syndrome). South Med J 1981;74:957–59.

Maurer K, Fenske A, Samii M. Carpal tunnel syndrome combined with trigger finger in early childhood (letter). J Neurol Neurosurg Psychiatry 1980;43:1148.

Maxwell JA, Clough CA, Reckling FW, Kelly CR. Carpal tunnel syndrome. A review of cases treated surgically. J Kans Med Soc 1973a;74:190–93.

Maxwell JA, Kepes JJ, Ketchum LD. Acute carpal tunnel syndrome secondary to thrombosis of a persistent median artery. Case report. J Neurosurg 1973b;38:774–77.

McArthur RG, Hayles AB, Gomez MR, Bianco AJ Jr. Carpal tunnel syndrome and trigger finger in childhood. Am J Dis Child 1969;117:463–69.

McClain EJ, Wissinger HA. The acute carpal tunnel syndrome: nine case reports. J Trauma 1976;16:75–78.

McDonnell JM, Makley JT, Horwitz SJ. Familial carpal-tunnel syndrome presenting in childhood. Report of two cases. J Bone Joint Surg 1987;69A:928–30.

McGrath MH, Polayes IM. Posttraumatic median neuroma: a cause of carpal tunnel syndrome. Ann Plast Surg 1979;3:227–30.

McKusick VA. Heritable disorders of connective tissue. 4th ed. Saint Louis: CV Mosby, 1972.

McMinn DJ. Carpal tunnel syndrome caused by a simple ganglion. J R Coll Surg Edinb 1985;30:325–26.

Mesgarzadeh M, Schneck CD, Bonakdarpour A, Mitra A, Conaway D. Carpal tunnel: MR imaging. Part II. Carpal tunnel syndrome. Radiology 1989;171:749–54.

Meyer FN, Pflaum BC. Median nerve compression at the wrist caused by a reversed palmaris longus muscle. J Hand Surg 1987;12A:369–71.

Michaud LJ, Hays RM, Dudgeon BJ, Kropp RJ. Congenital carpal tunnel syndrome: case report of autosomal dominant inheritance and review of the literature. Arch Phys Med Rehabil 1990;71:430–32.

Milroy BC, Aldred RJ, Vickers D. Digital avulsion injuries: the shish kebab effect of the fibrous flexor sheath. Aust NZ J Surg 1984;54:67–71.

Miner ME, Schimke RN. Carpal tunnel syndrome in pediatric mucopolysaccharidoses. Report of four cases. J Neurosurg 1975;43:102–3.

Mochizuki Y, Ohkubo H, Motomura T. Familial bilateral carpal tunnel syndrome (letter). J Neurol Neurosurg Psychiatry 1981;44:367–69.

Moneim MS. Unusually high division of the median nerve. J Hand Surg 1982;7:13–14.

Moneim MS, Gribble TJ. Carpal tunnel syndrome in hemophilia. J Hand Surg 1984; 9A:580–83.

Morgan LM. Acute median nerve compression (letter). Med J Aust 1985;142:620.

Muñoz-Gómez J, Gómez-Pérez R, Llopart-Buisán E, Solé-Arqués M. Clinical picture of the amyloid arthropathy in patients with chronic renal failure maintained on haemodialysis using cellulose membranes. Ann Rheum Dis 1987;46:573–79.

Murray WT, Meuller PR, Rosenthal DI, Jauernek RR. Fracture of the hook of the hamate. AJR 1979;133:899–903.

Nathan PA, Meadows KD. Ulna-minus variance and Kienbock's disease. J Hand Surg 1987;12A:777–78.

Nather A, Chong PY. A rare case of carpal tunnel syndrome due to tenosynovial osteochondroma. J Hand Surg 1986;11B:478–80.

Nather A, Pho RWH. Carpal tunnel syndrome produced by an organising haematoma within the anomalous second lumbrical muscle. Hand 1981;13:87–91.

Neviaser RJ. Flexor digitorum superficialis indicis and carpal tunnel syndrome. Hand 1974;6:155–56.

Nkele C. Acute carpal tunnel syndrome resulting from haemorrhage into the carpal tunnel in a patient on warfarin. J Hand Surg 1986;11B:455–56.

Oates GD. Median-nerve palsy as a complication of acute pyogenic infections of the hand. Br Med J 1960;1:1618–20.

Olerud C, Lonnquist L. Acute carpal tunnel syndrome caused by fracture of the scaphoid and the 5th metacarpal bones. Injury 1984;16:198–99.

Orfila C, Goffinet F, Goudable C, Eche JP, Ton-That H, Manuel Y, Suc JM. Unsuitable value of abdominal fat tissue aspirate examination for the diagnosis of amyloidosis in long-term hemodialysis patients. Am J Nephrol 1988;8:454–56.

Oster LH, Blair WF, Steyers CM. Large lipomas in the deep palmar space. J Hand Surg 1989;14:700–704.

Osterman AL. The double crush syndrome. Orthop Clin North Am 1988;19:147–55.

Owens DW, Garcia E, Pierce RR, Castrow II FF. Klippel-Trenaunay-Weber syndrome with pulmonary vein varicosity. Arch Dermatol 1973;108:111–13.

Paarlberg D, Linscheid RL, Soule EH. Lipomas of the hand. Including a case of lipoblasto-matosis in a child. Mayo Clin Proc 1972;47:121–24.

Paget J. Lectures on surgical pathology. Philadelphia: Lindsay & Blakiston, 1865. Third American.

Paley D, McMurtry RY. Median nerve compression by volarly displaced fragments of the distal radius. Clin Orthop 1987;215:139–47.

Patel MR, Desai SS, Gordon SL. Functional limb salvage with multimodality treatment in epithelioid sarcoma of the hand: a report of two cases. J Hand Surg 1986;11A:265–69.

Pecket P, Gloobe H, Nathan H. Variations in the arteries of the median nerve. Clin Orthop 1973;97:144–47.

Peterson DI, Bacchus H, Seaich L, Kelly TE. Myelopathy associated with Maroteaux-Lamy syndrome. Arch Neurol 1975;32:127–29.

Phalen GS. The carpal-tunnel syndrome. Seventeen years' experience in diagnosis and treatment of six hundred fifty-four hands. J Bone Joint Surg 1966;48A:211–28.

Poilvache P, Carlier A, Rombouts JJ, Partoune E, Lejeune G. Carpal tunnel syndrome in childhood: report of five new cases. J Pediatr Orthop 1989;9:687–90.

Potts F, Shahani BT, Young RR. A study of the coincidence of carpal tunnel syndrome and generalized peripheral neuropathy. Muscle Nerve 1980;3:440.

Primiano GA, Reef TC. Disruption of the proximal carpal arch of the hand. J Bone Joint Surg 1974;56A:328–32.

Prince H, Ispahani P, Baker M. A Mycobacterium malmoense infection of the hand presenting as carpal tunnel syndrome. J Hand Surg 1988;13B:328–30.

Pritsch M, Engel J, Horowitz A. Cystic change in the wrist, causing carpal tunnel syndrome. Plast Reconstr Surg 1980;65:494–95.

Probst CE, Hunter JM. A digastric flexor digitorum superficialis. Bull Hosp Joint Dis 1975;36:52–57.

Pronicka E, Tylki-Szymanska A, Kwast O, Chmielik J, Maciejko D, Cedro A. Carpal tunnel syndrome in children with mucopolysaccharidoses: needs for surgical tendons and median nerve release. J Ment Defic Res 1988;32:79–82.

Radford PJ, Matthewson MH. Hypoplastic scaphoid—an unusual cause of carpal tunnel syndrome. J Hand Surg 1987;12B:236–38.

Randall G, Smith PW, Korbitz B, Owen DR. Carpal tunnel syndrome caused by Mycobacterium fortuitum and Histoplasma capsulatum. Report of two cases. J Neurosurg 1982;56:299–301.

Reddy MP. Nerve entrapment syndromes in the upper extremity contralateral to amputation. Arch Phys Med Rehabil 1984;65:24–26.

Reicher MA, Kellerhouse LE. Carpal tunnel disease, flexor and extensor tendon disorders. In: Reicher MA, Kellerhouse LE, eds. MRI of the wrist and hand. New York: Raven Press, 1990;49–68.

Reimann AF, Daseler EH, Anson BJ, Beaton LE. The palmaris longus muscle and tendon. A study of 1600 extremities. Anat Rec 1944;89:495–505.

Robinson D, Aghasi M, Halperin N. The treatment of carpal tunnel syndrome caused by hypertrophied lumbrical muscles. Case reports. Scand J Plast Reconstr Surg 1989; 23:149–51.

Roos D, Thygesen P. Familial recurrent polyneuropathy. Brain 1972;95:235–48.

Rosenberg DB. Neurologic sequelae of minor electric burns. Arch Phys Med Rehabil 1989;70:914–15.

Rukavina JG, Block WD, Jackson CE, Falls HF, Carey JH, Curtis AC. Primary systemic amyloidosis: an experimental, genetic, and clinical study of 29 cases with particular emphasis on the familial form. Medicine (Baltimore) 1956;35:239–334.

Sahs AL, Helms CM, DuBois C. Carpal tunnel syndrome. Complication of toxic shock syndrome. Arch Neurol 1983;40:414–15.

Sainio K, Merikanto J, Larsen TA. Carpal tunnel syndrome in childhood. Dev Med Child Neurol 1987;29:794–97.

Sargent MA, Fleming SJ, Chattopadhyay C, Ackrill P, Sambrook P. Bone cysts and haemodialysis-related amyloidosis. Clin Radiol 1989;40:277–81.

Sarma DP, Weilbaecher TG, Rodriguez FH Jr. Fibroma of tendon sheath. J Surg Oncol 1986;32:230–32.

Scardapane D, Halter S, DeLisa JA, Sherrard DJ. Hand dysfunction due to carpal tunnel syndrome: a common sequela of dialysis. Proc Clin Dial Transplant Forum 1979;9:15–16.

Schlafly B, Lister G. Median nerve compression secondary to bifid reversed palmaris longus. J Hand Surg 1987;12A:371–73.

Schultz RJ, Endler PM, Huddleston HD. Anomalous median nerve and an anomalous muscle belly of the first lumbrical associated with carpal-tunnel syndrome. J Bone Joint Surg 1973;55A:1744–46.

Schwarz A, Keller F, Seyfert S, Poll W, Molzahn M, Distler A. Carpal tunnel syndrome: a major complication in long-term hemodialysis patients. Clin Nephrol 1984;22:133–37.

Schweitzer G, Lewis JS. Puff adder bite—an unusual cause of bilateral carpal tunnel syndrome. A case report. S Afr Med J 1981;60:714–15.

Schweitzer G, Miller RD. Carpal tunnel syndrome due to median nerve enlargement. S Afr Med J 1973;47:2222–24.

Selby RC, Neurosurgical aspects of leprosy. Surg Neurol 1974;2:165–77.

Shenoy KT, Saha PK, Ravindran M. Carpal tunnel syndrome: an unusual presentation of brachial hypertrophy. J Neurol Neurosurg Psychiatry 1980;43:82–84.

Sikka A, Kemmann E, Vrablik RM, Grossman L. Carpal tunnel syndrome associated with danazol therapy. Am J Obstet Gynecol 1983;147:102–3.

Smith RJ. Anomalous muscle belly of the flexor digitorum superficialis causing carpal-tunnel syndrome. Report of a case. J Bone Joint Surg 1971;53A:1215–16.

Solem L, Fischer RP, Strate RG. The natural history of electrical injury. J Trauma 1977;17:487–92.

Southworth SR, Hartwig RH. Foreign body in the median nerve: a complication of acupuncture. J Hand Surg 1990;15B:111–12.

Sparkes RS, Spence MA, Gottlieb NL, Gray RG, Crist M, Sparkes MC, Marazita M. Genetic linkage analysis of the carpal tunnel syndrome. Hum Hered 1985;35:288–91.

Spiegel PG, Ginsberg M, Skosey JL, Kwong P. Acute carpal tunnel syndrome secondary to pseudogout: case report. Clin Orthop 1976;120:185–87.

Sponsel KH, Palm ET. Carpal tunnel syndrome following Colles' fracture. Surg Gynecol Obstet 1965;121:1252–56.

Staal A, de Weerdt CJ, Went LN. Hereditary compression syndrome of peripheral nerves. Neurology 1965;15:1008–17.

Starreveld E, Ashenhurst EM. Bilateral carpal tunnel syndrome in childhood. A report of two sisters with mucolipidosis III (pseudo-Hurler polydystrophy). Neurology 1975; 25:234–38.

Sterling AP, Eshraghi A, Anderson WJ, Habermann ET. Acute carpal tunnel syndrome secondary to a foreign body within the median nerve. Bull Hosp Joint Dis 1972;33:130–34.

Stewart HD, Innes AR, Burke FD. The hand complications of Colles' fractures. J Hand Surg 1985;10B:103–6.

Stone DA, Laureno R. Handcuff neuropathies. Neurology 1991;41:145–47.

Stone WJ, Hakim RM. Beta-2-microglobulin amyloidosis in long-term dialysis patients. Am J Nephrol 1989;9:177–83.

Stratton CW, Lichtenstein KA, Lowenstein SR, Phelps DB, Reller LB. Granulomatous tenosynovitis and carpal tunnel syndrome caused by *Sporothrix schenckii*. Am J Med 1981;71:161–64.

Stratton CW, Phelps DB, Reller LB. Tuberculoid tenosynovitis and carpal tunnel syndrome caused by *Mycobacterium szulgai*. Am J Med 1978;65:349–51.

Strayer DS, Gutwein MB, Herbold D, Bresalier R. Histoplasmosis presenting as the carpal tunnel syndrome. Am J Surg 1981;141:286–88.

Sturim HS, Edmond JA. Carpal tunnel compression syndrome secondary to a retracted flexor digitorum sublimis tendon. Plast Reconstr Surg 1980;66:846–48.

Sukenik S, Horowitz J, Katz A, Henkin J, Buskila D. Quinidine-induced lupus erythematosus–like syndrome: three case reports and a review of the literature. Isr J Med Sci 1987;23:1232–34.

Suso S, Peidro L, Ramon R. Tuberculous synovitis with "rice bodies" presenting as carpal tunnel syndrome. J Hand Surg 1988;13A:574–76.

Sutro CJ. Carpal tunnel syndrome caused by calcification in the deep or volar radio-carpal ligament. Bull Hosp Joint Dis 1969;30:23–27.

Swift TR, McDonald TF. Peripheral nerve involvement in Hunter syndrome (mucopolysaccharidosis II). Arch Neurol 1976;33:845–46.

Teitz CC, DeLisa JA, Halter SK. Results of carpal tunnel release in renal hemodialysis patients. Clin Orthop 1985;198:197–200.

Thomas PK. Genetic factors in amyloidosis. J Med Genet 1975;12:317–26.

Thompson GR, Ferreyra A, Brackett RG. Acute arthritis complicating rubella vaccination. Arthritis Rheum 1971;14:19–26.

Tingle AJ, Chantler JK, Pot KH, Paty DW, Ford DK. Postpartum rubella immunization: association with development of prolonged arthritis, neurological sequelae, and chronic rubella viremia. J Infect Dis 1985;152:606–12.

Tompkins DG. Median neuropathy in the carpal tunnel caused by tumor-like conditions. Report of two cases. J Bone Joint Surg 1967;49A:737–40.

Touborg-Jensen A. Carpal-tunnel syndrome caused by an abnormal distribution of the lumbrical muscles. Case report. Scand J Plast Reconstr Surg 1970;4:72–74.

Trevaskis AE, Tilly D, Marcks KM, Heffernan AH. Loss of nerve function in the hand caused by ganglions. Plast Reconstr Surg 1967;39:97–100.

Ullian ME, Hammond WS, Alfrey AC, Schultz A, Molitoris BA. Beta-2-microglobulin-associated amyloidosis in chronic hemodialysis patients with carpal tunnel syndrome. Medicine (Baltimore) 1989;68:107–15.

Upton AR, McComas AJ. The double crush in nerve entrapment syndromes. Lancet 1973;2:359–62.

Vandenbroucke JM, Jadoul M, Maldague B, Huaux JP, Noël H, van Ypersele de Strihou C. Possible role of dialysis membrane characteristics in amyloid osteoarthropathy (letter). Lancet 1986;1:1210–11.

Vanwijck R, Bouillenne C. HL-A and carpal tunnel syndrome. Clin Rheumatol 1986;5:379–81.

Victor M. Polyneuropathy due to nutritional deficiency and alcoholism. In: Dyck PJ, Thomas PK, Lambert EH, Bunge R, eds. Peripheral neuropathy. 2nd ed. Philadelphia: WB Saunders, 1984;1899–1940.

Vinals-Torras M, Garcia AF, Barreiro-Tella P, Diez-Tejedor E, Cruz-Martínez A, Arpa-

Gutierrez J. Manifestation of Scheie mucopolysaccharidosis I: carpal tunnel syndrome in childhood. Case report. Arch Neurobiol (Madr) 1985;48:113–23.

Wallace MR, Conneally PM, Benson MD. A DNA test for Indiana/Swiss hereditary amyloidosis (FAP II). Am J Hum Genet 1988;43:182–87.

Walton S, Cutler CR. Carpal tunnel syndrome. Case report of unusual etiology. Clin Orthop 1971;74:138–40.

Warren DJ, Otieno LS. Carpal tunnel syndrome in patients on intermittent haemodialysis. Postgrad Med J 1975;51:450–52.

Watson-Jones R. Léri's pleonosteosis, carpal tunnel compression of the median nerves and Morton's metatarsalgia. J Bone Joint Surg 1949;31B:560–71.

Weiber H, Linell F. Tumoral calcinosis causing acute carpal tunnel syndrome. Case report. Scand J Plast Reconstr Surg 1987;21:229–30.

Weiland AJ, Lister GD, Villarreal-Rios A. Volar fracture dislocations of the second and third carpometacarpal joints associated with acute carpal tunnel syndrome. J Trauma 1976;16:672–75.

Wener MH, Metzger WJ, Simon RA. Occupationally acquired vibratory angioedema with secondary carpal tunnel syndrome. Ann Intern Med 1983;98:44–46.

Wilbourn AJ, Breuer AC. The double crush syndrome: a reappraisal. Neurology 1986;36:234–35.

Winkelman NZ. An accessory flexor digitorum profundus indicis. J Hand Surg 1983;8:70–71.

Wood KA, Jacoby RJ. Lithium induced hypothyroidism presenting with carpal tunnel syndrome (letter). Br J Psychiatry 1986;149:386–87.

Yeoman PM. Léri's pleonosteosis. Proc R Soc Med 1961;54:275.

Zamora JL, Rose JE, Rosario V, Noon GP. Double entrapment of the median nerve in association with PTFE hemodialysis loop grafts. South Med J 1986;79:638–40.

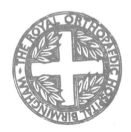

7

Electrodiagnostic Methods for Evaluation of Carpal Tunnel Syndrome

Electrodiagnostic tests are commonly used to aid in the diagnosis of carpal tunnel syndrome and to study its physiology (Table 7.1). Simpson (1958) stimulated the median nerve at the wrist and recorded a compound muscle action potential (CMAP) over the thenar eminence. He reported prolonged distal motor latency (DML) of the median nerve in 11 of 15 patients with carpal tunnel syndrome. Thomas (1960) found a similar diagnostic sensitivity in 95 patients. Gilliatt and Sears (1958) described the use of sensory nerve conduction measurements in the diagnosis of carpal tunnel syndrome. Subsequent authors have

Table 7.1 Abbreviations

CMAP	Compound muscle action potential
DML	Distal motor latency
DSL	Distal sensory latency
EMG	Electromyography
MLD	Maximum serial sensory latency difference
MNCV	Motor nerve conduction velocity
RF	Repeater F wave
%RF	Percent repeater F waves
RML	Residual motor latency
SNAP	Sensory nerve action potential
SNCV	Sensory nerve conduction velocity
SSEP	Somatosensory evoked potential
TLI	Terminal latency index

described a number of approaches to improving the diagnostic sensitivity of nerve conduction tests. Stevens (1987) has written a useful brief review of nerve conduction tests for carpal tunnel syndrome. Table 7.2 lists some of the more important variations, which are discussed in greater detail in this chapter.

Despite the abundant variety of available electrodiagnostic tests, carpal

Table 7.2 Electrodiagnostic tests for carpal tunnel syndrome

Motor Nerve Conduction Studies

Distal motor latency

Residual motor latency

Terminal latency index

CMAP amplitude and duration

Effects of ischemia

Lumbrical studies

Palmar stimulation

Palmar serial motor stimulation

Forearm motor nerve conduction velocity

Martin-Gruber anastomosis

Threshold distal motor latency

F-wave studies

Sensory Nerve Conduction Studies

Finger-to-wrist conduction

Palm-to-wrist conduction

Variability of digital nerves

Palmar serial sensory studies

Ipsilateral comparison methods
  Median-ulnar comparison
  Median-radial comparison
  SNAP amplitude and comparisons
  Hand-to-forearm comparison

Provocative tests

Minimum SNCV

Repetitive sensory stimulation

Electromyography

Evidence of axonal interruption

Repetitive neuronal firing

Somatosensory Evoked Potentials

tunnel syndrome is defined by symptoms and therefore remains a clinical diagnosis. Test results can support the diagnosis through documenting nerve fiber pathophysiology but can never make a definitive diagnosis by themselves. This chapter has a recurring theme: Laboratory evidence of impaired impulse conduction in the median nerve at the wrist does not prove that a patient's clinical symptoms are caused by the conduction abnormality.

There is no test that is always abnormal in every patient with carpal tunnel syndrome; normal tests in patients with clinical symptoms and signs of carpal tunnel syndrome are "false negatives." The sensitivity of a test for carpal tunnel syndrome is defined as the ratio of positive tests in patients with the syndrome (i.e., "true positives") to the total number of tested patients with the syndrome (Sackett et al. 1985; Riegleman and Hirsch 1989).

$$\text{Test sensitivity} = \frac{\text{True positives}}{\text{True positives} + \text{False negatives.}}$$

Any median nerve test will occasionally be abnormal in patients without clinical symptoms or signs of carpal tunnel syndrome; tests may be false positive in asymptomatic individuals, or they may be positive because of median nerve pathology outside the carpal tunnel syndrome.

Many clinicians will diagnose and initiate early treatment of carpal tunnel syndrome based on signs and symptoms before performing electrodiagnostic evaluation. Some hand surgeons will operate for carpal tunnel syndrome without obtaining electrodiagnostic tests (Duncan et al. 1987).

If their limitations are understood, the tests are very helpful in assessing carpal tunnel syndrome patients, particularly in difficult diagnostic cases. For a number of reasons, we favor electrodiagnostic evaluation of every patient before carpal tunnel surgery. First, electrodiagnosis offers information about the severity of dysfunction of the median nerve. Second, the electrodiagnostician, evaluating the patients with neuropathic arm symptoms, has the opportunity to obtain data on other diagnostic possibilities. Depending on the clinical setting, these possibilities might include other mononeuropathies, mononeuritis multiplex, disease of the median nerve outside the carpal tunnel, brachial plexopathy, cervical radiculopathy, anterior horn cell disease, or diffuse peripheral neuropathy. Third, preoperative electrodiagnostic studies provide baseline data necessary to adequately evaluate patients who may have persistent symptoms after surgery.

Devices are now commercially available that attempt to measure median nerve motor latencies automatically without showing the examiner the wave forms (and without training the examiner in full electrodiagnostic techniques and interpretation) (Feierstein 1988). These devices do a disservice both to diagnostician and patient by providing incomplete and potentially erroneous data on nerve function. Their use should be strongly discouraged.

In this chapter, we describe many of the available tests, including techniques, normal values, and findings in patients with carpal tunnel syndrome. This chapter will be better understood by those familiar with electrodiagnostic techniques. A number of good introductory texts are available (Aminoff 1987; Johnson 1988; Kimura 1989).

In the following chapter, "Interpretation of Electrodiagnostic Findings in Carpal Tunnel Syndrome," we review pathophysiology, diagnostic sensitivity and specificity, and prognostic value of electrodiagnostic tests. Chapter 8 also discusses interpretation of tests that are normal or only mildly abnormal.

MOTOR NERVE CONDUCTION STUDIES
Technique

The most commonly used median motor nerve conduction test measures conduction of the nerve to muscles of the thenar eminence (Ma and Liveson 1983). Surface recording electrodes should be on the thenar eminence with the active electrode over the motor point of the abductor pollicis brevis, two thirds of the way along a line running from the metacarpal-phalangeal joint to the carpal-metacarpal joint of the thumb (Figure 7.1). In this position, the electrode will detect potentials from multiple thenar muscles including the abductor pollicis

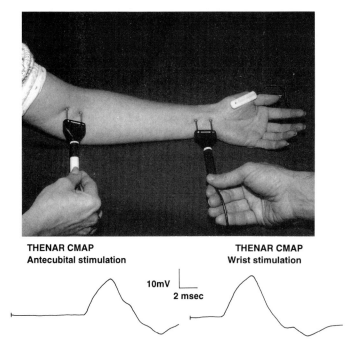

THENAR CMAP
Antecubital stimulation

THENAR CMAP
Wrist stimulation

10mV

2 msec

Figure 7.1 Electrode placement for studying median nerve motor conduction to the thenar muscles. The CMAPs obtained over the thenar muscles from stimulation at the wrist and at the antecubital space are shown. The wave forms shown in this chapter are an artist's renditions rather than pictures of actual recordings.

brevis, opponens pollicis, and flexor pollicis brevis, as well as from neighboring muscles such as the adductor pollicis and first dorsal interosseous. The reference electrode should be at the metacarpal-phalangeal joint of the thumb. The ground electrode may be on the dorsum of the hand. The stimulation sites are typically at the wrist, just medial to the tendon of flexor carpi radialis, and in the antecubital space just medial to the biceps tendon. The examiner records the latency in milliseconds between the time of stimulation and the onset of the CMAP. The amplitude of the CMAP is also recorded.

The distance from the wrist stimulation site to the active electrode should be measured and kept constant from study to study. Since the recurrent motor branch of the median nerve reaches the thenar muscles along a curved path, the measurement is only an approximation of nerve length. Some examiners measure directly between the stimulating and recording electrodes, whereas others bend the measuring tape, guessing at the course of the nerve. The measuring technique must be consistent from study to study.

The stimulus intensity is increased until the maximum amplitude CMAP is obtained to ensure that all motor nerve fibers in the median nerve are stimulated. When stimulating the median nerve at the wrist, the examiner must be careful to obtain supramaximal stimulation without stimulating the ulnar nerve. A thenar CMAP to median nerve stimulation at the wrist that is initially positive suggests volume-conducted contributions from ulnar-innervated muscles. A thenar CMAP to median stimulation at the wrist that is much larger than the CMAP to median stimulation in the antecubital space may be caused by volume-conducted ulnar stimulation at the wrist or by abnormal median nerve conduction in the forearm. To avoid inadvertent ulnar stimulation during median stimulation at the wrist, the stimulus can be decreased or the stimulator moved slightly radially. Sometimes use of a needle recording electrode in the abductor pollicis brevis is necessary to measure the median motor latencies accurately.

Normal Values

Ma and Liveson (1983) summarize the normal values from a number of different clinics. Typical values, shown in Table 7.3, are those from the Mayo Clinic, based on a 7-cm distance between the recording electrode and the wrist stimulation site (Stevens 1987).

Table 7.3 Median motor Conduction: normal values

DML *(msec)*		CMAP Amplitude *(mV)*		Forearm MNCV *(m/sec)*	
Mean	*Upper Normal*	*Mean*	*Lower Normal*	*Mean*	*Lower Normal*
3.2	4.7	10.7	3.7	59	49

(Data from Stevens 1987.)

Median DML is also considered abnormal by Mayo Clinic criteria if it is 1.0 msec longer than the contralateral median DML or 1.8 msec longer than the ipsilateral ulnar DML. Many laboratories use methods with lesser upper limits of normal, some as low as 4.0 msec, for the DML.

Findings in Carpal Tunnel Syndrome

In early published series of patients with carpal tunnel syndrome, two thirds to over four fifths of symptomatic hands had a prolonged median DML (Thomas 1960; Thomas et al. 1967; Kopell and Goodgold 1968; Buchthal et al. 1974). These are older series; the diagnostic sensitivity of median DML is probably lower in contemporary laboratories where it is common to test patients with relatively milder carpal tunnel syndrome. For example, in the series of Buchthal et al. (1974), 82% of the patients had abnormal median DML; in this series, one half the patients had clinical thenar weakness or atrophy—an incidence of clinical motor abnormality that would be quite high in contemporary clinics. In contrast, at the Mayo Clinic from 1961 to 1980, 51% of patients with clinical evidence of carpal tunnel syndrome who underwent electrodiagnostic studies had an abnormal median DML (Stevens 1987).

Residual Motor Latency

The normal median DML is too long to be explained solely by the conduction velocity of median myelinated fibers (Hodes et al. 1948). The median DML varies with (1) the length of nerve between sites of stimulation and recording, (2) the overall conduction velocity of the median nerve, (3) any delay in conduction attributable to focal nerve compression or disease, (4) any delay between arrival of the nerve action potential at the terminal unmyelinated axonal branches and activation of the muscle across the neuromuscular junction, and (5) systematic slowing of distal relative to proximal conduction (e.g., due to decrease in axon diameter distally or to distal temperature being less than proximal temperature). In normals, there is a relatively wide standard deviation and range of the median DML. Kraft and Halvorson (1983) corrected for the portion of this variation attributed to differences in distance between the stimulating and recording electrodes and to diffuse variations in conduction in the median nerve by calculating a residual motor latency (RML) using the following definition:

$$RML = DML - (10 \times D/MNCV),*$$

where RML = residual motor latency (msec)
DML = distal motor latency (msec)
D = distance from recording electrode to distal stimulating electrode (cm)
MNCV = motor nerve conduction velocity in the forearm (M/sec)

*The factor 10 in the formula corrects the dimensions so that although D is in centimeters and MNCV is in meters per second, the result is in milliseconds.

The recurrent median motor branch follows a curved and variable course in the palm, but D is measured on the surface; therefore, D is only an approximation of actual nerve length.

Kraft and Halvorson (1983) found an upper limit of normal median RML of 2.6 msec and gave examples of patients with clinical diagnoses of carpal tunnel syndrome who had normal median DML but prolonged median RML. One advantage of the RML over the DML is that the RML is less dependent on patient age.

Terminal Latency Index

Calculation of a terminal latency index (TLI) is another approach to correcting the DML for variations in the median forearm MNCV (Shahani et al. 1979). The TLI is defined by the following formula:

$$TLI = 10 \times D/(MNCV \times DML).$$

In normal subjects, the range of the TLI in one series was 0.36 to 0.55 (Shahani et al. 1979). Like the RML, the TLI may be abnormal in patients with carpal tunnel syndrome, even though the DML is normal (Evans and Daube 1984).

Compound Muscle Action Potential Amplitude and Duration

The normal amplitude and duration of the thenar CMAP to supramaximal stimulation have a large range and standard deviation (Hodes et al. 1948). Table 7.4 shows some sample values. The amplitude is influenced by technical factors such as electrode placement or amount of electrode paste used and by patient idiosyncracies such as local swelling, sweating, or callosity (Felsenthal 1978b). In a normal individual the thenar CMAP amplitude of one hand may be as low as 40% of the CMAP amplitude of the contralateral hand (Felsenthal 1978b).

In a population of patients with carpal tunnel syndrome, the mean thenar CMAP amplitude was 60% of the normal mean, but few individuals with carpal tunnel syndrome had CMAP amplitudes below the normal range (Thomas et al. 1967). There is a correlation between decrease in CMAP amplitude and slowing of forearm median MNCV (Thomas et al. 1967).

Table 7.4 CMAP amplitude and duration: normal values

	Mean	Standard Deviation	Range
Thenar CMAP amplitude (mV)	15.6	5.8	3.6–29.0
Thenar CMAP duration (msec)	12.23	1.64	9.0–16.0

(Data from Felsenthal 1978b.)

Effects of Ischemia on Nerve Conduction

Fullerton (1963) studied median motor conduction before and during ischemia of the forearm and hand, induced by a pneumatic cuff applied to the upper arm. Nerve conduction studies were repeated every two to five minutes after occlusion of blood flow. In control subjects, the amplitude and area of the thenar CMAP from median stimulation at the wrist remained unchanged for at least 20 minutes but fell as much as 50% by the thirtieth minute of ischemia. The thenar CMAP amplitude from median stimulation in the antecubital space often fell more quickly.

In two thirds of patients with carpal tunnel syndrome, the fall in thenar CMAP amplitude occurred more rapidly than in controls. There was a correlation in the patients between the severity of pain and paresthesias and the rate of fall in thenar CMAP amplitude during ischemia.

Sustained occlusion of blood flow by cuff on the upper arm also leads to gradual loss of amplitude of the median nerve sensory nerve action potential (SNAP) recorded at the wrist to digital stimulation (Cruz Martinez et al. 1980). In patients with carpal tunnel syndrome, SNAP amplitude falls faster than normal. In contrast, in patients with metabolic disturbances such as diabetes and chronic renal failure, SNAP amplitude may fall more slowly than normal.

Lumbrical Studies

Median motor conduction can also be measured to the second lumbrical. The active surface recording electrode is placed on the palm on the radial side of the third metacarpal, over the motor point of the lumbrical, approximately at the midpoint of the metacarpal (Figure 7.2). Alternatively, a needle recording electrode may be inserted into the lumbrical. The reference electrode is placed 3 cm distal to the active electrode (Logigian et al. 1987). In control patients, the median DML from the wrist is very similar whether measured to the abductor pollicis brevis or to the second lumbrical. In some patients with carpal tunnel syndrome, the DML to the abductor pollicis brevis is significantly longer than the DML to the second lumbrical. Logigian et al. (1987) classified patients with carpal tunnel syndrome as having "lumbrical sparing" if the DML to the abductor pollicis brevis was equal to or greater than 0.4 msec more than the DML to the ipsilateral second lumbrical. They found that four fifths of their carpal tunnel syndrome patients had lumbrical sparing. In 60 hands with carpal tunnel syndrome, the thenar DML was normal in 17. Of the 17 patients with normal thenar DML, 14 were classified as abnormal by demonstration of lumbrical sparing. Lumbrical sparing was noted in five patients with normal palm-to-wrist mixed nerve conduction velocity.

Lumbrical sparing may be detected in patients with severe carpal tunnel syndrome. When the thenar CMAP has an initial positive deflection with both wrist and antecubital stimulation, the source may be a volume-conducted CMAP from the median-innervated lumbricals (Yates et al. 1981). The median lumbrical

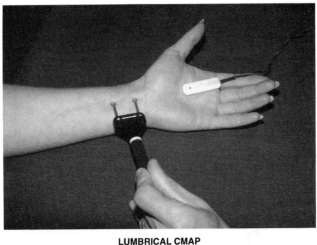

LUMBRICAL CMAP
Wrist stimulation

10mV
2 msec

Figure 7.2 Electrode placement recording for studying median nerve motor conduction to the lumbricals. The active surface recording electrode is placed on the radial side of the third metacarpal, over the motor point of the lumbrical, approximately at the midpoint of the metacarpal.

CMAP may be preserved when the thenar muscles are severely atrophic (Yates et al. 1981).

In the carpal tunnel, the median nerve fascicles that form the recurrent thenar motor branch are usually located on the anterior surface of the nerve, whereas the fascicles that form terminal branches to the lumbricals are farther from the surface of the nerve. Lumbrical sparing is hypothesized to reflect greater vulnerability to compression of the more superficial nerve fascicles.

Lumbrical sparing is not specific to carpal tunnel syndrome. It may also occur with injuries to the recurrent median motor nerve, true neurogenic thoracic outlet syndrome, partial median nerve transections, or median nerve injury in the axilla (Yates et al. 1981; Logigian et al. 1987).

Palmar Stimulation

Although the median DML is commonly obtained by stimulating the nerve at the wrist and recording over the thenar muscles, the median nerve can be stimulated more distally, in the palm (Figure 7.3). The site for palmar stimulation is traditionally approximated by asking the patient to flex the ring finger; the flexed finger points to the point in the palm that is chosen for stimulation. A more exact site of stimulation can be determined by starting slightly distal to this point

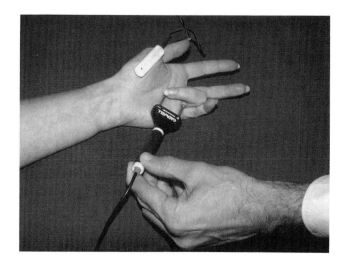

Figure 7.3 The site of palmar stimulation of the median nerve for motor conduction testing is found by asking the patient to flex the ring finger; the flexed finger points to the approximate stimulation site. The stimulating electrode may need to be moved until the optimal stimulation site is found.

in the palm and slowly moving the stimulating cathode proximally until a twitch of the median thenar muscles is elicited. The anode is distal to the cathode (Pease et al. 1988).

Kimura (1979) measured wrist-to-palm motor conduction in 122 control hands and 172 hands with symptomatic carpal tunnel syndrome. He obtained the results shown in Table 7.5. In this series, 61% of carpal tunnel syndrome patients had prolonged median DML (wrist-to-muscle). In an additional 23% of carpal tunnel syndrome patients, the wrist-to-palm motor conduction velocity was greater than two standard deviations below the mean of the normal controls.

In normals the amplitude of the CMAP from palmar stimulation is slightly larger than the amplitude of the CMAP from wrist stimulation. In many patients with carpal tunnel syndrome, loss of CMAP amplitude with the more proximal wrist stimulation is substantial, suggesting that in these patients conduction block (neurapraxia) is causing at least part of the loss of CMAP amplitude (Kimura 1979; Pease et al. 1988). Table 7.6 gives illustrative data.

Table 7.5 Wrist-to-palm median motor nerve conduction

	Velocity Mean (m/sec)	Standard Deviation
Controls	49.0	5.7
Carpal tunnel syndrome	28.2	7.5

(Data from Kimura 1979.)

Table 7.6 Thenar CMAP amplitude: wrist versus palmar stimulation

	CMAP Amplitude from Wrist (mV)		CMAP Amplitude from Palm minus CMAP Amplitude from Wrist (mV)	
	Mean	Standard Deviation	Mean	Range
Controls	8.8	3.1	0.6	0.0–2.0
Carpal tunnel syndrome patients	4.2	1.7	2.2	–1.0–6.0

(Data from Pease et al. 1988.)

The presence of conduction block suggests that the blocked axons are probably intact as they run through the carpal tunnel and that improvement may be relatively rapid following treatment of the nerve compression.

Palmar Serial Motor Stimulation

Median motor conduction in the palm can be further studied by "inching," that is, serially stimulating the nerve at 1-cm increments in an effort to find localized nerve segments with excessive slowing of conduction. The technique is difficult because of the recurrent course of the motor branch to the thenar muscles, which makes it hard to stimulate only the median nerve in the palm without also stimulating the recurrent motor branch. Kimura (1979) found that motor inching was often impossible to perform accurately.

White et al. (1988) took care to stimulate in the palm as far medially as possible in an effort to stimulate the median nerve without also stimulating the recurrent motor branch. They discuss criteria for ensuring the technical accuracy of the stimulation. They found an abnormal 1-cm motor segment in 72% of *asymptomatic* hands in patients with contralateral unilateral carpal tunnel syndrome. They also describe a technique for performing median nerve palmar inching studies with recording over the second lumbrical.

Forearm Motor Nerve Conduction Velocity

In some patients with carpal tunnel syndrome and prolonged median DML, the median forearm MNCV will be mildly slowed (Thomas 1960). Table 7.7 shows the incidence of this finding in selected series. Slowed median forearm MNCV is evidence of more severe median nerve compression in the carpal tunnel. The series with higher incidences of slowing included more patients with severe carpal tunnel syndrome. Patients with decreased amplitude of the thenar CMAP or prolonged median DML are more likely to have slowing of median forearm MNCV (Stoehr et al. 1978; Kimura and Ayyar 1985).

Table 7.7 Incidence of forearm MNCV slowing in carpal tunnel syndrome patients

Reference	%
Buchthal and Rosenfalck 1971	50–65
Thomas et al. 1967	43
Kimura and Ayyar 1985	23
Stevens 1987	11

One hypothesized mechanism of proximal slowing is retrograde axonal atrophy in more severely compressed nerve fibers. In a group of patients with carpal tunnel syndrome and prolonged median DML, the mean amplitude of the mixed nerve action potential recorded at the antecubital space after median nerve stimulation at the wrist was decreased compared with controls (Stoehr et al. 1978). The median sensory nerve conduction velocity (SNCV) in the forearm is also reduced for a group of carpal tunnel syndrome patients compared with controls (Kimura and Ayyar 1985).

Martin-Gruber Anastomosis

The anatomy of the Martin-Gruber anastomosis is discussed in Chapter 1 (Figure 7.4). The fibers participating in the Martin-Gruber anastomosis are components of the median nerve at the level of the antecubital space. These fibers then cross to the ulnar nerve in the forearm, usually via the anterior interosseous nerve. The fibers cross the wrist with the ulnar nerve and may then innervate hypothenar, thenar, or interosseous muscles.

Sun and Streib (1983) searched systematically for the Martin-Gruber anastomosis in 150 arms by comparing the amplitude of the thenar, hypothenar, and first dorsal interosseous CMAPs from median nerve stimulation at the wrist and at the antecubital space. The electrodiagnostic criteria for the anomaly were:

1. a thenar CMAP that was larger with median nerve stimulation at the antecubital space than at the wrist
2. a thenar CMAP that was at least 25% smaller with ulnar stimulation above the elbow compared by ulnar stimulation at the wrist
3. a hypothenar CMAP with initial negative deflection obtained by median stimulation at the antecubital space
4. a first dorsal interosseous CMAP that was at least 25% larger with median stimulation at the antecubital space than with median stimulation at the wrist

Note that application of criterion 2 assumes that there is no coexisting ulnar conduction block between the two stimulating sites. Figure 7.4 shows typical CMAPs obtained over the thenar eminence in a patient with Martin-Gruber anastomosis. Table 7.8 shows the incidence of detection of Martin-Gruber anastomosis at different recording sites (Sun and Streib 1983).

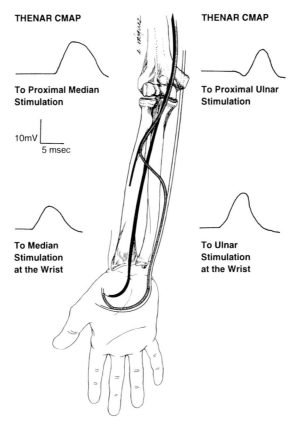

THENAR CMAP

To Proximal Median
Stimulation

10mV | 5 msec

To Median
Stimulation
at the Wrist

THENAR CMAP

To Proximal Ulnar
Stimulation

To Ulnar
Stimulation
at the Wrist

Figure 7.4 Martin-Gruber anastomosis. The CMAPs recorded over the thenar eminence to median and to ulnar nerve stimulation are shown. This patient meets Sun and Streib's (1983) criteria 1 and 2 for presence of the anastomosis.

Even in the absence of Martin-Gruber anastomosis, a volume-conducted response from thenar muscles is routinely recorded over the first dorsal interosseous and the hypothenar eminence after median nerve stimulation. To eliminate the effect of volume-conducted responses, Kimura et al. (1976) used a

Table 7.8 Incidence of Martin-Gruber anastomosis

Muscle Innervated by Anastomotic Fibers	%
Overall	34
First dorsal interosseous	34
Thenar	12
Hypothenar	16

(Data from Sun and Streib 1983.)

collision technique, stimulating the median nerve at the wrist, followed by a paired stimulus in the antecubital space. Using this technique and recording from thenar and hypothenar muscles but not from the first dorsal interosseous, they found a Martin-Gruber anastomosis of 17% of arms.

Patients who have both carpal tunnel syndrome and a Martin-Gruber anastomosis may show distinctive findings on nerve conduction studies. The median latency to thenar muscles after antecubital stimulation may not be prolonged despite prolongation of the DML [Figure 7.5, example *a*] (Iyer and Fenichel 1976). The result may be an erroneously high calculated forearm MNCV. At the extreme, the median DML may be longer than the latency from antecubital stimulation to the thenar CMAP [Figure 7.5, example *b*]. Another variation is a bifid or double-humped thenar CMAP to median nerve stimulation in the antecubital area (Lambert 1962).

When carpal tunnel syndrome and Martin-Gruber anastomosis coexist, the thenar CMAP from median nerve stimulation at the wrist may have an initial negative deflection, whereas the thenar CMAP from median nerve stimulation at the antecubital space has an initial positive deflection [Figure 7.5, example *c*)] (Gutmann 1977). The positive deflection is explained by volume-conducted

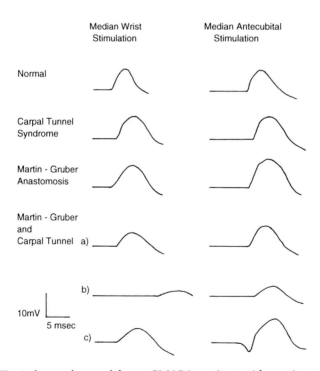

Figure 7.5 Typical wave forms of thenar CMAP in patients with coexistent carpal tunnel syndrome and Martin-Gruber anastomosis. The stimulation sites are shown in Figure 7.4.

potentials from thenar or first dorsal interosseous muscles that are innervated via fibers in the median nerve at the antecubital space, then cross with the anastomosis, and enter the hand in the ulnar nerve. Fibers that cross in the anastomosis do not go through the carpal tunnel, and conduction in these fibers is not slowed in carpal tunnel syndrome. This finding may be present even when median DML and transcarpal sensory conduction are normal (Gutmann et al. 1986).

Threshold Distal Motor Latency

Preswick (1963) proposed measuring conduction in other than the fastest median motor fibers. He recorded in the abductor pollicis brevis with a needle electrode while stimulating the median nerve at the wrist. Rather than using supramaximal nerve stimulation, he gradually increased stimulus intensity until the first motor unit was recorded. He then measured latency to onset of this potential. In 25 control subjects, this latency, the "threshold distal motor latency," was shorter than or equal to 5.2 msec. Preswick studied 29 hands in which carpal tunnel syndrome was clinically suspected. Of these, 83% had a prolonged threshold DML, but only 38% had a prolonged supramaximal DML. Loong (1977), using surface recording electrodes, found that 52% of patients with a clinical diagnosis of carpal tunnel syndrome had prolonged median threshold DML, whereas only 35% had a prolonged supramaximal DML.

In vitro, the largest myelinated fibers have the lowest threshold to electrical stimulation, so that threshold conduction velocity is equal to supramaximal conduction velocity. In contrast, in human median nerve motor conduction studies, stimulating at the wrist, the supramaximal DML and threshold DML are unequal (Preswick 1963). This inequality implies that topographic factors, such as the proximity of fibers to the stimulating electrode, influence the selection of fibers responding to threshold stimulus.

Some patients with carpal tunnel syndrome have a larger-than-normal range between threshold stimulation voltage (i.e., voltage of the stimulator, not CMAP amplitude) and the maximal stimulation voltage (Brismar 1985). This is not a useful diagnostic test for carpal tunnel syndrome (1) because of low sensitivity and (2) because the effect is also observed in neuropathies such as those caused by diabetes or uremia (Brismar 1985).

F-Wave Studies

The F wave is a late response recorded in muscle following mixed nerve stimulation. It can be recorded in the median-innervated thenar muscles following median nerve stimulation. The nerve stimulation is performed with the cathode proximal to the anode—the reverse of the normal electrode orientation used for routine nerve conduction studies. A nerve stimulus does not always evoke an F response. Moreover, the nerve stimulus evokes an F response in only a fraction of the stimulated motor neurons; therefore, the amplitude of the F wave is only a fraction of the amplitude of the CMAP from supramaximal stimulation. The configuration and latency of the F wave vary from stimulus to stimulus. Multiple stimuli are needed to evaluate the range of F-wave responses from an individual nerve. Most studies measure the minimum F-wave latency, but some authors favor use of the mean F-wave latency in diagnosis of carpal tunnel syndrome (Reiners et al. 1984).

In some patients with carpal tunnel syndrome and prolonged median DML, the minimum F-wave latency from the wrist is proportionately prolonged (Eisen et al. 1977). In other patients, the DML is prolonged out of proportion to the F-wave latency (Kimura 1983). Table 7.9 shows representative data.

In carpal tunnel syndrome patients who have normal motor and sensory conduction studies, median minimum F latency to thenar muscles is sometimes abnormal by virtue of being prolonged over 2.0 msec in comparison to the ulnar minimum F latency to abductor digiti minimi (Egloff-Baer et al. 1980). A prolonged median F-wave latency with a normal median DML does not distinguish between carpal tunnel syndrome and a proximal median neuropathy or brachial plexopathy. Nerves in addition to the median must be studied since a prolonged F latency can also be seen in peripheral neuropathies.

Another way to use the F wave to evaluate conduction through the carpal tunnel is to compare the median minimum F-wave latency with palmar stimulation to the median minimum F-wave latency with wrist stimulation. In one series, the difference between these two latencies was abnormal in 64% of patients with carpal tunnel syndrome, including some cases with normal median DML and distal sensory latency (DSL) (Maccabee et al. 1980).

Macleod (1987) recorded 100 consecutive F waves in the thenar muscles evoked by stimulation of an individual median nerve. He defined a repeater F wave (RF) as an F wave that was identical in configuration, amplitude, and latency to the F wave elicited by the preceding stimulus (Figure 7.6). He calculated the ratio of RF responses to total elicited F waves to obtain a percent repeater F wave (%RF) value. In 90% of controls, the %RF was less than 37; in 84% of carpal tunnel syndrome patients, the %RF was greater than 37. In patients with carpal tunnel syndrome, the %RF may be abnormal when the DML and palm-to-wrist sensory latency are normal. The %RF may also be abnormal in other disorders of the alpha motor neuron.

Table 7.9 Median nerve F-wave latency in patients with carpal tunnel syndrome

| | Median DML (msec) | | Minimum F-latency (wrist) (msec) | |
	Mean	S.D.	Mean	S.D.
Controls	3.4	0.4	26.6	2.2
Carpal tunnel syndrome patients	5.4	1.2	30.8	3.3

(Data from Eisen et al. 1977.)

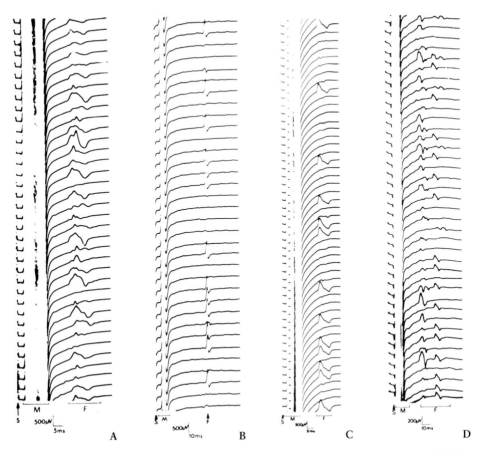

Figure 7.6 **A**, F-wave sweeps from a healthy median nerve. Two F waves recur; %RF value = 12%. **B–D**, Median nerve F-wave sweeps from patients with carpal tunnel syndrome. **B**, RF follows the majority of supramaximal stimuli at a delayed latency. **C**, Two RFs predominate. **D**, RFs firing "in series." Two individual RFs repeatedly follow the initial F response. (Reproduced with permission of the author and the publisher, from Macleod WN. Repeater F waves: a comparison of sensitivity with sensory antidromic wrist-to-palm latency and distal motor latency in the diagnosis of carpal tunnel syndrome. Neurology 1987;37:773–78.)

SENSORY NERVE CONDUCTION STUDIES
Technique

Median nerve sensory conduction can be assessed by a number of different techniques (Ma and Liveson 1983). Figure 7.7 illustrates typical electrode placement. The technical details of papers on sensory conduction must be read carefully. Variations of technique between laboratories often make it difficult to compare the results of one study with those of another.

For median sensory antidromic stimulation, the nerve is stimulated at the wrist or palm while recording with ring electrodes on any of the first four digits.

For median sensory orthodromic stimulation, the nerve is stimulated on a median-innervated digit or at the palm. The recording electrodes are placed over the median nerve at the wrist or more proximally along its course, such as in the antecubital fossa or in the axilla. Some examiners use needle rather than surface electrodes for stimulation or recording (Johnson and Melvin 1967; Buchthal and Rosenfalck 1971). Latency to negative peak varies with distance between recording electrodes. By changing the positions of the recording electrodes, slight differences can be detected between orthodromic and antidromic latencies (Murai and Sanderson 1975). Whether orthodromic or antidromic approaches are used has little practical effect on normal or pathologic values (Ludin et al. 1977; Goddard et al. 1983).

To assess conduction velocity in the fastest myelinated sensory fibers, the latency is measured to onset of the SNAP. The SNAP amplitude is measured in microvolts (μV), and an averager is often needed to obtain accurately measurable latencies and amplitudes. Many examiners measure latency to initial positive peak or initial negative peak rather than to onset of SNAP; this decreases measurement error, but a conduction velocity calculated from peak latency will

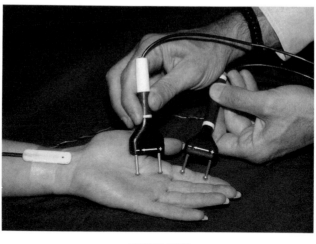

MEDIAN SNAP
at Wrist

Stimulate Index Finger   Stimulate Palm

20μV

2 msec

Figure 7.7 Typical electrode placement for measuring sensory nerve conduction between the wrist and index finger. The example shown is an orthodromic study with the stimulating electrodes on the index finger and in the palm and the recording electrode over the wrist.

not reflect the velocity of the fastest fibers. Calculations can use latency data obtained with a constant distance between stimulating and recording electrodes; alternatively, conduction velocity can be calculated from distance and latency measurements.

Some examiners measure SNAP amplitude from negative peak to positive peak; others measure from baseline to negative peak. Amplitudes are greater with antidromic than with orthodromic stimulation and greater with needle than with surface recording electrodes. Amplitude, duration, and configuration will depend on the distance between the recording electrodes (Gilliatt et al. 1965).

Di Benedetto et al. (1986) emphasize that the upper limit of normal for median DSL can be decreased, and the diagnostic sensitivity can be increased, with attention to details such as temperature control and careful distance measurement. Table 7.10 shows examples of normal limits for median sensory nerve conduction studies.

Finger-to-Wrist Conduction

In patients with carpal tunnel syndrome, median sensory conduction studies are more likely to be abnormal than median DML (Kopell and Goodgold 1968). Thomas et al. (1967) found that 85% of their carpal tunnel syndrome patients had sensory conduction abnormalities. They did not use an averager, and the most common abnormality was an unobtainable or undiscernible SNAP. Melvin et al. (1973) found a prolonged latency from wrist to index finger in 88% of their 17 carpal tunnel syndrome patients. In contrast, only 76% of their patients had a prolonged median DML, and only 6% had an abnormally low SNAP amplitude.

Transcarpal Conduction

Sensory conduction time in the segment of the median nerve in the carpal tunnel can be assessed by stimulating at the wrist and at the midpalm while recording the SNAP from a digit. The transcarpal sensory conduction time is the difference between the two measured latencies (Wiederholt 1970). Transcarpal nerve conduction can also be studied by stimulating the median nerve in the palm and recording over the nerve at the wrist or more proximally (Eklund 1975; Mills 1985). In this technique, both motor and sensory fibers are stimulated, and a

Table 7.10 Median sensory nerve conduction: examples of normal values

Source	Technique	Normal Limits
Gilliatt and Sears (1958)	Orthodromic digit II	Peak latency ≤4.0 msec Amplitude ≥9 μV
Mayo Clinic Stevens (1987)	Antidromic digit II	Peak latency ≤3.5 msec Amplitude ≥25 μV

mixed nerve action potential is recorded. Both techniques give similar latency values (Tackmann et al. 1981; Monga et al. 1985). In normal subjects the median SNCV between digit and palm and between palm and wrist is the same (Buchthal and Rosenfalck 1971).

In carpal tunnel syndrome patients, conduction in the palm-to-wrist segment of the median nerve is often disproportionately slowed; these patients may have normal digit-to-wrist conduction but abnormally slow palm-to-wrist conduction (Buchthal and Rosenfalck 1971).

In some patients with carpal tunnel syndrome, the SNCV is slowed in both the digit-to-palm and palm-to-wrist segment of the nerve. Patients with diffuse peripheral neuropathies, such as diabetic neuropathy, may also have slowing of both digit-to-palm and palm-to-wrist conduction (Casey and Le-Quesne 1972).

Variability of Digital Nerves

In most cases of carpal tunnel syndrome, sensory fibers in all median digital nerves are affected. This can be demonstrated by measuring conduction to each digit separately from the wrist or by calculating a transcarpal SNCV for each digit. Table 7.11 shows data from an antidromic study (Toyonaga and DeFaria 1978). Note that the index finger is slightly less likely to show abnormal values.

Cioni et al. (1989), using ring electrodes for orthodromic sensory studies, also found that index finger-to-wrist SNCV was less likely than middle finger-to-wrist SNCV to be abnormal in carpal tunnel syndrome patients. The ring finger-to-wrist median SNAP was the most likely to be absent.

When ring electrodes are used for orthodromic sensory studies, both digital nerves in a digit are stimulated. Macdonell et al. (1990) used a pair of stimulating electrodes held against the lateral or medial side of the digit in an effort to stimulate individual digital nerves. They recorded with surface electrodes at the wrist. In hands of women with a clinical diagnosis of carpal tunnel syndrome, abnormalities varied in frequency from one digital nerve to the next, as shown in Figure 7.8. This data is from 29 dominant hands; similar findings were recorded

Table 7.11 Variation in SNCV results by finger tested in 30 patients with carpal tunnel syndrome

Result	Thumb	Index	Middle	Ring
Unobtainable	2	1	0	3
Wrist-to-digit slow	18	16	21	21
Palm-to-wrist slow (wrist-digit normal)	7	9	8	4
Normal	3	4	1	2

(Data from Toyonaga and DeFaria 1978.)

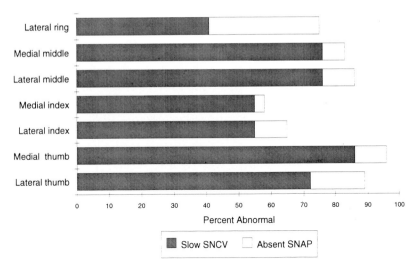

Figure 7.8 The results of digital nerve stimulation in patients with carpal tunnel syndrome. The site of stimulation is shown at the *left*; recordings were made at the wrist. (Data from Macdonell et al. 1990.)

in nondominant hands. Again, the index finger was least likely to yield abnormal results. The SNAP from the ring finger was most often absent, perhaps because of ulnar nerve supply of this digital nerve in some patients or perhaps because in the other digits volume-conducted stimulation of the adjoining digital nerve was more likely to give a higher-amplitude SNAP.

Palmar Serial Sensory Studies

Kimura (1979) standardized a technique for studying conduction in the median nerve, centimeter by centimeter. He used ring recording electrodes on the index finger and stimulated the nerve at 1-cm intervals along the distal forearm and palm. He measured latency to onset of negative deflection and subtracted successive latencies to obtain a latency difference for each centimeter of the nerve. In controls, the mean latency difference was 0.2 msec/cm. The latency differences for the portions of the nerve under the carpal ligament, 1 to 4 cm distal to the distal wrist crease, were slightly greater than for the adjacent distal and proximal segments of the nerve. For example, the mean latency difference was 0.22 msec for the segment 3 to 4 cm past the distal wrist crease and 0.17 msec for the segment 4 to 5 cm past the distal wrist crease.

About one half of patients with carpal tunnel syndrome showed slowing of sensory conduction distributed fairly evenly along the palm-to-wrist portion of the nerve; the other one half of patients showed localized conduction delay in one segment. Kimura used delay of *greater* than 0.5 msec over 1 cm as abnormal. In 4 of 172 hands with symptoms of carpal tunnel syndrome, he found a delayed conduction latency difference over 1 cm even though wrist-to-palm latencies were normal.

Other authors have proposed increasing the diagnostic sensitivity of serial palmar sensory studies by using a latency difference over 1 cm of greater than or equal to 0.4 msec as abnormal. For example, Seror (1988) found this measure abnormal in each of 45 cases of carpal tunnel syndrome and initially thought this criterion could "suppress" false negatives; later, Seror (1990) found cases with typical carpal tunnel syndrome symptoms but no abnormality on palmar median serial sensory latency studies.

Nathan et al. (1988b) studied segmental sensory latency values over 1 cm in 70 hands of 38 controls without clinical suggestion of carpal tunnel syndrome and in 54 hands with carpal tunnel syndrome. Using criteria for carpal tunnel syndrome that relied heavily on classical clinical history, they found that the maximum segmental latency difference (MLD) was greater than or equal to 0.4 msec in 81% and greater than or equal to 0.5 msec in 54% of hands with carpal tunnel syndrome.

Ipsilateral Comparison Methods

Comparing conduction in the median nerve to conduction in ipsilateral radial or ulnar nerves minimizes confounding personal factors—such as age and temperature—that decrease diagnostic sensitivity by increasing the variation in normals.

Median-Ulnar Comparison

When median wrist-to-index finger and ulnar wrist-to-little finger sensory latencies are obtained over identical distances in the same hand, they are normally within 0.4 msec of each other (Felsenthal 1977). When median wrist-to-ring finger and ulnar wrist-to-ring finger sensory latencies are compared over 14 cm in the same normal hand, the difference in latencies is 0.3 msec or less (Johnson et al. 1981). One disadvantage of using the ring finger for studies is the lower amplitude of the ring finger SNAP for either nerve compared with the amplitudes from other digits. Another disadvantage is the possibility of anomalous sensory patterns so that ring finger innervation might be solely median or solely ulnar (Monga and Laidlow 1982). Felsenthal (1978a) studied 82 hands with carpal tunnel syndrome and found that 17 had a prolonged median minus ulnar latency difference even though the median wrist-to-index finger sensory latency was normal. Uncini et al. (1989, 1990) also found that comparing ulnar and median nerve responses to ring finger stimulation was a sensitive test for carpal tunnel syndrome.

In some series, patients with carpal tunnel syndrome were more likely than controls to show abnormalities of ulnar nerve conduction. Sedal et al. (1973) found low-amplitude ulnar SNAPs in 39% and delayed ulnar DSL in 5% of hands that had both clinical and nerve conduction evidence of carpal tunnel syndrome. Patients with generalized peripheral neuropathy or illness such as diabetes that might predispose to neuropathy were excluded. Harrison (1978) disagreed, finding normal ulnar SNAP amplitude in 60 consecutive patients with carpal tunnel syndrome. Cassvan et al. (1986) found an ulnar DSL equal to or greater than 3.7 msec in 46% of patients with carpal tunnel syndrome. Mortier et al. (1988) found a prolonged ulnar DML in 18% of patients with carpal tunnel syndrome. The mechanism underlying these ulnar nerve conduction abnormalities may vary from patient to patient. If ulnar abnormalities are present, they may decrease the sensitivity of median-ulnar comparison methods.

Median-Radial Comparison

With stimulation of the thumb, a SNAP can be recorded over the median nerve at the wrist or over the superficial radial nerve as it crosses the extensor pollicis longus tendon to course along the lateral aspect of the radius (Figure 7.9). For comparison, the distance for the two nerves from the stimulating to the recording electrodes should be the same (Carroll 1987). Alternatively, ring recording electrodes can be placed on the thumb at the metacarpal-phalangeal and interphalangeal joints, and the median or radial nerves may be stimulated 10 cm proximally (Johnson et al. 1987). Measured orthodromically or antidromically, the difference between the sensory latencies of the two nerves normally should be less than 0.5 msec (Carroll 1987; Johnson et al. 1987).

Carroll (1987) found that 49% of 161 patients with a clinical diagnosis of carpal tunnel syndrome had abnormal thumb-to-wrist median sensory latencies. An additional 21% of patients showed abnormal median nerve conduction demonstrated by a prolonged median-radial sensory latency difference. Pease et al. (1989) and Cassvan et al. (1988) also noted high sensitivity for median-radial comparisons.

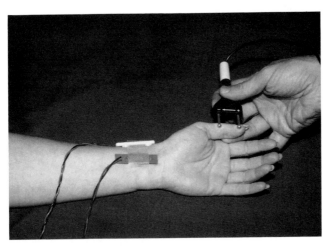

Figure 7.9 Typical electrode placement for comparing orthodromic nerve conduction in the radial and median nerves between the thumb and the wrist.

Sensory Nerve Action Potential Amplitude Comparisons

The median SNAP amplitude, whether antidromically or orthodromically determined, is normal in most patients with carpal tunnel syndrome. Diagnostic sensitivity can be increased by comparing it to the ulnar SNAP amplitude. For example, Table 7.12 shows the results of Loong and Seah (1971, 1972) using surface electrodes and the orthodromic technique.

Of their 23 patients with carpal tunnel syndrome, only 37% had a subnormal median SNAP amplitude, but 91% had a median-ulnar SNAP amplitude ratio below the normal range. In four of the patients, the digit-to-wrist median sensory latency was normal, but the median-ulnar SNAP amplitude ratio was abnormal.

Felsenthal (1978a) extended this approach to antidromic studies, comparing SNAP amplitudes in the index finger from median wrist stimulation and in the ring finger from ulnar wrist stimulation. He found that the normal range of ratios of median to ulnar SNAP amplitudes was from 0.67 to 2.0. A ratio less than 0.67 was more sensitive than median SNAP amplitude alone in identifying carpal tunnel syndrome patients.

**Hand to Forearm Sensory Nerve Conduction
Velocity Comparison**

Kimura and Ayyar (1985) calculated median sensory conduction velocity from wrist to index finger and from antecubital space to wrist, based on latencies to negative peak. They found that in patients with carpal tunnel syndrome, but never in controls, the ratio of hand SNCV to forearm SNCV was always less than 0.75. This ratio was abnormal even in carpal tunnel syndrome patients with normal DSLs and SNCVs.

Provocative Tests

Marin et al. (1983) tested median DML and DSL with the wrist in neutral position and after 5 and 10 minutes of sustained maximum wrist flexion or extension. In normal controls, the DML and DSL increased slightly with this

Table 7.12 Ratio of median to ulnar SNAP amplitude in controls and patients with carpal tunnel syndrome

	Median SNAP Amplitude (μV)		Ratio of Median to Ulnar Amplitude	
	Mean	*Range*	*Mean*	*Range*
Controls	28.6	9–48	1.5	1.1–2.4
Carpal tunnel syndrome patients		0–18		0.4–1.3

(Data from Loong and Seah 1971, 1972.)

procedure; for example, the mean DML increased by 0.13 msec after 10 minutes of wrist extension. Smaller changes in mean DML were noted with wrist flexion or with briefer wrist extension. In patients with carpal tunnel syndrome, the changes in DML were often greater. Of five patients with normal DML and DSL in the neutral position, three developed prolonged DSL after five minutes of sustained wrist flexion or extension.

Two other papers reported median DML and DSL after two minutes of wrist flexion (Schwartz et al. 1980; White et al. 1988). In some patients with carpal tunnel syndrome, DML may increase 0.2 msec or more with this test. On rare occasions, median DML after wrist flexion will be abnormal when DML and DSL with the wrist in the neutral position are normal.

Minimum Sensory Nerve Conduction Velocity

Buchthal et al. (1974) used near-nerve needle recording electrodes and averaged the responses to between 500 and 1,000 stimuli. They measured the latencies to the last peak distinguishable from noise to calculate a minimum detectable SNCV. In normals, the mean minimum SNCV was 16 M/sec with lower limits of normal of 12 M/sec. The amplitude of the slowest component was 0.05 to 0.1 μV.

In patients with carpal tunnel syndrome, the SNAP often showed temporal dispersion over as long as 30 msec. Fibers conducting at 16 M/sec created a potential of 0.2 to 3 μV—much higher than the amplitude from the slowest fibers in normal nerve.

Minimum SNCV is less sensitive than maximum SNCV in diagnosis of carpal tunnel syndrome. Of 11 patients with carpal tunnel and abnormal median maximum SNCV or SNAP amplitude, only 3 had reduced median minimum SNCV (Shefner et al. 1991).

The duration of the SNAP is a measure of temporal dispersion between conduction in fastest and slower fibers. The value measured for duration is very dependent on technical factors such as filter and gain settings, surface versus needle electrodes, and whether an averager is used. Using surface electrodes for antidromic recording without an averager, Bhala and Thoppil (1981) found a prolonged SNAP duration in 64% of their carpal tunnel patients.

Repetitive Sensory Stimulation

Repetitive sensory stimulation is another technique that increases diagnostic sensitivity in patients with carpal tunnel syndrome. Lehmann and Tackmann (1974) studied the response of median sensory fibers to trains of stimuli. They stimulated the index finger with ring electrodes and recorded from the median nerve at the wrist with needle electrodes. They stimulated the nerve with trains of stimuli at 100 to 500 Hz, compared the latencies and amplitudes of the first and tenth responses, and found differences in the responses of normal and carpal tunnel syndrome subjects. Table 7.13 gives representative data from 500-Hz stimulation.

Lehmann and Tackmann also found an increase in latency of the tenth response, compared with the first. For example, at 200 Hz the mean latency of the tenth response in carpal tunnel syndrome patients was 109% of the latency of the first response, but no prolongation of mean latency was noted in control patients. For both latency and amplitude comparisons, the abnormalities were noted at 100-Hz stimulation, and differences between controls and patients increased as stimulation frequency increased to 500 Hz.

All patients with clinical history suggesting carpal tunnel syndrome had abnormal responses to trains of stimuli, even though 5 of 24 patients with carpal tunnel syndrome had normal routine DML and DSL. Tackmann and Lehmann (1974) also compared responses to paired stimuli spaced 1.0 to 50 msec apart and found abnormal "Relative refractory period of median sensory fibers in the carpal tunnel syndrome."

Gilliatt and Meer (1990) studied the refractory period of transmission by stimulating the median nerve at the wrist with paired stimuli at intervals of 0.8 to 1.0 msec. They recorded nerve action potentials over the index or middle fingers and over the median nerve at the antecubital space. Controls always showed transmission of paired responses at both the distal and proximal recording sites. Eleven of 14 patients with carpal tunnel syndrome showed an impaired or absent response to the second stimulus at the distal recording site. Two of these patients had normal transcarpal SNCVs. Gilliatt and Meer discussed the possibility that refractory period of transmission might normalize following remyelination even if SNCV remained abnormal.

PERSONAL FACTORS AFFECTING NERVE CONDUCTION
Temperature

Median motor and sensory latencies increase, and SNAP amplitudes decrease, as limb temperature increases (Buchthal and Rosenfalck 1966; Bolton et al. 1981). For example, Halar et al. (1983) measured wrist skin temperature and found that median DSL or DML increased 0.2 msec for each degree Celsius decrease in temperature. In the forearm, median MNCV decreased 1.5 M/sec and median SNCV decreased 1.4 M/sec for each degree Celsius decrease in temperature.

Table 7.13 Repetitive index finger stimulation* amplitude ratio of tenth to first SNAP

	Mean	Range
Controls	0.70	0.50–0.89
Hands with carpal tunnel syndrome	0.31	0.19–0.40

*500 Hz. (Data from Lehmann and Tackmann 1974.)

Table 7.14 Effect of age on median nerve conduction

	Decade of Age						
	Third	Fourth	Fifth	Sixth	Seventh	Eighth	Ninth
Mean SNAP amplitude (μV)	55	47	44	36	36	18	23
Mean DSL (msec)	3.15	3.19	3.43	3.67	3.82	3.96	4.08
Mean DML (msec)	3.45	3.44	3.71	3.81	3.91	3.77	3.98

(Data from LaFratta and Canestrari 1966, and LaFratta, 1972.)

A pathologic nerve may respond to temperature changes differently than a normal nerve. In one study, patients with carpal tunnel syndrome did not display the same relation of median SNCV to temperature change that had been found in normal median nerves (Fine and Wongjirad 1985).

Age

In normals median nerve conduction velocity falls with increasing age. The amplitude of the median SNAP decreases, the DML and DSL increase, and MNCV and SNCV decrease with age. For example, Table 7.14 and Figure 7.10 show data from LaFratta (LaFratta and Canestrari 1966; LaFratta 1972) obtained using surface electrodes, stimulating at the wrist, and recording at the index finger for sensory studies and at the thenar eminence for motor studies.

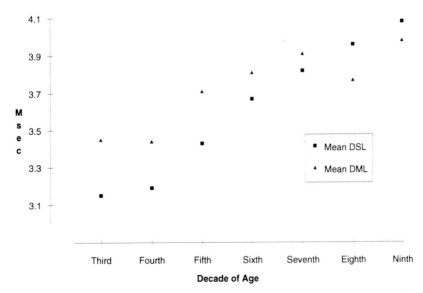

Figure 7.10 Effect of age on DSL and DML. (Data from LaFratta 1972, 1978b.)

Kraft and Halvorson (1983) found that RML did not increase with age, whereas DML did.

The slowing of nerve conduction with age is more marked in the portion of the median nerve in the carpal tunnel than in the digital nerves or in the palmar portion of the ulnar nerve. Cruz Martínez et al. (1978a) measured orthodromic SNCV in median and ulnar nerves in an asymptomatic population. They compared digit-to-palm and palm-to-wrist SNCV in both nerves. In all segments, the mean SNCV was lower in subjects over 50 years old than in younger subjects. The drop in SNCV with age was most marked in the palm-to-wrist segment of the median nerve. Regardless of age, the ulnar palm-to-wrist SNCV remained faster than the ulnar digit-to-palm SNCV. In contrast, in the group over age 50, the median palm-to-wrist SNCV fell slightly below the median digit-to-palm SNCV. The median transcarpal MLD also increases with age (Nathan et al. 1988a).

The decrease in SNAP amplitude with age, using finger stimulation and recording at the wrist, is greater in median-innervated digits than in ulnar-innervated digits. Table 7.15 shows representative data (Cruz Martínez et al. 1978b). This may be important if the SNAP amplitude ratio is used as a diagnostic test.

Gender

The mean median thenar CMAP amplitude was slightly smaller in a group of normal women (15.0 mV) than in a group of normal men (17.1 mV); the mean antidromic median SNAP amplitude recorded at the index finger with ring electrodes after wrist stimulation was higher in a group of normal women (62.1 μV) than in a group of normal men (45.3 μV) (Felsenthal 1978b). The standard deviations for both CMAP amplitude and SNAP amplitude are large, so there is a large overlap in amplitudes comparing individual men and women.

Handedness

Mean median DSL and DML do not vary with handedness in groups of normals (Felsenthal 1978b). The amplitudes of the median thenar CMAP and antidromic SNAP recorded with surface electrodes at the index finger are slightly smaller in the right than in the left hand of asymptomatic right handers (Felsen-

Table 7.15 Effect of age on SNAP amplitude

| Age (years) | SNAP Amplitude (μV) | | |
	Middle	Little	Ratio
≤30	22.2	11.5	1.93
31–49	18.0	11.0	1.64
≥50	12.0	7.5	1.60

(Data from Cruz Martinez et al. 1978b.)

thal 1978b). The amplitude differences might reflect differences in hand callosity. The opposite effect on SNAP amplitude is reported with orthodromic stimulation (Cruz Martínez et al. 1978b).

Hand Position

The median nerve slides with wrist motion so that the length of nerve between surface stimulating and recording electrodes will vary unless wrist position is kept constant from test to test (Gordan 1977).

Height

Normal median DML increases with the height of the subject. Rivner et al. (1990) found that each centimeter of height added 0.0156 msec to the normal DML but that height had no significant correlation with median forearm MNCV.

NEEDLE ELECTROMYOGRAPHY

Electromyographic (EMG) examination of thenar muscles is normal in most patients with carpal tunnel syndrome. The early Mayo Clinic series found fibrillations in 44% of patients (Thomas et al. 1967). Fasciculations were found in about 12% of patients.

The series from Buchthal et al. (1974) examined patients whose carpal tunnel syndrome was often clinically severe; half of the patients had wasting or severe weakness of abductor pollicis brevis. As expected, the patients in the series had a high incidence of EMG abnormalities in abductor pollicis brevis: Only one third of patients had a full interference pattern; the mean motor unit potential duration was prolonged in one half the patients; one half the patients had fibrillations or positive sharp waves. The probability of finding an EMG abnormality increased, as median DML increased.

The later Mayo series covering 1961 to 1980 found fibrillations in only 18% of patients (Stevens 1987). Decreased recruitment or abnormal motor units were present in 41% of patients. As shown in Table 7.16, Kimura and Ayyar

Table 7.16 EMG abnormalities in abductor pollicis brevis in 585 hands with carpal tunnel syndrome (in %)

	Fibrillations Sharp Waves	Fascicu- lations	Decreased Recruitment	Increased Polyphasics
Total (585 hands)	22	6	31	18
DML <4.7 msec (279 hands)	13	3	19	10
DML ≥7.7 msec (37 hands)	46	14	60	43

(Data from Kimura and Ayyar 1985.)

(1985) found a similar incidence of electromyographic abnormalities in 585 abductor pollicis brevis muscles of patients with carpal tunnel syndrome and confirmed that electromyographic abnormalities were more common in patients with prolonged median DML.

Repetitive Nerve Fiber Discharge

Simpson (1958) used a needle electrode in the abductor pollicis brevis for his pioneering motor nerve conduction studies. In patients with carpal tunnel syndrome, he noted occasional repetitive firing of individual motor units, particularly of the unit elicited by threshold stimulation.

By EMG, Spaans (1982) found spontaneous rhythmic firing of motor unit potentials in the thenar muscles in 8% of hands with carpal tunnel syndrome (Figure 7.11). Single-fiber EMG supported the hypothesis that these rhythmic discharges originated in the motor axon rather than in muscle fibers. The spontaneously discharging motor units were found in mild or severe cases of carpal tunnel syndrome; in contrast, fibrillations and positive sharp waves were much more common in severe cases. When spontaneously discharging motor units were present, they became more abundant after one or two minutes of forearm ischemia. They were not abolished by local anesthetic block of the median nerve in the antecubital space. Other authors have not reported a similar incidence of spontaneous motor unit potential firing; for example, Kimura and Ayyar (1985) found myokymia in the abductor pollicis brevis only four times out of 585 muscles tested. Another example of compression-induced irritability of median nerve motor fibers is that median nerve stimulation with a linearly rising current evokes repetitive firing in the abductor pollicis brevis more easily in patients with carpal tunnel syndrome than in controls (Simpson and Thomaides 1988).

Electromyography and Differential Diagnosis

The EMG is particularly important in searching for other neuropathic conditions that might mimic or coexist with carpal tunnel syndrome. When EMG

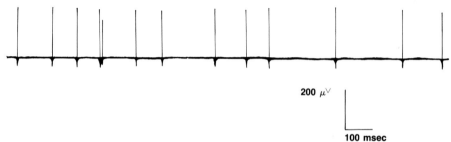

200 $\mu^\vee$

100 msec

Figure 7.11 In this patient with carpal tunnel syndrome, EMG done with a needle electrode in the abductor pollicis brevis shows spontaneous rhythmic firing at rest; there were no fibrillations or changes in configuration of voluntary motor units. Median sensory latencies were abnormal. Median DML was normal. (Courtesy of Dr. Patrick Radecki.)

examination of abductor pollicis brevis is abnormal or when otherwise clinically indicated, the EMG should be extended to more proximal median-innervated muscles, ulnar-innervated muscles, and additional muscles as needed to search for mononeuritis multiplex, brachial plexopathy, or cervical radiculopathy.

SOMATOSENSORY EVOKED POTENTIALS

Somatosensory evoked potentials (SSEPs) recorded over the contralateral cerebral cortex to median nerve stimulation of the index finger are sometimes abnormal in carpal tunnel syndrome patients (Constantinovici 1989). In these patients, comparison of latencies measured over the contralateral scalp to stimulation at the wrist and at the index finger can demonstrate distal slowing, and the cerebral SSEP can sometimes be obtained when a SNAP is unobtainable (Desmedt et al. 1966).

Cortical somatosensory potentials evoked by painful stimuli to the middle finger using argon laser stimulation may also be abnormal in patients with carpal tunnel syndrome (Arendt-Nielsen et al. 1991). This is unlikely to be a sensitive diagnostic test for carpal tunnel syndrome because of the relative resistance of pain fibers to compression.

REFERENCES

Aminoff MJ. Electromyography in clinical practice: electrodiagnostic aspects of neuro-muscular disease. 2nd ed. New York: Churchill Livingstone, 1987.

Arendt-Nielsen L, Gregersen H, Toft E, Bjerring P. Involvement of thin afferents in carpal tunnel syndrome: evaluated quantitatively by argon laser stimulation. Muscle Nerve 1991;14:508–14.

Bhala RP, Thoppil E. Early detection of carpal tunnel syndrome by sensory nerve conduction. Electromyogr Clin Neurophysiol 1981;21:155–64.

Bolton CF, Sawa GM, Carter K. The effects of temperature on human compound action potentials. J Neurol Neurosurg Psychiatry 1981;44:407–13.

Brismar T. Changes in electrical threshold in human peripheral neuropathy. J Neurol Sci 1985;68:215–23.

Buchthal F, Rosenfalck A. Evoked action potentials and conduction velocity in human sensory nerves. Brain Res 1966;3:1–122.

Buchthal F, Rosenfalck A. Sensory conduction from digit to palm and from palm to wrist in the carpal tunnel syndrome. J Neurol Neurosurg Psychiatry 1971;34:243–52.

Buchthal F, Rosenfalck A, Trojaborg W. Electrophysiological findings in entrapment of the median nerve at wrist and elbow. J Neurol Neurosurg Psychiatry 1974;37:340–60.

Carroll GJ. Comparison of median and radial nerve sensory latencies in the electro-physiological diagnosis of carpal tunnel syndrome. Electroencephalogr Clin Neurophysiol 1987;68:101–6.

Casey EB, Le-Quesne PM. Digital nerve action potentials in healthy subjects, and in carpal tunnel and diabetic patients. J Neurol Neurosurg Psychiatry 1972;35:612–23.

Cassvan A, Ralescu S, Shapiro E, Moshkovski FG, Weiss J. Median and radial sensory latencies to digit I as compared with other screening tests in carpal tunnel syndrome. Am J Phys Med Rehabil 1988;67:221–24.

Cassvan A, Rosenberg A, Rivera LF. Ulnar nerve involvement in carpal tunnel syndrome. Arch Phys Med Rehabil 1986;67:290–92.

Cioni R, Passero S, Paradiso C, Giannini F, Battistini N, Rushworth G. Diagnostic specificity of sensory and motor nerve conduction variables in early detection of carpal tunnel syndrome. J Neurol 1989;236:208–13.

Constantinovici A. The diagnostic value of somatosensory evoked potentials in the diseases of peripheral nervous system. Neurol Psychiatr (Bucur) 1989;27:111–25.

Cruz Martínez A, Barrio M, Pérez Conde MC, Gutiérrez AM. Electrophysiological aspects of sensory conduction velocity in healthy adults. 1. Conduction velocity from digit to palm, from palm to wrist, and across the elbow as a function of age. J Neurol Neurosurg Psychiatry 1978a;41:1092–96.

Cruz Martínez A, Barrio M, Pérez Conde MC, Ferrer MT. Electrophysiological aspects of sensory conduction velocity in healthy adults. 2. Ratio between the amplitude of sensory evoked potentials at the wrist on stimulating different fingers in both hands. J Neurol Neurosurg Psychiatry 1978b;41:1097–1101.

Cruz Martinez A, Perez Conde MC, Ferrer MT. Effect of ischaemia on sensory evoked potentials. 2. Study in patients with diabetes mellitus, alcoholism, chronic renal failure, carpal tunnel syndrome and hyperparathyroidism. Electromyogr Clin Neurophysiol 1980;20:193–203.

Desmedt JE, Manil J, Borenstein S, Debecker J, Lambert C, Franken L, Danis A. Evaluation of sensory nerve conduction from averaged cerebral evoked potentials in neuropathies. Electromyography 1966;6:263–69.

Di Benedetto M, Mitz M, Klingbeil GE, Davidoff D. New criteria for sensory nerve conduction especially useful in diagnosing carpal tunnel syndrome. Arch Phys Med Rehabil 1986;67:586–89.

Duncan KH, Lewis RC Jr, Foreman KA, Nordyke MD. Treatment of carpal tunnel syndrome by members of the American Society for Surgery of the Hand: results of a questionnaire. J Hand Surg 1987;12A:384–91.

Egloff-Baer S, Shahani BT, Young RR. Usefulness of late response studies in diagnosis of entrapment neuropathies. Electroencephalogr Clin Neurophysiol 1980;45:16P.

Eisen A, Schomer D, Melmed C. The application of F-wave measurements in the differentiation of proximal and distal upper limb entrapments. Neurology 1977;27:662–68.

Eklund G. A new electrodiagnostic procedure for measuring sensory nerve conduction across the carpal tunnel. Ups J Med Sci 1975;80:63–64.

Evans BA, Daube JR. A comparison of three electrodiagnostic methods of diagnosing carpal tunnel syndrome. Muscle Nerve 1984;7:565.

Feierstein MS. The performance and usefulness of nerve conduction studies in the orthopedic office. Ortho Clin North Am 1988;19:859–66.

Felsenthal G. Median and ulnar distal motor and sensory latencies in the same normal subject. Arch Phys Med Rehabil 1977;58:297–302.

Felsenthal G. Comparison of evoked potentials in the same hand in normal subjects and in patients with carpal tunnel syndrome. Am J Phys Med 1978a;57:228–32.

Felsenthal G. Median and ulnar muscle and sensory evoked potentials. Am J Phys Med 1978b;57:167–82.

Fine EJ, Wongjirad C. The fallacy of temperature correction in carpal tunnel syndrome. Muscle Nerve 1985;8:628.

Fullerton PM. The effect of ischaemia on nerve conduction in the carpal tunnel. J Neurol Neurosurg Psychiatry 1963;26:385–397.

Gilliatt RW, Meer J. The refractory period of transmission in patients with carpal tunnel syndrome. Muscle Nerve 1990;13:445–50.

Gilliatt RW, Melville ID, Velate AS, Willison RG. A study of normal nerve action potentials using an averaging technique (barrier grid storage tube). J Neurol Neurosurg Psychiatry 1965;28:191–200.

Gilliatt RW, Sears TA. Sensory nerve action potentials in patients with peripheral nerve lesions. J Neurol Neurosurg Psychiatry 1958;21:109–18.

Goddard DH, Barnes CG, Berry H, Evans S. Measurement of nerve conduction—

a comparison of orthodromic and antidromic methods. Clin Rheumatol 1983;2:169–74.

Gordan DS. Nerve sliding and conduction velocity (letter). J Neurol Neurosurg Psychiatry 1981;44:457.

Gutmann L. Median-ulnar nerve communications and carpal tunnel syndrome. J Neurol Neurosurg Psychiatry 1977;40:982–86.

Gutmann L, Gutierrez A, Riggs JE. The contribution of median-ulnar communications in diagnosis of mild carpal tunnel syndrome. Muscle Nerve 1986;9:319–21.

Halar EM, DeLisa JA, Soine TL. Nerve conduction studies in upper extremities: skin temperature corrections. Arch Phys Med Rehabil 1983;64:412–16.

Harrison MJ. Lack of evidence of generalised sensory neuropathy in patients with carpal tunnel syndrome. J Neurol Neurosurg Psychiatry 1978;41:957–59.

Hodes R, Larrabee MG, German W. The human electromyogram in response to nerve stimulation and the conduction velocity of motor axons. Arch Neurol Psychiat (Chicago) 1948;60:340–365.

Iyer V, Fenichel GM. Normal median nerve proximal latency in carpal tunnel syndrome: a clue to coexisting Martin-Gruber anastomosis. J Neurol Neurosurg Psychiatry 1976;39:449–52.

Johnson EW. Practical electromyography. 2nd ed. Baltimore: Williams & Wilkins, 1988.

Johnson EW, Kukla RD, Wongsam PE, Piedmont A. Sensory latencies to the ring finger: normal values and relation to carpal tunnel syndrome. Arch Phys Med Rehabil 1981;62:206–8.

Johnson EW, Melvin JL. Sensory conduction studies of median and ulnar nerves. Arch Phys Med Rehabil 1967;48:25–30.

Johnson EW, Sipski M, Lammertse T. Median and radial sensory latencies to digit I: normal values and usefulness in carpal tunnel syndrome. Arch Phys Med Rehabil 1987;68:140–41. (published erratum appears in Arch Phys Med Rehabil 1987;68:388)

Kimura I, Ayyar DR. The carpal tunnel syndrome: electrophysiological aspects of 639 symptomatic extremities. Electromyogr Clin Neurophysiol 1985;25:151–64.

Kimura J. The carpal tunnel syndrome: localization of conduction abnormalities within the distal segment of the median nerve. Brain 1979;102:619–35.

Kimura J. F-wave determination in nerve conduction studies. Adv Neurol 1983;39:961–75.

Kimura J. Electrodiagnosis in diseases of nerve and muscle: principles and practice. 2nd ed. Philadelphia: FA Davis, 1989.

Kimura J, Murphy MJ, Varda DJ. Electrophysiological study of anomalous innervation of intrinsic hand muscles. Arch Neurol 1976;33:842–44.

Kopell HP, Goodgold J. Clinical and electrodiagnostic features of carpal tunnel syndrome. Arch Phys Med Rehabil 1968;49:371–75.

Kraft GH, Halvorson GA. Median nerve residual latency: normal value and use in diagnosis of carpal tunnel syndrome. Arch Phys Med Rehabil 1983;64:221–26.

LaFratta CW. Relation of age to amplitude of evoked antidromic sensory nerve potentials: a supplemental report. Arch Phys Med Rehabil 1972;53:388–89.

LaFratta CW, Canestrari RE. A comparison of sensory and motor nerve conduction velocities as related to age. Arch Phys Med Rehabil 1966;47:286–90.

Lambert EH. Diagnostic value of electrical stimulation of motor nerves. Electroencephalogr Clin Neurophysiol Suppl 1962;22:9–16.

Lehmann HJ, Tackmann W. Neurographic analysis of trains of frequent electric stimuli in the diagnosis of peripheral nerve diseases. Investigations in the carpal tunnel syndrome. Eur Neurol 1974;12:293–308.

Logigian EL, Busis NA, Berger AR, Bruyninckx F, Khalil N, Shahani BT, Young RR. Lumbrical sparing in carpal tunnel syndrome: anatomic, physiologic, and diagnostic implications. Neurology 1987;37:1499–1505.

Loong SC. The carpal tunnel syndrome: a clinical and electrophysiological study of 250 patients. Proc Aust Assoc Neurol 1977;14:51–65.

Loong SC, Seah CS. Comparison of median and ulnar sensory nerve action potentials in the diagnosis of the carpal tunnel syndrome. J Neurol Neurosurg Psychiatry 1971;34:750–54.

Loong SC, Seah CS. A sensitive diagnostic test for carpal tunnel syndrome. Singapore Med J 1972;13:249–55.

Ludin HP, Lütschg J, Valsangiacomo F. Comparison of orthodromic and antidromic sensory nerve conduction. 1. Normals and patients with carpal tunnel syndrome (in German). EEG EMG 1977;8:173–79.

Ma DM, Liveson JA. Nerve conduction handbook. Philadelphia: FA Davis, 1983.

Maccabee PJ, Shahani BT, Young RR. Usefulness of double simultaneous recording (DSR) and F response studies in the diagnosis of carpal tunnel syndrome (CTS). Electroencephalogr Clin Neurophysiol 1980;49:18P.

Macdonell RA, Schwartz MS, Swash M. Carpal tunnel syndrome: which finger should be tested? An analysis of sensory conduction in digital branches of the median nerve. Muscle Nerve 1990;13:601–6.

Macleod WN. Repeater F waves: a comparison of sensitivity with sensory antidromic wrist-to-palm latency and distal motor latency in the diagnosis of carpal tunnel syndrome. Neurology 1987;37:773–78.

Marin EL, Vernick S, Friedmann LW. Carpal tunnel syndrome: median nerve stress test. Arch Phys Med Rehabil 1983;64:206–8.

Melvin JL, Schuchmann JA, Lanese RR. Diagnostic specificity of motor and sensory nerve conduction variables in the carpal tunnel syndrome. Arch Phys Med Rehabil 1973;54:69–74.

Mills KR. Orthodromic sensory action potentials from palmar stimulation in the diagnosis of carpal tunnel syndrome. J Neurol Neurosurg Psychiatry 1985;48:250–55.

Monga TN, Laidlow DM. Carpal tunnel syndrome. Measurement of sensory potentials using ring and index fingers. Am J Phys Med 1982;61:123–29.

Monga TN, Shanks GL, Poole BJ. Sensory palmar stimulation in the diagnosis of carpal tunnel syndrome. Arch Phys Med Rehabil 1985;66:598–600.

Mortier G, Deckers K, Dijs H, Vander Auwera JC. Comparison of the distal motor latency of the ulnar nerve in carpal tunnel syndrome with a control group. Electromyogr Clin Neurophysiol 1988;28:75–77.

Murai Y, Sanderson I. Studies of sensory conduction. J Neurol Neurosurg Psychiatry 1975;38:1187–89.

Nathan PA, Meadows KD, Doyle LS. Relationship of age and sex to sensory conduction of the median nerve at the carpal tunnel and association of slowed conduction with symptoms. Muscle Nerve 1988a;11:1149–53.

Nathan PA, Meadows KD, Doyle LS. Sensory segmental latency values of the median nerve for a population of normal individuals. Arch Phys Med Rehabil 1988b;69:499–501.

Pease WS, Cannell CD, Johnson EW. Median to radial latency difference test in mild carpal tunnel syndrome. Muscle Nerve 1989;12:905–9.

Pease WS, Cunningham ML, Walsh WE, Johnson EW. Determining neurapraxia in carpal tunnel syndrome. Am J Phys Med Rehabil 1988;67:117–19.

Preswick G. The effect of stimulus intensity on motor latency in the carpal tunnel syndrome. J Neurol Neurosurg Psychiatry 1963;26:398–401.

Reiners K, Jackowski M, Toyka KV. F response latency determinations (letter). Muscle Nerve 1984;7:338–39.

Riegleman RK, Hirsch RP. Studying a study and testing a test. 2nd ed. Boston: Little, Brown, 1989.

Rivner MH, Swift TR, Crout BO, Rhodes KP. Toward more rational nerve conduction interpretations: the effect of height. Muscle Nerve 1990;13:232–39.

Sackett DL, Haynes RB, Tugwell P. Clinical epidemiology. Boston: Little, Brown, 1985.

Schwartz MS, Gordon JA, Swash M. Slowed nerve conduction with wrist flexion in carpal tunnel syndrome. Ann Neurol 1980;8:69–71.

Sedal L, McLeod JG, Walsh JC. Ulnar nerve lesions associated with the carpal tunnel syndrome. J Neurol Neurosurg Psychiatry 1973;36:118–23.

Seror P. The centrimetric test: a diagnostic test of certainty in carpal tunnel syndrome (letter) (in French). Presse Med 1988;17:588.

Seror P. The centimeter test: diagnostic test for beginning carpal tunnel syndrome (in French). Neurophysiol Clin 1990;20:137–44.

Shahani BT, Young RR, Potts F, Maccabee P. Terminal latency index (TLI) and late response studies in motor neuron disease (MND), peripheral neuropathies and entrapment syndromes. Acta Neurol Scand 1979;60(Sup. 73):118.

Shefner JM, Buchthal F, Krarup C. Slowly conducting myelinated fibers in peripheral neuropathy. Muscle Nerve 1991;14:534–42.

Simpson JA. Electrical signs in the diagnosis of carpal tunnel and related syndromes. J Neurol Neurosurg Psychiatry 1958;19:275–80.

Simpson JA, Thomaides T. Fasciculation and focal loss of nerve accommodation in peripheral neuropathies. Acta Neurol Scand 1988;77:133–41.

Spaans F. Spontaneous rhythmic motor unit potentials in the carpal tunnel syndrome. J Neurol Neurosurg Psychiatry 1982;45:19–28.

Stevens JC. AAEE minimonograph #26: the electrodiagnosis of carpal tunnel syndrome. Muscle Nerve 1987;10:99–113.

Stoehr M, Petruch F, Scheglmann K, Schilling K. Retrograde changes of nerve fibers with the carpal tunnel syndrome. An electroneurographic investigation. J Neurol 1978; 218:287–92.

Sun SF, Streib EW. Martin-Gruber anastomosis: electromyographic studies. Electromyogr Clin Neurophysiol 1983;23:271–85.

Tackmann W, Kaeser HE, Magun HG. Comparison of orthodromic and antidromic sensory nerve conduction velocity measurements in the carpal tunnel syndrome. J Neurol 1981;224:257–66.

Tackmann W, Lehmann HJ. Relative refractory period of median nerve sensory fibres in the carpal tunnel syndrome. Eur Neurol 1974;12:309–16.

Thomas JE, Lambert EH, Cseuz KA. Electrodiagnostic aspects of the carpal tunnel syndrome. Arch Neurol 1967;16:635–41.

Thomas PK. Motor nerve conduction in the carpal tunnel syndrome. Neurology 1960;10:1045–50.

Toyonaga K, DeFaria CR. Electromyographic diagnosis of the carpal tunnel syndrome. Arq Neuropsiquiatr 1978;36:127–34.

Uncini A, Di Muzio A, Cutarella R, Awad J, Gambi D. Orthodromic median and ulnar fourth digit sensory conductions in mild carpal tunnel syndrome. Neurophysiol Clin 1990;20:53–61.

Uncini A, Lange DJ, Solomon M, Soliven B, Meer J, Lovelace RE. Ring finger testing in carpal tunnel syndrome: a comparative study of diagnostic utility. Muscle Nerve 1989;12:735–41.

White JC, Hansen SR, Johnson RK. A comparison of EMG procedures in the carpal tunnel syndrome with clinical-EMG correlations. Muscle Nerve 1988;11:1177–82.

Wiederholt WC. Median nerve conduction velocity in sensory fibers through carpal tunnel. Arch Phys Med Rehabil 1970;51:328–30.

Yates SK, Yaworski R, Brown WF. Relative preservation of lumbrical versus thenar motor fibres in neurogenic disorders. J Neurol Neurosurg Psychiatry 1981;44:768–74.

8

Interpretation of Electrodiagnostic Findings in Carpal Tunnel Syndrome

UNDERSTANDING ELECTRODIAGNOSTIC FINDINGS
Test Sensitivity in Carpal Tunnel Syndrome

The relative sensitivity of different techniques for electrodiagnosis of carpal tunnel syndrome is shown in Table 8.1 (Evans and Daube 1984; White et al. 1988; Cruz Martinez 1991). Exact comparison of techniques is difficult because each published study uses a unique population of patients, and methodology and interpretation may vary from laboratory to laboratory.

A less sensitive test may be occasionally abnormal when a more sensitive test is normal. For example, in carpal tunnel syndrome patients, median distal motor latency (DML) is less likely to be abnormal than median distal sensory latency (DSL). However, cases with carpal tunnel syndrome in which DML is abnormal, but DSL is normal, do rarely occur and raise the question of selective fascicular damage (Stevens 1987).

There is conflicting data on the relative sensitivity of different sensory techniques. Felsenthal and Spindler (1979) found that median-ulnar sensory latency comparison and median transcarpal sensory conduction values were equally sensitive in diagnosing mild median sensory conduction abnormalities. Median-radial and median-ulnar sensory latency comparisons are probably equally sensitive in detecting mild median nerve conduction slowing (Pease et al. 1989). Pease et al. (1989) and Cassvan et al. (1988) both found median-radial latency comparisons more sensitive than median palmar conduction studies. Monga et al. (1985) found median palmar studies slightly more sensitive than median-ulnar latency studies.

The Contralateral Asymptomatic Median Nerve

In patients with unilateral symptomatic carpal tunnel syndrome, the median nerve in the contralateral asymptomatic hand will frequently be abnormal on nerve conduction tests. The frequency of abnormality varies with the test used.

Table 8.1 Relative sensitivity of electrodiagnostic tests for carpal tunnel syndrome

Most Sensitive

Serial motor studies

Serial sensory studies

Repetitive sensory stimulation

Transcarpal motor conduction

Transcarpal sensory conduction

Ipsilateral nerve comparisons

Threshold distal motor latency

Distal sensory latency

Less Sensitive

Residual motor latency

Terminal latency index

Distal motor latency

Insensitive

Electromyographic evidence of axonal interruption

Rare

Electromyographic evidence of spontaneous repetitive discharges

Those tests that are more sensitive to abnormalities in the symptomatic hand are more likely to be abnormal in the asymptomatic hand. Table 8.2 gives representative data for asymptomatic hands in patients with unilateral symptoms.

Using repetitive stimulation of sensory fibers at 500 Hz, Lehmann and Tackmann (1974) found abnormalities in seven of eight contralateral asymptomatic hands in patients with unilateral carpal tunnel syndrome.

Table 8.2 Nerve conduction abnormalities in asymptomatic hand contralateral to a hand with carpal tunnel syndrome

	% Abnormal
DML	9
DSL	19
Sensory serial stimulation (MLD ≥0.5 msec)	23
Median-radial sensory latency difference	34
Transcarpal sensory latency	56
TLI	58
Motor serial stimulation	72

DML = Distal motor latency. DSL = Distal sensory latency. MLD = Maximum serial sensory latency difference. TLI = Terminal latency index. (Data from White et al. 1988.)

False-Positive Electrodiagnostic Tests

Electrodiagnostic abnormalities are found in many limbs that do not have symptoms of carpal tunnel syndrome. In the asymptomatic hand that is contralateral to a symptomatic hand, one can argue the semantics of whether to classify a detected abnormality as "false positive." Since the hand is asymptomatic, the abnormality would by definition be a false-positive indicator of carpal tunnel syndrome. However, in many, but probably not all, contralateral asymptomatic hands, the abnormal electrodiagnostic test is a true-positive sign of structural median nerve pathology. Another example of the same dichotomy is persistence of abnormalities of nerve conduction after carpal tunnel surgery that successfully relieves symptoms; the abnormal test signifies persisting neuropathology that is no longer symptomatic.

Abnormal median nerve conduction values may also be present in individuals who have no history of carpal tunnel syndrome. In some, these abnormalities may reflect asymptomatic or presymptomatic nerve pathology; in others, the abnormalities may reflect statistical overlap of the test result between the normal and pathologic population. The overlap is caused both by biologic variability of the normal population and by experimental error inherent in nerve conduction techniques. As illustrated by the data from contralateral asymptomatic hands, the more sensitive the diagnostic test, the higher the incidence of false-positive test responses.

Despite the inevitability of false-positive responses, there is a dearth of data on the false-positive rate of various electrodiagnostic tests. Table 8.3 shows false-positive rates in 50 subjects with no history of neurologic disease and no signs or symptoms of carpal tunnel syndrome (Redmond and Rivner 1988). For each test, the incidence of false positives could be decreased by using more stringent criteria for abnormality, but such more stringent criteria would decrease the diagnostic sensitivity of the test.

As shown in Table 8.4, the relationship between increasing diagnostic sensitivity and increased incidence of false positives is also evident for median nerve palmar serial sensory stimulation studies (Nathan et al. 1988b).

The maximum serial sensory latency difference (MLD) increases with age.

Table 8.3 Incidence of abnormal nerve conduction tests in normal subjects

	%
DML >4.5 msec	2
Median-ulnar palmar sensory latency difference >0.3 msec	8
RML >2.6 msec	14
Median-ulnar SNAP amplitude ratio <1.1	30
Abnormality on at least one of above tests	46

DML = Distal motor latency. RML = Residual motor latency. SNAP = Sensory nerve action potential. (Data from Redmond and Rivner 1988.)

Table 8.4 Serial sensory stimulation sensitivity and false positives vary with diagnostic criteria

Definition of Abnormal	Sensitivity (%)	False Positives (%)
MLD ≥0.5 msec	54	3
MLD ≥0.4 msec	81	19

MLD = Maximum serial sensory latency difference. (Data from Nathan et al. 1988b.)

Table 8.5 shows data for one group of workers randomly chosen without regard to symptoms (Nathan et al. 1988a). Is an MLD greater than 0.5 msec abnormal in sexagenarians? The incidence of carpal tunnel syndrome is lower after age 65 than between the ages of 45 and 64 (Stevens et al. 1988). If normal limits are not adjusted upward for age, the incidence of false-positive results increases with age.

Need for Disease Controls

Development of a test for carpal tunnel syndrome begins with data from normal controls and from patients with carpal tunnel syndrome. Validation of the diagnostic value of the test requires "disease controls": data from patients with illnesses that may be confused with, or coexist with, carpal tunnel syndrome (Nierenberg and Feinstein 1988). So far, published disease control data are inadequate for most electrodiagnostic tests for carpal tunnel syndrome. For example, what are the ranges of median nerve conduction findings for patients with soft tissue abnormalities of the arm such as De Quervain's tenosynovitis? If the ranges of values for these conditions differ from normals, do the abnormalities bespeak coexistent symptomatic carpal tunnel syndrome or asymptomatic deterioration of median nerve conduction? The answers require very careful clinical assessment and long-term follow-up. Appropriate data is not yet available in the literature.

Results in Patients with Coexistent Neuropathy

Normative studies of nerve conduction techniques in patients with carpal tunnel syndrome routinely exclude patients with diffuse neuropathy. Interpretation of nerve conduction values across the carpal tunnel in patients with neuropathies requires appropriate disease control data.

Table 8.5 Variation with age of median serial sensory MLD (in %)

	18–29 Years	30–39 Years	40–49 Years	50–69 Years
Men with MLD >0.5	8	9	23	32
Women with MLD >0.5	15	20	28	35

MLD = Maximum serial sensory latency difference. (Data from Nathan et al. 1988a.)

Diabetic peripheral neuropathy is the best-studied example. There is an increased incidence of symptoms of carpal tunnel syndrome in patients with diabetic peripheral neuropathy (Dieck and Kelsey 1985). Ozaki et al. (1988) compared ulnar and median nerve conduction in insulin-dependent diabetics, most of whom had clinical evidence of peripheral neuropathy. The population was carefully screened to *exclude* patients with symptoms of carpal tunnel syndrome. As expected, in diabetic neuropathy, the median and ulnar nerves of the patient group had abnormal DSL, DML, motor nerve conduction velocity (MNCV), and sensory nerve conduction velocity (SNCV) compared with controls. In addition, median DSL and DML were often more abnormal than ulnar DSL and DML, suggesting that the median nerve in the carpal tunnel was more vulnerable than the ulnar nerve in the hand to developing conduction abnormality. For example, 14 of 49 asymptomatic diabetic hands (29%) had a median DML equal to or greater than 2.0 msec longer than the ipsilateral ulnar DML. Focal median nerve abnormalities across the carpal tunnel were more common in women than in men.

The high incidence of asymptomatic focal slowing of median nerve conduction across the carpal tunnel in patients with diabetic neuropathy creates a diagnostic paradox: Symptomatic carpal tunnel syndrome is common in diabetics; nonetheless, the presence of a focal abnormality of median nerve conduction may be less helpful in diabetics than in nondiabetics in determining whether or not hand symptoms are caused by carpal tunnel syndrome.

Guillain-Barré syndrome provides another example of the propensity of the median nerve to show asymptomatic focal abnormalities across the çarpal tunnel in patients with diffuse neuropathy. Patients with Guillain-Barré syndrome often show a prolonged median DSL when sensory conduction is normal in the sural nerve (Albers et al. 1985).

Asymptomatic focal median nerve conduction slowing in patients with neuropathy might signify vulnerability of diseased nerve to entrapment. Alternatively, nerve fiber demyelination or dropout may unmask preexisting focal nerve entrapment.

Clinical-Electrodiagnostic Correlation

In patients with carpal tunnel syndrome, the correlation between symptoms, signs, and electrodiagnostic findings is imperfect. Patients with pain and paresthesias with normal nerve conduction studies, or with abnormal nerve conduction in an asymptomatic hand, are commonplace. The presence or absence of pain and paresthesias correlates poorly with electrodiagnostic abnormalities (Wilbourn et al. 1980; Shivde et al. 1981). Nonetheless, there are general associations between the severity of clinical disease and severity of electrodiagnostic abnormalities.

Nerve conduction is more likely to be abnormal in patients with longer duration of symptoms. In one series, only one half of patients with symptoms for less than three months had a prolonged median DML; in contrast, three quarters of patients with symptoms for greater than one year had a prolonged median DML (Thomas et al. 1967). Similar differences are noted for median sensory nerve action potential (SNAP) amplitude or median sensory latencies across the carpal tunnel (Loong 1977). Clinical thenar weakness is more likely to be present if there is prolonged median DML, low-amplitude thenar compound muscle action potential (CMAP), or neuropathic abnormalities on electromyography (EMG) (Wilbourn et al. 1980; Shivde et al. 1981; Pavesi et al. 1986).

The clinical sensory exam is often normal despite mild to moderate abnormalities of sensory conduction. If the clinical sensory exam is abnormal, sensory studies usually show slowed conduction, often with decreased amplitude of the SNAP (Thomas et al. 1967; Pavesi et al. 1986). Patients with constant rather than intermittent symptoms are more likely to have abnormal nerve conduction findings (White et al. 1988). Results will depend on both the nerve conduction test used and the clinical sensory test used.

Spindler and Dellon (1982) divided carpal tunnel syndrome patients into those with intermittent and those with constant symptoms. Motor conduction was considered abnormal if the median DML was greater than 4.0 msec or greater than the ulnar DML plus 1.0 msec. Sensory conduction was considered abnormal if the DSL measured to onset was greater than 3.1 msec or greater than the ulnar DSL plus 0.4 msec. Sensory tests were perception of a vibrating tuning fork head or two-point discrimination. Figure 8.1 shows the correlation between sensory symptoms, sensory exam, and nerve conduction results.

Electrodiagnosis and Response to Therapy

Median nerve conduction may improve following successful treatment of carpal tunnel syndrome, but the time course of improvement in nerve conduction often does not match the pace of symptomatic improvement. Treatment of carpal

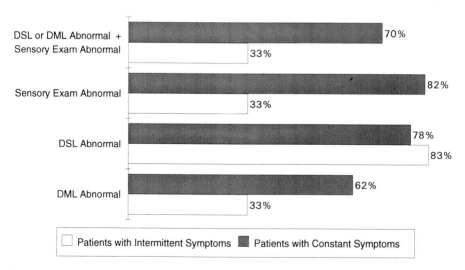

Figure 8.1 Correlating symptoms, signs, and nerve conduction in patients with carpal tunnel syndrome. (Data from Spindler and Dellon 1982.)

tunnel syndrome with splinting or with steroid injection into the carpal tunnel leads to improvement in median DML in some cases (Goodman and Gilliatt 1961; Goodwill 1964). However, individual patients may have relief of symptoms without improvement in DML or may have normalization of DML despite persistent symptoms.

Following carpal tunnel surgery, changes in median nerve conduction go through a number of phases.

Immediate Postoperative Changes

In many patients with carpal tunnel syndrome, some improvement in nerve conduction can be demonstrated intraoperatively within minutes of division of the flexor retinaculum (Hongell and Mattsson 1971). Regardless of whether or not there is intraoperative improvement in nerve conduction, further improvement usually occurs over the ensuing months (Luchetti et al. 1988).

Eversmann and Ritsick (1978) measured median DML in 51 hands before surgery and within 10 minutes of wound closure. DML improved in 44 of the hands. The most dramatic improvement was from 10.8 msec preoperatively to 5.8 msec after surgery. Four patients with high normal DML before surgery showed a drop of DML following surgery. A few patients had a prolongation of DML immediately after surgery; the worst deterioration was an increase from 4.0 to 5.1 msec.

The effect of neurolysis on intraoperative changes in nerve conduction is discussed in Chapter 15.

Long-Term Postoperative Changes

Both sensory and motor conduction across the carpal tunnel improve gradually following successful surgery (Goodman and Gilliatt 1961; Hongell and Mattsson 1971; Shurr et al. 1986). The greatest rate of improvement is seen during the first few months. Patients with more severe preoperative abnormalities have a greater relative improvement. Goodman and Gilliatt (1961) found that in patients with preoperative median DML greater than 10 msec, DML improved 40% or more within five months of surgery; in patients with preoperative DML between 5 and 7 msec, DML improved 20% or more within the same period. Patients who have high normal median DML preoperatively may have postoperative decrease in DML toward the normal mean. Patients often become asymptomatic long before nerve conduction has returned to normal. A few patients with clinically satisfactory responses to surgery will have persistent mild abnormalities of nerve conduction even when examined a year or more after surgery (Goodwill 1964; Melvin et al. 1968).

Sensory conduction in median digital nerves may be abnormal in patients with carpal tunnel syndrome. This abnormal conduction distal to the site of compression usually remains abnormal if checked six to eight weeks after surgery. By 12 to 18 weeks after surgery, both digital SNCV and SNAP amplitude may improve (Le-Quesne and Casey 1974).

ELECTRODIAGNOSTIC PITFALLS

Various techniques are available to study median nerve conduction. The majority of these measure some aspect of nerve impulse transmission in the fastest-conducting myelinated fibers. These large myelinated fibers are the most likely to be damaged in carpal tunnel syndrome, yet nerve conduction studies are imperfect diagnostic tools in carpal tunnel syndrome for a number of reasons.

1. *Biologic variability creates an overlap of normal and abnormal.* Conduction of normal nerves varies with a number of factors. Some personal factors, such as age and temperature, are known, and allowances can be made for them. Other factors, such as individual variation in nerve fiber size or anomalous variations in nerve length or course (e.g., the variety of possible courses of the recurrent thenar motor branch), inevitably widen the normal range.

One way to partially correct for biologic variability is by comparing conduction across the carpal tunnel against conduction in another nerve segment in the same individual. The residual motor latency (RML) and the terminal latency index (TLI) use the proximal median nerve for this purpose. The radial and ulnar comparison tests also decrease the normal range by using the individual as his or her own control for some factors of individual biologic variation. The rationale of these tests is defeated if the nerve segment being used for comparison is also abnormal.

2. *Experimental error increases with increased attention to a short abnormal segment of nerve.* Errors in measuring latencies and conduction distances add to the uncertainty of the results of nerve conduction tests. For example, size of the stimulating electrode, spread of stimulating current through electrode paste, and volume conduction of the stimulus all blur the exact site of nerve stimulation when surface stimulating electrodes are used. Variations in nerve course and sliding of the nerve with changes of hand or arm position increase the error of measurement. Sensory nerve conduction techniques have evolved from examining 13 or 14 cm of nerve between wrist and finger to examining the nerve in 1-cm segments. With longer nerve lengths, sensitivity is lower; biologic variability in normal nerve may mask abnormalities in a short segment of compressed nerve. With shorter nerve lengths, a few millimeters of imprecision in localizing site of stimulation can introduce a large relative variation in the measured latency. This imprecision is amplified when using latency differences to compare conduction in adjacent segments. A mismeasured stimulation site will result in a longer latency adjacent to a shorter latency.

The ratio of experimental error to conduction velocity increases as both the distance and latency differences decrease, so conduction measured over shorter distances with shorter latency differences has a larger experimental error and hence a larger scatter of normal values (Maynard and Stolov 1972). A large experimental error not only increases the difficulty of separating normal from abnormal but also decreases the reproducibility of a test repeated in the same subject.

3. *The probability of an abnormal result increases if multiple tests are done on the same patient.* When routine studies such as DML and DSL are normal in a patient suspected of having carpal tunnel syndrome, many examiners will proceed to increasingly more sensitive tests and will often find abnormalities by doing so. Unfortunately, adding extra tests increases the probability of false-positive results. If each test has a probability of positives in a few percent of the normal population, the probability of a false positive increases with the number of different tests performed.

4. *Symptoms of carpal tunnel syndrome may occur whether or not nerve conduction is measurably impaired.* The telltale early symptoms of carpal tunnel syndrome, intermittent pain and paresthesias, are symptoms not of slowed nerve conduction but rather of abnormal nerve impulse generation that is not detected by nerve conduction techniques (see Chapter 12) (Ochoa and Torebjörk 1979). Figure 8.2 illustrates the pattern of sensory symptoms for a patient in whom abnormal median nerve impulses were recorded by microneurography. Any study

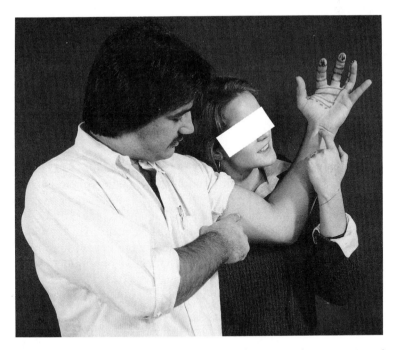

Figure 8.2 This patient developed constant tingling paresthesias projected to the cutaneous territory of the left median nerve after he fell, landing on his wrist. Mild tactile sensory loss was limited to the tips of index and ring fingers. A witness is pointing to the location of Tinel's sign. Conventional median nerve conduction studies were normal, but microneurographic recording through a microelectrode, inserted where he is pointing, revealed abnormal, continual spontaneous bursting unitary discharges in a median nerve fascicle that supplied the skin of the index finger.

for conduction slowing, no matter how refined, is unlikely to correlate perfectly with the phenomena that are causing the patient's symptoms.

Some papers overlook this dissociation between symptoms and nerve conduction findings and demand nerve conduction abnormalities as a criterion for the diagnosis of carpal tunnel syndrome. For example, Katz et al. (1990) relied on a nerve conduction–based definition of carpal tunnel syndrome and came to the erroneous, but self-fulfilling, conclusion that nocturnal paresthesias were not a diagnostic feature of carpal tunnel syndrome.

Patients with carpal tunnel syndrome occasionally show abnormal impulse generation in motor neurons. Examples include fasciculations or repetitive firing on EMG and, probably, the repeater F wave. Unfortunately, these phenomena are observed too infrequently to be amenable to sensitive diagnostic tests. There is no data on how they correlate with symptomatic abnormal impulse generation in sensory neurons.

5. *Nerve conduction slowing or loss of evoked potential amplitude does not actually measure clinical disruption of nerve function.* Examples of asymptomatic slowing of conduction have been given above. Abnormal signs on sensory examination correlate particularly poorly with nerve conduction studies because only a minority of sensory fibers need to function for the patient to perform normally on common clinical sensory tests. An electrical stimulus is perceptible when it activates only 1 of the approximately 600 median sensory fibers to the normal finger (Johansson and Vallbo 1979; Ochoa and Torebjörk 1983). When the median nerve recovers from local anesthesia, normal sensitivity to two-point discrimination and to von Frey's hairs returns when SNAP amplitude is only about 20% of normal (Buchthal and Rosenfalck 1966).

6. *Mild nerve compression is a common finding in the asymptomatic population.* Microscopic evidence of median nerve compression was found in over 40% of cadavers examined in one autopsy series (Neary et al. 1975). About 20% of asymptomatic control subjects have serial segmental maximum latency differences of 0.4 msec or greater: Many of these control subjects may have asymptomatic focal median nerve pathology; some may have normal median nerves but false-positive results because of measurement error or biologic variability. Little is known of the natural history of mild asymptomatic nerve compression or of mild asymptomatic nerve conduction abnormalities. However, given the much lower incidence of symptoms of carpal tunnel syndrome in the population, overattention to asymptomatic electrical abnormalities will usually be misleading.

7. *Axonal interruption is a late manifestation of carpal tunnel syndrome.* The best measures of axonal interruption in patients with carpal tunnel syndrome are the EMG, amplitude of the CMAP and the SNAP, and the forearm MNCV and SNCV. Note that the amplitudes following proximal stimulation may also be reduced as a consequence of conduction block; the differentiation between conduction block and axonal disease requires data on amplitudes from stimulation distal to the carpal tunnel. In patients with carpal tunnel syndrome, distortion of myelin precedes axonal disruption, so the measures of axonal interruption are

rarely abnormal in early or mild cases; conversely, electromyographic signs of axonal interruption are evidence of more severe median nerve injury.

TESTING IN SUSPECTED CARPAL TUNNEL SYNDROME

Electrodiagnostic testing for carpal tunnel syndrome customarily starts with motor and sensory conduction studies of the symptomatic median nerve. Each laboratory should use a selection of the available tests and need not perform every known variation. The electrodiagnostic report must consider CMAP amplitudes and configurations to avoid overlooking coexistent Martin-Gruber anastomosis or more proximal median neuropathies.

If median nerve conduction is normal, the clinical setting will dictate appropriate electrodiagnostic evaluation for alternative diagnoses.

If median nerve conduction is abnormal, the ipsilateral ulnar nerve and contralateral median nerve should also be studied. If these nerves are abnormal, testing must be extensive enough to distinguish between a diffuse peripheral neuropathy and multiple mononeuropathies.

In addition, if median nerve conduction is abnormal, electromyographic needle examination should be done on at least one median thenar muscle. If this muscle is abnormal, other median and C-8 to T-1 muscles must be studied to consider radiculopathy, plexopathy, or more proximal median neuropathy.

The American Association of Electrodiagnostic Medicine (1992) makes similar recommendations for evaluation of any suspected mononeuropathy.

REFERENCES

Albers JW, Donofrio PD, McGonagle TK. Sequential electrodiagnostic abnormalities in acute inflammatory demyelinating polyradiculoneuropathy. Muscle Nerve 1985;8:528–39.

American Association of Electrodiagnostic Medicine. Guidelines in electrodiagnostic medicine. Muscle Nerve 1992;15:229–253.

Buchthal F, Rosenfalck A. Evoked action potentials and conduction velocity in human sensory nerves. Brain Res 1966;3:1–122.

Cassvan A, Ralescu S, Shapiro E, Moshkovski FG, Weiss J. Median and radial sensory latencies to digit I as compared with other screening tests in carpal tunnel syndrome. Am J Phys Med Rehabil 1988;67:221–24.

Cruz Martínez A. Diagnostic yield of different electrophysiological methods in carpal tunnel syndrome. Muscle Nerve 1991;14:183–84.

Dieck GS, Kelsey JL. An epidemiologic study of the carpal tunnel syndrome in an adult female population. Prev Med 1985;14:63–69.

Evans BA, Daube JR. A comparison of three electrodiagnostic methods of diagnosing carpal tunnel syndrome. Muscle Nerve 1984;7:565.

Eversmann WW Jr, Ritsick JA. Intraoperative changes in motor nerve conduction latency in carpal tunnel syndrome. J Hand Surg 1978;3:77–81.

Felsenthal G, Spindler H. Palmar conduction time of median and ulnar nerves of normal subjects and patients with carpal tunnel syndrome. Am J Phys Med 1979;58:131–38.

Goodman HV, Gilliatt RW. The effect of treatment on median nerve conduction in patients with the carpal tunnel syndrome. Ann Phys Med 1961;6:137–55.

Goodwill CJ. The carpal tunnel syndrome—long-term follow-up showing relation of latency measurements to response to treatment. Ann Phys Med 1965;8:12–21.

Hongell A, Mattsson HS. Neurographic studies before, after, and during operation for median nerve compression in the carpal tunnel. Scand J Plast Reconstr Surg 1971;5:103–9.

Johansson RS, Vallbo B. Detection of tactile stimuli. Thresholds of afferent units related to psychophysical thresholds in the human hand. J Physiol [Lond] 1979;297:405–22.

Katz JN, Larson MG, Sabra A, Krarup C, Stirrat CR, Sethi R, Eaton HM, Fossel AH, Liang MH. The carpal tunnel syndrome: diagnostic utility of the history and physical examination findings. Ann Intern Med 1990;112:321–27.

Lehmann HJ, Tackmann W. Neurographic analysis of trains of frequent electric stimuli in the diagnosis of peripheral nerve diseases. Investigations in the carpal tunnel syndrome. Eur Neurol 1974;12:293–308.

Le Quesne PM, Casey EB. Recovery of conduction velocity distal to a compressive lesion. J Neurol Neurosurg Psychiatry 1974;37:1346–51.

Loong SC. The carpal tunnel syndrome: a clinical and electrophysiological study of 250 patients. Proc Aust Assoc Neurol 1977;14:51–65.

Luchetti R, Schoenhuber R, Landi A. Assessment of sensory nerve conduction in carpal tunnel syndrome before, during and after operation. J Hand Surg 1988;13B:386–90.

Maynard FM, Stolov WC. Experimental error in determination of nerve conduction velocity. Arch Phys Med Rehabil 1972;53:362–72.

Melvin JL, Johnson EW, Duran R. Electrodiagnosis after surgery for the carpal tunnel syndrome. Arch Phys Med Rehabil 1968;49:502–7.

Monga TN, Shanks GL, Poole BJ. Sensory palmar stimulation in the diagnosis of carpal tunnel syndrome. Arch Phys Med Rehabil 1985;66:598–600.

Nathan PA, Meadows KD, Doyle LS. Relationship of age and sex to sensory conduction of the median nerve at the carpal tunnel and association of slowed conduction with symptoms. Muscle Nerve 1988a;11:1149–53.

Nathan PA, Meadows KD, Doyle LS. Sensory segmental latency values of the median nerve for a population of normal individuals. Arch Phys Med Rehabil 1988b;69:499–501.

Neary D, Ochoa J, Gilliatt RW. Sub-clinical entrapment neuropathy in man. J Neurol Sci 1975;24:282–98.

Nierenberg AA, Feinstein AR. How to evaluate a diagnostic marker test. JAMA 1988;259:1699–1702.

Ochoa J, Torebjörk E. Abnormal impulse generation in human sensory nerve fibers during paraesthesiae. Acta Neurol Scand 1979;60(Sup. 73):113.

Ochoa J, Torebjörk E. Sensations evoked by intraneural microstimulation of single mechanoreceptor units innervating the human hand. J Physiol [Lond] 1983;342:633–54.

Ozaki I, Baba M, Matsunaga M, Takebe K. Deleterious effect of the carpal tunnel on nerve conduction in diabetic polyneuropathy. Electromyogr Clin Neurophysiol 1988;28:301–6.

Pavesi G, Olivieri MF, Misk A, Mancia D. Clinical-electrophysiological correlations in the carpal tunnel syndrome. Ital J Neurol Sci 1986;7:93–96.

Pease WS, Cannell CD, Johnson EW. Median to radial latency difference test in mild carpal tunnel syndrome. Muscle Nerve 1989;12:905–9.

Redmond MD, Rivner MH. False positive electrodiagnostic tests in carpal tunnel syndrome. Muscle Nerve 1988;11:511–18.

Shivde AJ, Dreizin I, Fisher MA. The carpal tunnel syndrome. A clinical-electrodiagnostic analysis. Electromyogr Clin Neurophysiol 1981;21:143–53.

Shurr DG, Blair WF, Bassett G. Electromyographic changes after carpal tunnel release. J Hand Surg 1986;11A:876–80.

Spindler HA, Dellon AL. Nerve conduction studies and sensibility testing in carpal tunnel syndrome. J Hand Surg 1982;7:260–63.

Stevens JC. AAEE minimonograph #26: the electrodiagnosis of carpal tunnel syndrome. Muscle Nerve 1987;10:99–113.

Stevens JC, Sun S, Beard CM, O'Fallon WM, Kurland LT. Carpal tunnel syndrome in Rochester, Minnesota, 1961 to 1980. Neurology 1988;38:134–38.

Thomas JE, Lambert EH, Cseuz KA. Electrodiagnostic aspects of the carpal tunnel syndrome. Arch Neurol 1967;16:635–41.

White JC, Hansen SR, Johnson RK. A comparison of EMG procedures in the carpal tunnel syndrome with clinical-EMG correlations. Muscle Nerve 1988;11:1177–82.

Wilbourn AJ, Hanson MR, Lederman RJ, Salanga VD. Carpal tunnel syndrome: clinical-electrodiagnostic correlations. Electroencephalogr Clin Neurophysiol 1980;49:18P.

9

Quantitative Sensory Testing

In the evaluation of nerve function, "conventional electrophysiological testing falls short in two major areas. One concerns sensory phenomena of positive character and another one, dysfunction of small caliber fiber systems, both afferent and sympathetic efferent" (Ochoa 1987, page 121). Supplementary information concerning these two areas of dysfunction may be obtained with quantitative sensory testing and thermography (see Chapter 10).

The bedside sensory examination must be supplemented if a standardized measure of somatosensory function is desired. In quantitative sensory tests, defined amounts of stimulus energy are applied, and the sensory response is measured. Precise assessment of subjective responses is achieved through standard determination of perception thresholds or through estimation of the psychophysical suprathreshold magnitude function. Precise delivery of stimuli is possible through instruments that generate finite mechanical or thermal energies, noxious or nonnoxious, to sensory receptors. Instruments such as the vibrameter, the thermostimulator, and the mechanical algometer have proven to be valuable and sometimes indispensable aids in clinical assessment of certain sensory parameters (Lindblom 1981; Lindblom and Ochoa 1986; Triplett and Ochoa 1990; Verdugo and Ochoa 1992).

QUANTITATIVE SENSORY THERMOTESTING

Quantitative sensory thermotesting is a key method for evaluation of four sensory submodalities served by small-caliber fiber afferent channels (Verdugo and Ochoa 1992). The method applies measured ramps of ascending or descending temperature to the skin through a thermode based on the Peltier principle. The subjective response is measured by recording detection thresholds; the subject signals onset of a specific sensation (Figure 9.1). The Marstock method (Fruhstorfer et al. 1976) allows assessment in a noninvasive and yet rigorous fashion of receptor encoding, nerve transmission, and central subjective decoding of cold sensation, warm sensation, pain induced by low temperature, and pain induced by heat. Other methods confine their assessment to cold and warm sensations; measurement of cold and heat pain multiplies the sensitivity of the

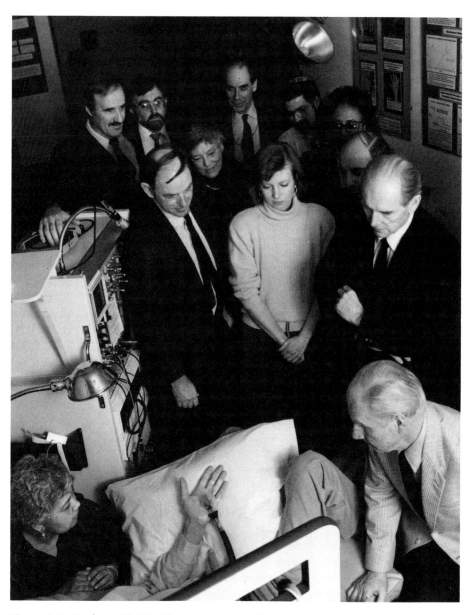

Figure 9.1 Professor U. Lindblom oversees performance of the quantitative thermotest with Marstock apparatus in a patient while a distinguished crowd attends. Peltier thermoprobe is on left palm of subject who is instructed to signal onset of a specified sensory quality by pressing a switch that reverses the direction of excursion of the temperature record in the plotter. The examiner starts the stimulus ramp by pressing a separate switch unknown to the subject.

method so that not only sensory deficits but also sensory exaggeration, or release, such as heat hyperalgesia or cold hyperalgesia, are detected.

After measuring all four functions, the abnormal patterns may be segregated into three main groups: (1) cold or warm hypoesthesia; (2) heat or cold pain hyperalgesia; and (3) combination of thermal hypoesthesia with thermal hyper-algesia (Figures 9.2 and 12.1). These abnormal thermotest profiles may occur in the absence of hypoesthesia for tactile submodalities served by large-caliber fibers. Moreover, hypoesthesia for low temperature may dissociate from warm hypoesthesia, and thermal hyperalgesia may occur in the absence of deficit of cold or warm sensations. Furthermore, thermal hyperalgesia for heat may dissociate from hyperalgesia for cold. Unfortunately, unlike electrophysiological methods for testing large-caliber afferent fibers, these psychophysical tests do not specify the level between skin and brain where the abnormality resides. Moreover, abnormal tests may result from pure psychological dysfunction (Verdugo and Ochoa 1992).

Methodologic Aspects

A contact thermode of standard surface area, based on the Peltier principle, is applied to tested skin. Depending on the direction of electrical current passed through the semiconductor elements within the thermode, a ramp of increasing or

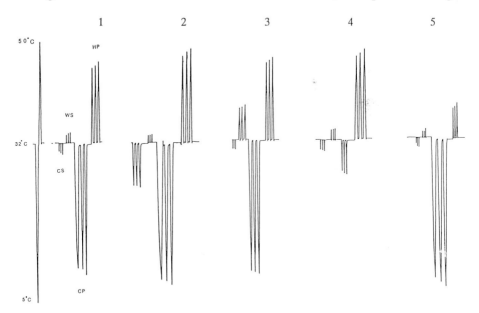

Figure 9.2 Marstock thermotest records of typical pure sensory patterns found in the clinic. Adapting temperature = 32° C. *CS*, cold sensation; *WS*, warm sensation; *CP*, cold pain; *HP*, heat pain; *1*, normal pattern; *2*, cold hypoesthesia; *3*, warm hypoesthesia; *4*, cold hyperalgesia; *5*, heat hyperalgesia. Thermal hypoesthesia, thermal hyperalgesia, and thermal hypoalgesia may combine in various other patterns.

decreasing temperature will be generated. The slope of the changing temperature generated is determined by the intensity of current applied. Temperature at the surface of the stimulator probe is measured through a thermocouple in the probe. The ramps of applied temperature are displayed graphically by a calibrated pen recorder connected to the apparatus. The subject is instructed to signal onset of a given sensation by pressing the switch, which automatically reverses the temperature ramp to baseline adapting temperature. The turning point reflects in degrees centigrade the threshold signaled by the individual for a particular sensation.

A typical normal profile of quantitative thermotest for cold, warm, heat pain, and cold pain sensation is shown in Figure 9.2. Examples of profiles of the three major abnormal categories—namely, pure temperature-specific hypoesthesia, pure thermal hyperalgesia, and combinations of hypoesthesia and hyperalgesia—are shown in Figures 9.2 and 12.1.

Warm Hypoesthesia

In peripheral nerve disease, this abnormal pattern implies dropout of unmyelinated C fibers. Commonly, warm hypoesthesia occurs in the absence of hypoesthesia to pain induced by heat, even though heat pain is also mediated by an afferent system using unmyelinated C fibers. Thus, threshold function remains normal for heat pain but is deficient for warm sensation in the presence of significant depopulation of unmyelinated afferent fibers. This occurs because warm sensation has a marked requirement for spatial summation, whereas heat pain does not. Distal warm hypoesthesia in lower limbs is a "normal" phenomenon in aging.

Cold Hypoesthesia

In peripheral nerve disease, cold hypoesthesia correlates with loss of small-caliber A-delta fibers. Cold hypoesthesia will tend to associate with cold hyperalgesia since deficit of cold-specific input releases pain induced by low temperature (Wahrén et al. 1989; Yarnitsky and Ochoa 1990). Pure cold hypoesthesia is an exceptionally rare finding in organic disease (Verdugo and Ochoa 1992). Cold hypoesthesia from experimental block of A-delta fibers naturally releases hyperalgesia with a paradoxical burning quality in response to low temperature stimuli (Wahrén et al. 1989; Yarnitsky and Ochoa 1990).

Heat and Cold Hyperalgesias

Detection of cold and heat hyperalgesias is an important part of the evaluation of sensory dysfunction of peripheral nerve origin. Fully developed heat and/or cold hyperalgesia may occur in absence of deficit of warm or cold sensations and in absence of deficit of tactile modalities of any kind.

Clinical Use

The quantitative sensory thermotest is valuable for evaluation of polyneuropathies involving small caliber fibers, nerve injuries, and neuropathic pain syndromes. Like thermography, it is of limited value in assessing patients with carpal tunnel syndrome, in whom small-fiber dysfunction is a late and unusual consequence of nerve compression.

VIBRATION SENSE AND VIBRAMETRY

Sensibility to vibration is a defined normal skill of the nervous system that has long attracted the interest of neurophysiologists (Lindblom and Lund 1966; Talbot et al. 1968; Merzenich and Harrington 1969), clinicians (Goff et al. 1965; Calne and Pallis 1966; Goldberg and Lindblom, 1979), and psychophysicists (Verrillo 1980). Vibrating mechanical stimuli excite specifically sensitive receptors encapsulated in Pacinian corpuscles. These connect with somatotopic and modality-specific loci in the somatosensory cortex through large-caliber myelinated fibers in nerves, posterior columns, lemniscal system, and thalamic relays.

The Pacini system is very sensitive in mechanoreception and transmission of high-frequency sustained vibration. This sensitivity derives from the very low mechanical thresholds and rapid adaptation of Pacinian corpuscles. Indeed, they sensitively fire one action potential per mechanical stimulus and adapt to become instantaneously available to respond to further incoming stimuli. The characteristics that make Pacini organs suitable to respond to repetitive mechanical stimuli disable them from responding in a sustained fashion to a slow deformation or to constant pressure.

Intraneural selective microstimulation of identified Pacinian (PC) units in humans using repetitive electrical stimuli at various frequencies typically evokes a sensation of vibration with a minimal frequency of 10 Hz for conscious detection. In contrast, slowly adapting (SA-I) units evoke a sustained sensation of pressure in response to intermittent electrical stimuli applied to their nerve fibers in isolation (Ochoa and Torebjörk 1983). "In everyday tasks of the exploring hand the PC system seems suited to provide an overall idea of very fine textures, without providing the more exact spatio-temporal detail that the rapidly adapting (RA) system probably gives" (Ochoa and Torebjörk 1983, p. 650).

Clinical abnormalities of vibration sense correlate with impaired function of afferent pathways served by large-caliber myelinated fibers. Typically, large-caliber axonal polyneuropathies, demyelinating polyneuropathies, and demyelinating disease in posterior columns affect vibration sense early or predominantly. The traditionally acknowledged loss of vibration sense with aging probably relates to cumulative functional impairment all along the sensory pathway, between receptor and brain (Pearson 1928; Critchley 1956; Steiness 1957; Verrillo 1980; Spencer and Ochoa 1981).

Measurement of vibration sense is an important part of the routine clinical neurologic examination and is usually conducted with a tuning fork delivering mechanical oscillations at 128 Hz. In the clinical evaluation of peripheral nerve injuries, some surgeons view impaired vibration sense as indicative of complete nerve division and therefore of the need for surgical intervention (Dellon 1980). While this concept applies to nerve lacerations, it does not apply to acute closed injuries in which nerve block may well occur in the absence of anatomic interruption of nerve trunks (axonotmesis) or fibers (neurapraxia).

Quantitative vibrametry through electromagnetic devices introduces precision to assessment of vibration sense both at the level of stimulus delivery and at the level of measurement of sensory response (Goldberg and Lindblom 1979). Lindblom (1981) rates vibrametry as less reliable for assessment of mononeuropathy than for polyneuropathy because of stimulus spread to areas innervated by neighboring intact nerves. However, when the stimulus can be confined to a specific territory, vibrametry can be quite sensitive. This is the case when stimuli are applied to some individual fingers (Borg and Lindblom 1986). Reference values for vibration sense, as determined through thresholds during vibrametry, are available for carpal, tibial, and tarsal stimulus sites (Goldberg and Lindblom 1979). In patients with various neurologic disorders, Dyck et al. (1987) and Gerr et al. (1991) found statistically significant correlations between vibrotactile thresholds and electrophysiologic status, particularly sensory nerve action potential parameters.

Gelberman et al. (1983) subjected 12 volunteers to controlled external compression of the median nerve at the carpal tunnel to levels between 40 and 70 mm of mercury. Nerve compression was applied externally through a specially designed device, and fluid pressure within the carpal tunnel was registered by a wick catheter. Vibration sense accurately reflected gradual decreases in nerve function as expressed by subjective sensation and by electrodiagnostic testing. Two-point discrimination threshold was insensitive. Median amplitude of the sensory nerve action potential (SNAP) was 87% of the baseline value at the time when paresthesias in the distribution of the median nerve were first experienced. Median amplitude of the SNAP was 75% of normal when abnormalities in vibration sense were first noticed. Declines in amplitudes of the SNAP and compound muscle action potential constituted the first objective median nerve impairment in each subject.

Vibration sense has been specifically studied in carpal tunnel syndrome. Dellon (1980) evaluated 36 patients with a history of carpal tunnel syndrome and found abnormal perception of vibratory stimuli in 72%, testing with the head of a tuning fork. Within that subpopulation, electrodiagnostic studies were abnormal in only 63%. The 256-Hz tuning fork appeared to be more specific than a 30-Hz tuning fork for detection of abnormalities in patients with carpal tunnel syndrome. Following surgical release for treatment of carpal tunnel syndrome, vibratory perception returned to normal in all those patients who were tested. "This study demonstrates that the tuning fork is an acceptable, convenient, simple, and quick test instrument for use in emergencies; the patient in pain is not further discomforted, the child views it as a non-threatening toy, and the intoxicated patient perceives the vibration through his stupor" (Dellon 1980, 472). Subsequently, Dellon (1983), applying an electromagnetic vibrometer, evaluated

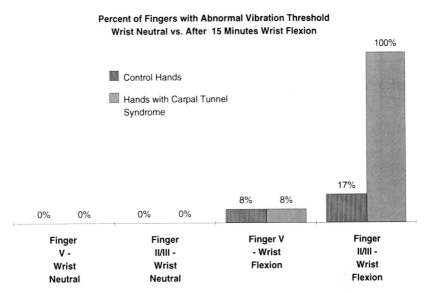

Figure 9.3 Effect of 15 minutes of wrist flexion on vibration perception threshold in patients with carpal tunnel syndrome confirmed by nerve conduction studies compared with control patients with hand paresthesias and normal nerve conduction studies. (Data from Borg and Lindblom 1986.)

34 patients with carpal tunnel syndrome. He found that threshold, as detected by quantitative electromagnetic vibrametry, was no better than the patient's perception of tuning fork stimulus in diagnosing carpal tunnel syndrome. Increased thresholds were observed in 55% of patients with "moderate" and 85% of patients with "severe" carpal tunnel syndrome in this study.

Using provocation with sustained wrist flexion, Borg and Lindblom (1986) showed that many patients with carpal tunnel syndrome develop an abnormally increased vibration perception threshold in skin of fingers supplied by the median nerve but not in fingers supplied by the ulnar nerve. The patients flexed their wrists as for Phalen's test but sustained the flexed position for up to 15 minutes. Figure 9.3 compares the results in control patients with hand paresthesias and normal nerve conduction studies and in patients with carpal tunnel syndrome and abnormal median nerve conduction across the carpal tunnel. Borg and Lindblom concluded that quantitative sensory testing during provocation increases the sensitivity of quantitative sensory testing in diagnosis of carpal tunnel syndrome.

REFERENCES

Borg C, Lindblom U. Increase of vibration threshold during wrist flexion in patients with carpal tunnel syndrome. Pain 1986; 26:211–19.

Calne DB, Pallis CA. Vibratory sense: a critical review. Brain 1966;4:723–46.

Critchley M. Neurological changes in the aged. In: Moore JE, Merritt HH, Masserlink RJ, eds. The neurologic and psychiatric aspects of the disorders of aging. Proc Assoc Res Nervous Ment Dis 1956;35:198.

Dellon AL. Clinical use of vibratory stimuli to evaluate peripheral nerve injury and compression neuropathy. Plast Reconstr Surg 1980;65:466–76.

Dellon AL. The vibrometer. Plast Reconstr Surg 1983;71:427–31.

Dyck PJ, Bushek W, Spring EM, Karnes JL, Litchy WJ, O'Brien PC, Service FJ. Vibratory and cooling detection thresholds compared with other tests in diagnosing and staging diabetic neuropathy. Diabetes Care 1987;10:432–40.

Fruhstorfer H, Lindblom U, Schmidt WG. Method for quantitative estimation of thermal thresholds in patients. J Neurol Neurosurg Psychiatry 1976;39:1071–75.

Gelberman RH, Szabo RM, Williamson RV, Dimick MP. Sensibility testing in peripheral-nerve compression syndromes. An experimental study in humans. J Bone Joint Surg 1983;65A:632–38.

Gerr F, Letz R, Hershman D, Farraye J, Simpson D. Comparison of vibrotactile thresholds with physical examination and electrophysiological assessment. Muscle Nerve 1991;14:1059–66.

Goff GD, Rosner BS, Detre T, Kennard D. Vibration perception in normal man and medical patients. J Neurol Neurosurg Psychiatry 1965;28:305–509.

Goldberg JM, Lindblom U. Standardized method of determining vibratory perception thresholds of diagnosis and screening in neurological investigation. J Neurol Neurosurg Psychiatry 1979;42:793–803.

Lindblom U. Quantitative testing of sensibility including pain. In: Stalberg E, Young RR, eds. Clinical neurophysiology. London: Butterworths, 1981;168–90.

Lindblom U, Lund L. The discharge from vibration-sensitive receptors in the monkey foot. Exp Neurol 1966;15:401–17.

Lindblom U, Ochoa JL. Somatosensory function and dysfunction. In: Asbury AK, McKhann GM, McDonald WI, eds. Diseases of the nervous system. Vol 1. Philadelphia: Ardmore Medical Books, 1986;283–98.

Merzenich MM, Harrington T. The sense of flutter-vibration evoked by stimulation of the hairy skin of primates: comparison of human sensory capacity with the responses of mechanoreceptive afferents innervating the hairy skin of monkeys. Exp Brain Res 1969;9:236–60.

Ochoa JL. Mechanisms of symptoms in neuropathy. The London symposia. EEG Suppl 1987;39:121–27.

Ochoa JL, Torebjörk HE. Sensations evoked by intraneural microstimulation of single mechanoreceptor units innervating the human hand. J Physiol (Lond) 1983;342:633–54.

Pearson GHJ. Effect of age on vibratory sensibility. Arch Neurol Psychiatry 1928;20:482.

Spencer PS, Ochoa J. The mammalian peripheral nervous system in old age. In: Johnson JE, ed. Aging and cell structure. Vol. 1. New York: Plenum Press, 1981;35–103.

Steiness I. Vibratory perception in normal subjects. Acta Med Scand 1957;158:315.

Talbot WH, Darian-Smith I, Kornhuber HH, Mountcastle VB. The sense of flutter-vibration: comparison of the human capacity with response patterns in mechanoreceptive afferents from the monkey hand. J Neurophysiol 1968;31:301–34.

Triplett B, Ochoa JL. Contemporary techniques in assessing peripheral nervous system function. Am J EEG Technol 1990;30:29–44.

Verdugo R, Ochoa JL. Quantitative somatosensory thermotest. A key method for functional evaluation of small caliber afferent channels. Brain 1992; 115:893–913.

Verrillo RT. Age related changes in the sensitivity to vibration. J Gerontol 1980;35:185–93.

Wahrén LK, Torebjörk E, Jörum E. Central suppression of cold-induced C fibre pain by myelinated fibre input. Pain 1989;38:313–19.

Yarnitsky D, Ochoa JL. Release of cold-induced burning pain by block of cold-specific afferent input. Brain 1990;113:893–902.

10

Thermography

Conventional nerve conduction studies (see Chapters 7 and 8) exclusively test nerve impulse conduction in large-caliber, myelinated sensory and motor fibers. Thermography provides noninvasive insights into the functional status of small-caliber, mostly unmyelinated, nociceptor and sympathetic vasomotor nerve fibers. Thermography is not well suited for routine diagnosis of nerve entrapment at the carpal tunnel or elsewhere, because nerve compression predominantly affects myelinated fibers. However, the method is useful in evaluating painful diseases of peripheral nerves of all kinds. Thermography sensitively detects and precisely delineates variations of skin temperature. When used in conjunction with local anesthetic nerve blocks, thermography can objectively document the cutaneous distribution of nerve fibers in specific nerve trunks, thus providing data that may be critical in clinical assessment (Colorplate 10.1A; Colorplates 16.2 and 16.4).

Thermography is best combined with quantitative sensory testing of function of small-caliber sensory channels (see Chapter 9), so that function of small-caliber sensory fibers and small-caliber sympathetic fibers can be correlated. Details of methodology and general interpretation of thermography are beyond the scope of this chapter (for reviews, see Aarts et al. 1975; Houdas and Ring 1982; Engel et al. 1985; Abernathy and Uematsu 1986).

ABNORMAL PATTERNS

Abnormal thermographic patterns may result from neuropathic abnormalities and also, of course, from focal inflammation or vascular disease. Four elementary thermographic patterns of neuropathic origin can be defined: two are "hot," and two are "cold" (Ochoa 1986b).

1. *Hot pattern I: sympathoparalytic vasodilatation.* If sympathetic vasomotor tone is acutely removed, for example, through sympathetic blockade, sympathectomy, somatic nerve block, or neurectomy, the skin acutely warms. The mechanism is increased blood flow as a consequence of arteriolar vasodilatation after removal of sympathetic-mediated vasoconstrictor tone (Colorplate 10.1A is

an infrared thermogram displaying hyperthermia in the median nerve territory of the palm and digits during local anesthetic median nerve block).

2. *Cold pattern I: denervation supersensitivity vasospasm.* Chronic interruption of the postganglionic sympathetic neuron that supplies skin eventually leads to reduced blood flow, resulting in hypothermia of the denervated areas. The blood flow reduction by vasospasm in arteriolar smooth muscle is caused by sympathetic denervation supersensitivity (Cannon and Rosenblueth 1949). Since cold pattern I results from a postsynaptic abnormality in the smooth muscle proper, the vasospasm and the resulting skin cooling cannot be reversed by conventional sympathetic ganglion blocks, sympathectomy, nerve blocks, or neurectomy (Colorplate 10.1B is an infrared thermogram displaying hypothermia in the median nerve territory of the palm and digits present chronically, corresponding to denervation supersensitivity after severe injury to the median nerve at the forearm level).

3. *Cold pattern II: somatosympathetic reflex vasoconstriction.* Excitation of sensory receptors (at least from the skin), or "irritation" of a sensory nerve, normally elicits rapid cooling of the skin, mostly in the territory from which afferent input emanates. This phenomenon is easily reproduced by electrical stimulation of a nerve trunk. It is a reflex, like a tendon reflex, but the afferent input activates sympathetic rather than lower motor units in the efferent limb of the reflex arc (see Colorplate 16.4 where baseline hypothermia (Colorplate 16.4B) is reversed after median nerve block (Colorplate 16.4D) attesting to maintenance of the vasoconstriction through sympathetic neural outflow, even in the partially denervated half of the index finger). See case 2, page 296.

In the clinic, sympathetic denervation supersensitivity vasospasm can be distinguished from neurally sustained somatosympathetic reflex vasoconstriction through somatic local nerve block. Vasodilatation after nerve block attests to neural mediation of the vasoconstriction. However, this does not resolve whether the exaggerated vasoconstrictor tone is an innocent sympathetic response to abnormal afferent input or whether it depends on primarily up-modulated central sympathetic control. An experimental animal preparation illustrates that abnormal afferent activity generated in myelinated fibers proximal to a local nerve lesion elicits, via spinal reflex connections, sympathetic efferent activity that reaches peripheral targets along uninjured small-caliber fibers. Under these circumstances, neurectomy immediately reverses the local vasoconstriction (see figure 2 in Bennett and Ochoa 1991).

4. *Hot pattern II: antidromic vasodilatation.* This interesting pattern is also caused by changes in neurosecretory function of peripheral nerve fibers. However, here the hyperthermia resulting from vasodilatation is independent of sympathetic activity. The pattern relates to enhanced neurosecretion of vasodilator substances released from nerve endings of sensory nociceptor units in response to nerve action potentials. These nerve impulses are either conducted antidromically from parent axon, or reflected antidromically when afferent impulses initiated in dichotomized nerve terminals of nociceptor endings reach branching points.

A familiar example of this phenomenon is the flare component of the triple response of Lewis (1927) elicitable by intradermal injection of histamine. The chemical agent stimulates chemoreceptors in the excitable membrane of C-nociceptor units and fires afferent orthodromic volleys of nerve impulses. Impulses that reflect at branching points will, under normal circumstances, trigger cutaneous neurosecretion and vasodilatation.

Stimulation of nerve trunks at intensity sufficient to excite propagated nerve impulses in midaxons of nociceptors endowed with this neurosecretory property will elicit antidromic vasodilatation. This is strikingly confined to the skin territory supplied by the nerve trunk or the individual nerve fascicles stimulated (Ochoa et al. 1987) (Colorplate 10.1D is an infrared thermogram displaying hyperthermia in the cutaneous territory of a median nerve fascicle. The hatched area of skin shown in Colorplate 10.1C marks the territory of projection of painful paresthesias induced by intense repetitive intrafascicular stimulation of the median nerve at elbow level. This thermogram was taken shortly after prolonged stimulation was stopped. If stimulation were resumed, the focal hyperthermia would be replaced by hypothermia, because during stimulation, the evoked somatosympathetic reflex vasoconstriction (cold pattern II) overrides antidromic vasodilatation).

Direct evidence that cutaneous vasodilatation in a particular case is caused by antidromic neurosecretion rather than by sympathoparalytic vasodilatation is often unavailable. An indirect differential strategy is to demonstrate that the symptomatic vasodilated skin retains capacity for reflex sympathetic vasoconstriction. This clinical stratagem is viable because sympathetic-mediated vasoconstriction overrides nociceptor-mediated antidromic vasodilatation (Ochoa et al. 1990). This occurrence also warns the clinician about the possibility that states of abnormal primary nociceptor activity, leading to pain and associated antidromic vasodilatation, might be partially masked by superimposed and predominant sympathetic reflex vasoconstriction.

In certain natural disease states, antidromic neurogenic vasodilatation, either localized or diffuse, may be prominent and is best detected by thermographic monitoring (Ochoa 1986a; Cline et al. 1989).

In summary, patients with hyperthermic symptomatic limbs do not necessarily have paralysis of sympathetic efferent activity. Conversely, patients with hypothermic symptomatic limbs do not necessarily have exaggerated neural sympathetic outflow; they may actually have ablated sympathetic postganglionic outflow.

OBJECTIVE THERMOGRAPHIC DELINEATION OF CUTANEOUS INNERVATION

Figure 16.3 and Colorplate 16.4 illustrate the cutaneous innervation pattern, as reflected in the thermogram, following local anesthetic block of the median nerve in patients. The block causes acute paralysis of sympathetic vasomotor fibers and results in vasodilatation in the cutaneous distribution of the blocked fibers. The thermogram shows increased temperature in this distribution (hot pattern I). Both sympathetic sudomotor (Guttmann 1940) and vasomotor fibers distribute over the same area of skin as cutaneous sensory fibers, so determination of the area of sympathetic supply provides a valid measure of the area of sensory distribution.*

This technique is more objective than other methods of measuring sensory patterns, such as mapping paresthesias following percutaneous electrical stimulation or mapping sensory deficit following nerve block, which rely on the patient for subjective sensory witnessing (Highet 1942; Schady et al. 1983; Marchettini et al. 1990). Similar data can be obtained by the relatively more cumbersome technique of measuring sympathetic sudomotor function with a "sweat test" (Moberg 1958).

THERMOGRAPHY AND POSITIVE SENSORY SYMPTOMS

Thermography is very useful in the evaluation of patients expressing positive sensory symptoms, specifically pains and hyperalgesias, that originate from dysfunction of nerve fibers. In painful median mononeuropathy, including rare instances of painful carpal tunnel syndrome, any of the four abnormal patterns described earlier may be seen, depending on the acuteness and mechanism of the neuropathy.

Ill-conceived use of thermography can prove misleading. The most common level of misuse is considering the simple physical sign that is quantified by thermography as if it were diagnostic of a syndrome. An unfortunate example is diagnosing "reflex sympathetic dystrophy" simply by documenting a hypothermic symptomatic limb; this may condemn the patient to repetitive sympathetic blocks and sometimes to ultimate sympathectomy, an itinerary that characteristically meets therapeutic failure. This ill-advised practice stems from misperceiving in thermography an illusion of pathophysiology, when in reality it only records spectacularly a clinical sign: deviation of temperature.

THERMOGRAPHY IN CARPAL TUNNEL SYNDROME

Thermography is not useful for the routine diagnosis of carpal tunnel syndrome. Like other entrapment neuropathies, carpal tunnel syndrome primarily affects larger myelinated fibers (see Chapter 12). Median nerve autonomic vasomotor dysfunction is demonstrable in only a minority of cases of carpal tunnel syndrome (Aminoff 1979). Fowler and Ochoa (1975), using a baboon model of *acute* focal compression neuropathy, found pathologic damage in unmyelinated fibers only if Wallerian degeneration was occurring in myelinated fibers. Marotte (1974) found that unmyelinated fiber structure remained intact until late in the course of *chronic* animal nerve entrapment. Thus, the pathophysiology of carpal tunnel syndrome is such that thermographic determination of small-fiber function is a relatively insensitive test for its diagnosis. Clinical data support this conclusion. Thermography may show abnormalities in

*Wang, Sonnad, and Ochoa 1992: unpublished.

median nerve distribution in severe cases of carpal tunnel syndrome (Harway 1986). However, in clinical series, many patients with carpal tunnel syndrome diagnosed on clinical and electrophysiologic criteria have normal thermographic studies; for example, So et al. (1989) found abnormal thermograms in only 55% of their patients with carpal tunnel syndrome. Another series reported similar results (Myers et al. 1988).

When thermographic abnormalities are present in patients with carpal tunnel syndrome, interpretation is complicated by the nonspecific nature of the abnormalities. In a given patient the thermogram may not distinguish which side is abnormal and may not differentiate between ulnar and median nerve dysfunction (Reilly et al. 1989; So et al. 1989).

REFERENCES

Aarts NJM, Gautherie M, Ring EFJ, eds. Thermography. Proceedings of the 1st European Congress on Thermography, organized by the European Thermographic Association with the collaboration of the American Thermographic Society, Amsterdam, June 1974. Basel: S Karger, 1975.

Abernathy M, Uematsu S, eds. Medical thermology. Washington, DC: American Academy of Thermology, 1986.

Aminoff MJ. Involvement of peripheral vasomotor fibres in carpal tunnel syndrome. J Neurol Neurosurg Psychiatry 1979;42:649–55.

Bennett GJ, Ochoa JL. Thermographic observations on rats with experimental neuropathic pain. Pain 1991;45:61–67.

Cannon WB, Rosenblueth A. The supersensitivity of denervated structures: a law of denervation. New York: Macmillan, 1949.

Cline MA, Ochoa JL, Torebjörk HE. Chronic hyperalgesia and skin warming caused by sensitized C nociceptors. Brain 1989;112:621–47.

Engel JM, Flesch U, Stüttgen G. Applied thermology. Thermological methods. Weinheim, Germany: VCH Verlagsgesellschaft, 1985.

Fowler TJ, Ochoa JL. Unmyelinated fibres in normal and compressed peripheral nerves of the baboon; a quantitative electron microscopic study. Neuropathol Appl Neurobiol 1975;1:247–65.

Guttmann L. Topographic studies of disturbances of sweat secretion after complete lesions of peripheral nerves. J Neurol Psychiatry 1940;3:197–210.

Harway RA. Precision thermal imaging of the extremities. Orthopedics 1986;9:379–82.

Highet WB. Procaine nerve block in the investigation of peripheral nerve injuries. J Neurol Psychiatry 1942;5:101–16.

Houdas Y, Ring EFJ. Human body temperature. Its measurement and regulation. New York and London: Plenum Press, 1982.

Lewis T. The blood vessels of the human skin and their responses. London: Shaw and Sons, 1927.

Marchettini P, Cline M, Ochoa JL. Innervation territories for touch and pain afferents of single fascicles of the human ulnar nerve. Mapping through intraneural microrecording and microstimulation. Brain 1990;113:1491–1500.

Marotte LR. An electron microscope study of chronic median nerve compression in the guinea-pig. Acta Neuropathol (Berl) 1974;27:69–82.

Moberg E. Objective methods for determining the functional value of sensibility in the hand. J Bone Joint Surg 1958;40B:454–76.

Myers S, Vermeire P, Sherry B, Cros D. Liquid crystal thermography: quantitative studies of abnormalities in the carpal tunnel syndrome. Neurology (Minneap) Suppl 1988; 38:200.

Ochoa JL. The newly recognized painful ABC syndrome: thermographic aspects. Thermology 1986a;2:65–107.

Ochoa JL. Unmyelinated fibers, microneurography, thermography and pain. American Association of Electromyography and Electrodiagnosis; ninth annual continuing education course B. Rochester: AAEE, 1986b;29–34.

Ochoa JL, Comstock WJ, Marchettini P, Nizamuddin G. Intrafascicular nerve stimulation elicits regional skin warming that matches the projected field of evoked pain. In: Schmidt RF, Schaible H-G, Vahle-Hinz C, eds. Fine afferent nerve fibers and pain. Weinheim, Germany: VCH Verlagsgesellschaft, 1987.

Ochoa JL, Yarnitsky D, Marchettini P, Dotson R, Cline M. Antidromic vasodilatation overridden by somatosympathetic reflexes in man. Intraneural stimulation and thermography (abstract). Soc Neurosci 1990;16(2):1280.

Reilly PA, Clarke AK, Ring EF. Thermography in carpal tunnel syndrome (CTS) (letter). Br J Rheumatol 1989;28:553–54.

Schady W, Ochoa JL, Torebjörk HE, Chen LS. Peripheral projections of fascicles in the human median nerve. Brain 1983;106:745–60.

So YT, Olney RK, Aminoff MJ. Evaluation of thermography in the diagnosis of selected entrapment neuropathies. Neurology (Minneap) 1989;39:1–5.

11

Imaging the Carpal Tunnel

WRIST RADIOGRAPHS

In patients with carpal tunnel syndrome, wrist radiographs occasionally give clues to the cause of the nerve compression. Examples are evidence of old trauma, deformities of the carpal bones or distal radius or ulna, or unexpected calcifications in the canal.

Wrist radiographs may provide a rough estimate of size of the carpal tunnel. Gelmers (1981) took vertical wrist radiographs of the boundaries of the tunnel, approximating the flexor retinaculum as a straight line from the navicular tuberosity to the pisiform bone. Table 11.1 shows his data comparing the cross-sectional area of the carpal tunnel in women with carpal tunnel syndrome and in controls. Symptomatic women had a statistically significant ($p < 0.001$ compared with female controls) smaller mean cross-sectional area of the carpal tunnel.

COMPUTED TOMOGRAPHY SCANNING

The anatomy of the carpal canal can be imaged in vivo by computed tomography (CT) (see Figures 1.11a–1.13a). Serial cross sections show the carpal bones, flexor tendons, synovium, and median nerve (Zucker-Pinchoff et al. 1981). Good detail is obtained with 3-mm thick slices. The flexor tendons (attenuation coefficient about 100 HU [Hounsfield units]) have higher attenuation than their surrounding synovium. The median nerve blends with the synovium. The flexor retinaculum is visible as a thin soft tissue line (Merhar et al. 1986).

Measurements by CT of the cross-sectional area of the canal have given conflicting results in patients with carpal tunnel syndrome. Table 11.2 compares carpal canal cross-sectional area measured by CT in women with carpal tunnel syndrome and in controls (Dekel et al. 1980). Symptomatic women had a statistically significant ($p < 0.001$ proximally, $p < 0.05$ distally, compared with female controls) smaller mean cross-sectional area of the carpal tunnel. Male controls had larger tunnel cross-sectional areas. There was a large overlap between the

Table 11.1 Carpal tunnel cross-sectional area by wrist radiographs

	Area (mm²)	Standard Error
Female controls (19)	206.6	12.4
Females with carpal tunnel syndrome (11)	153.8	11.8
Male controls (17)	234.1	14.3

(Data from Gelmers 1981.)

areas for individual patients and individual controls; so this technique does not provide a diagnostic test for individual patients. There was no correlation between patient age and tunnel area, suggesting that tunnel area is determined by age 20 years and does not decline with age.

Bleecker et al. (1985) studied all 14 male electricians in an electrical shop. They classified the workers as (1) symptomatic carpal tunnel syndrome, (2) asymptomatic with abnormal median nerve conduction, or (3) normal. Using 5-mm contiguous CT slices through the canal, they identified the slice in each patient with the smallest cross-sectional area. In most cases, the smallest area was 2.0 to 2.5 cm distal to the distal wrist crease. In four cases, the minimum area was more proximal. For both the workers with carpal tunnel syndrome and the workers with asymptomatic median nerve conduction abnormalities, the mean of the smallest tunnel cross-sectional area was lower than for the normal workers.

Merhar et al. (1986), however, found no significant difference in canal areas comparing patients to controls. They used a 3-mm section technique that visualized the flexor retinaculum. Dekel et al. (1980) had not visualized the retinaculum and approximated it for measurement purposes by a straight line connecting the scaphoid tubercle to the pisiform or trapezium to the hook of the hamate. The flexor retinaculum is actually slightly curved, so that the canal is oval. As expected, the areas reported by Merhar et al. were slightly larger than those reported by Dekel et al. Merhar et al. also measured the relative amount of synovium in the canal, the attenuation coefficient of the canal, and the thickness of the flexor retinaculum and found that these did not differ significantly between patients and controls.

Table 11.2 Carpal tunnel cross-sectional area by CT scan

	Proximal Area (mm²)	Standard Error	Distal Area (mm²)	Standard Error
Female controls (19)	213.7	4.8	209.3	7.7
Females with carpal tunnel syndrome (26) (42 hands)	184.1	4.0	188.0	6.5
Male controls (14)	279.9	8.3	254.1	7.8

(Data from Dekel et al. 1980.)

Jessurun et al. (1987) compared CT scans of the carpal tunnel in patients and controls with the wrist neutral, flexed 70°, or extended 70°. They found that the normal median nerve moves away from the flexor retinaculum during wrist flexion. In one fifth of hands with carpal tunnel syndrome, this nerve movement relative to the flexor retinaculum did not occur with flexion. The cross-sectional areas of the tunnel did not change significantly among the three positions in patients or controls. There was no significant difference in the areas of the tunnels between patients and controls. The tunnel area was smallest 6 mm proximal to the distal border of the hook of the hamate. At this level, the proportion of the tunnel occupied by tendons was larger in female patients than in female controls; however, male patients and controls matched female patients in the proportion of their tunnels occupied by tendons. Winn and Habes (1990) found that patients with carpal tunnel syndrome had *larger* minimum tunnel areas as measured by CT than did sex-matched controls.

In summary, there are conflicting data on the relationship between tunnel size, as measured by CT scan, and development of carpal tunnel syndrome. Even in the studies that found smaller mean tunnel sizes in groups of patients with carpal tunnel syndrome, the differences are insufficient to provide useful diagnostic information in most individual patients.

On rare occasion, CT scan of the wrist might reveal other wrist pathology or anomalies of diagnostic importance (Hindman et al. 1989). Nonetheless, in most cases of carpal tunnel syndrome, wrist CT scan is not a necessary part of the diagnostic evaluation. Strict criteria for its use await further experience.

MAGNETIC RESONANCE IMAGING

Magnetic resonance imaging (MRI) of the wrist using surface coils can give excellent high-resolution images of the hands and wrists (see Figures 1.11b–1.13b) (Weiss et al. 1986b; Middleton et al. 1987; Mesgarzadeh et al. 1989a). Normal anatomy varies with wrist position (Zeiss et al. 1989; Skie et al. 1990).

Details of a variety of hand pathology such as ganglia, fractures, tendon ruptures, vascular malformations, and rheumatoid deformities are visible by MRI (Weiss et al. 1986a). MRI often demonstrates asymptomatic anatomic variations in the tunnel such as proximal extension of lumbricals into the tunnel, persistent median artery, or anomalous relation of the median nerve to the flexor tendons (Middleton et al. 1987).

A variety of MRI abnormalities may be found in patients with carpal tunnel syndrome (Mesgarzadeh et al. 1989b):

1. swelling of the median nerve at the level of the pisiform
2. flattening of the median nerve (best evaluated at the level of the hamate)
3. abnormally high signal intensity of the median nerve on T2-weighted images (Weiss et al. 1986a; Middleton et al. 1987)

Table 11.3 Gross appearance of the median nerve at the time of carpal tunnel surgery

Nerve Appearance at Surgery	Number of Patients
No visible change	3
Slight nerve compression	3
Nerve narrowing, normal blood supply	19
Nerve narrowing, reduced blood supply	30

(Data from Leblhuber et al. 1986.)

4. abnormally low signal intensity of the median nerve on T2-weighted images (Reicher and Kellerhouse 1990)
5. palmar bowing of the flexor retinaculum

In one series 3 of 10 wrists with carpal tunnel syndrome had abnormally large median nerve area proximally with normal area distally, and in 3 other symptomatic wrists, the median nerve appeared diffusely enlarged (Middleton et al. 1987). In some cases of carpal tunnel syndrome, the median nerve appears normal on MRI, but the flexor tendon sheaths are thickened, or the synovium and flexor retinaculum may be poorly delineated (Middleton et al. 1987; Healy et al. 1990).

Little published data exists on tunnel size estimated by MRI. Healy et al. (1990) propose using a "carpus/tunnel index" as a guide to tunnel stenosis but provide no objective data on the meaning of this index.

The literature on MRI scanning in carpal tunnel syndrome is growing. To date, reports are chiefly small series in the radiologic journals. No data is yet available on the diagnostic sensitivity or specificity of MRI scanning in carpal tunnel syndrome.

Extrapolating from the gross appearance of the median nerve at the time of carpal tunnel surgery may provide some insight into the potential accuracy of MRI scanning as a diagnostic test for carpal tunnel syndrome. In surgical series, the gross appearance of the nerve may vary considerably, as shown by the data in Table 11.3.

Although MRI might show abnormalities in a nerve that appeared grossly normal to inspection by the surgeon, this variability in gross nerve appearance suggests that MRI is likely to have false-negative findings, particularly in mild cases of carpal tunnel syndrome. Clinical detail is largely lacking in the MRI series reported to date.

REFERENCES

Bleecker ML, Bohlman M, Moreland R, Tipton A. Carpal tunnel syndrome: role of carpal canal size. Neurology (Minneap) 1985;35:1599–1604.

Dekel S, Papaioannou T, Rushworth G, Coates R. Idiopathic carpal tunnel syndrome caused by carpal stenosis. Br Med J 1980;280:1297–99.

Gelmers HJ. Primary carpal tunnel stenosis as a cause of entrapment of the median nerve. Acta Neurochir (Wien) 1981;55:317–20.

Healy C, Watson JD, Longstaff A, Campbell MJ. Magnetic resonance imaging of the carpal tunnel. J Hand Surg 1990;15B:243–48.

Hindman BW, Kulik WJ, Lee G, Avolio RE. Occult fractures of the carpals and metacarpals: demonstration by CT. AJR 1989;153:529–32.

Jessurun W, Hillen B, Zonneveld F, Huffstadt AJ, Beks JW, Overbeek W. Anatomical relations in the carpal tunnel: a computed tomographic study. J Hand Surg 1987; 12B:64–67.

Leblhuber F, Reisecker F, Witzmann A. Carpal tunnel syndrome: neurographical parameters in different stages of median nerve compression. Acta Neurochir (Wien) 1986;81:125–27.

Merhar GL, Clark RA, Schneider HJ, Stern PJ. High-resolution computed tomography of the wrist in patients with carpal tunnel syndrome. Skeletal Radiol 1986;15:549–52.

Mesgarzadeh M, Schneck CD, Bonakdarpour A. Carpal tunnel: MR imaging. Part I. Normal anatomy. Radiology 1989a;171:743–48.

Mesgarzadeh M, Schneck CD, Bonakdarpour A, Mitra A, Conaway D. Carpal tunnel: MR imaging. Part II. Carpal tunnel syndrome. Radiology 1989b;171:749–54.

Middleton WD, Kneeland JB, Kellman GM, Cates JD, Sanger JR, Jesmanowicz A, Froncisz W, Hyde JS. MR imaging of the carpal tunnel: normal anatomy and preliminary findings in the carpal tunnel syndrome. AJR 1987;148:307–16.

Reicher MA, Kellerhouse LE. Carpal tunnel disease, flexor and extensor tendon disorders. In: Reicher MA, Kellerhouse LE, eds. MRI of the wrist and hand. New York: Raven Press, 1990;49–68.

Skie M, Zeiss J, Ebraheim NA, Jackson WT. Carpal tunnel changes and median nerve compression during wrist flexion and extension seen by magnetic resonance imaging. J Hand Surg 1990;15A:934–39.

Weiss KL, Beltran J, Lubbers LM. High-field MR surface-coil imaging of the hand and wrist. Part II. Pathologic correlations and clinical relevance. Radiology 1986a;160:147–52.

Weiss KL, Beltran J, Shamam OM, Stilla RF, Levey M. High-field MR surface-coil imaging of the hand and wrist. Part I. Normal anatomy. Radiology 1986b;160:143–46.

Winn FJ Jr, Habes DJ. Carpal tunnel area as a risk factor for carpal tunnel syndrome. Muscle Nerve 1990;13:254–58.

Zeiss J, Skie M, Ebraheim N, Jackson WT. Anatomic relations between the median nerve and flexor tendons in the carpal tunnel: MR evaluation in normal volunteers. AJR 1989;153:533–36.

Zucker-Pinchoff B, Hermann G, Srinivasan R. Computed tomography of the carpal tunnel: a radioanatomical study. J Comput Assist Tomogr 1981;5:525–28.

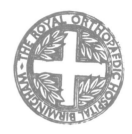

12

Acute and Chronic Mechanical Nerve Injury: Pathologic, Physiologic, and Clinical Correlations

The subject of mechanical nerve injury is more complex than often assumed, even by skilled practitioners. Substantial scientific data is available on the basic underlying phenomena and permits intelligible clinical-pathologic-electro-physiologic correlations.

Among the multiple risks for physical injury to nerves, the incidence of mechanical trauma far outweighs electrical, cold, heat, injection, or radiation nerve damage. Particularly in the median nerve, chronic local mechanical compression and entrapment are much more common than transection, percussion and stretch injury, or acute neurapraxia.

To explain the pathophysiology of carpal tunnel syndrome, the archetype of chronic focal nerve entrapment, we begin with a general discussion of the consequences of acute and chronic nerve ischemia and acute and chronic nerve compression.

ACUTE ISCHEMIA AND NERVE FIBER DYSFUNCTION

Acute episodes of nerve compression and ischemia are ostensibly superimposed on chronic entrapment of the median nerve at the carpal tunnel. This pathogenic overlap probably applies to mechanically entrapped nerves in general. Local compression affects nerve trunk microcirculation and nerve fiber metabolism, and ischemia provokes transient clinical manifestations similar to those commonly experienced by patients with carpal tunnel syndrome. However, as clarified later, ischemia does not cause the distinctive pathology of myelinated fibers found in locally entrapped nerves.

Acute compression of a limb above systolic pressure leads to a stereotyped sequence of sensory and motor, negative and positive manifestations (for general review, see Sivak and Ochoa 1987). Paresthesias and mild fasciculations usually develop within a few minutes of onset of ischemia. Acroparesthesias are central to this topic, since they are commonplace in carpal tunnel syndrome and other entrapment neuropathies. The *intraischemic* paresthesias reflect ectopic impulse generation in sensory fibers caused by transient disruption of membrane excitability (Kugelberg 1944; Merrington and Nathan 1949; Nathan 1958; Bergmans 1973; Bergmans 1982a, 1982b). Fasciculations, from ectopic impulse generation in motor nerve fibers, are less common than paresthesias because motor fibers accommodate better than sensory fibers to ischemia (Erlanger and Blair 1938). This difference in accommodation is a reflection of differences in concentration of potassium channels found in those two types of fibers (see Culp and Ochoa 1982).

Approximately 20 minutes after onset of ischemia, muscle weakness and sensory loss ensue, following a characteristically centripetal pattern. These are expressions of nerve conduction block in motor and sensory nerve fibers. Initially, nerve impulse conduction fails selectively in large-caliber myelinated fibers. Indeed, while light touch is lost, sympathetic function and "temperature sensation" remain unaffected (Lewis et al. 1931; Gasser 1935; Sinclair and Hinshaw 1950). Preferential involvement of large-caliber fiber functions is a reflection of differential susceptibility of nerve fibers to anoxia (Lewis et al. 1931; Gasser and Grundfest 1936).

Quantitative measurement of thermal thresholds allows specific testing of submodalities of "temperature sensation" (see Chapter 9). Warm sensation, mediated by unmyelinated fibers, is relatively resistent to ischemia (Yarnitsky and Ochoa 1991), whereas cold sensation, mediated by small-caliber myelinated fibers, fails much earlier (Yarnitsky and Ochoa 1990) (Figure 12.1). Furthermore, warm sensation behaves differently from pain induced by heat, which is much more resistent to ischemia, even though both sensations are served by subsets of unmyelinated fibers. The explanation for this puzzling phenomenon is that warm sensation requires much spatial summation; that is, a critical population of nerve fibers must be activated for warmth to be perceptible. Pain induced by heat requires a lesser degree of spatial summation (Yarnitsky and Ochoa 1991).

Deficit of motor and sensory nerve fiber function recovers almost immediately upon reestablishment of circulation, provided ischemia is not sustained beyond about two hours. In the case of acute ischemia induced by local limb compression above systolic pressure, the situation is complicated by the possibility that local compression might mechanically deform and thus affect function of nerve fibers. Lewis et al. (1931) discounted the role of acute local mechanical compression in an ingeniously simple experiment: Once ascending paralysis and sensory loss were established after application to the arm of a pneumatic cuff inflated above systolic pressure, the authors placed a second suprasystolic cuff proximally and then released the first one. Although pressure on the first site was relieved by removal of the first cuff, anesthesia and paralysis did not recover until after the second site of compression had been released, indicating that the neural

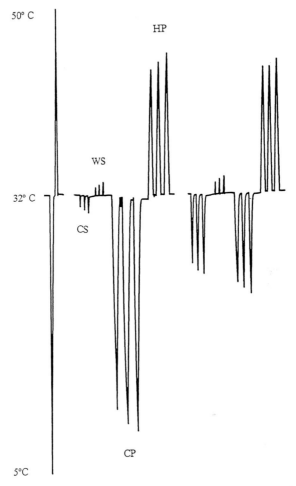

Figure 12.1 Quantitative Marstock thermotest comparing normal profile *(left)* against dissociated loss of cold sensation with sparing of warm sensation during ischemia *(right)*. Note that together with increased thresholds for cold sensation there are lowered thresholds for pain induced by low temperature, due to disinhibition as reported by Yarnitsky and Ochoa (1990). CS: Cold sensation; WS: Warm sensation; CP: Cold pain; HP: Heat pain.

deficits were sustained by unrelieved ischemia rather than by direct nerve fiber compression.

During acute ischemia, nerve fiber functions served by unmyelinated fibers are retained for about an hour, much longer than functions of myelinated fibers. The "neurapraxia" of severe local nerve compression also strikingly spares not only function but also structure of small-caliber nerve fibers (Fowler and Ochoa 1975). This and other coincidences misled pioneers to attribute erroneously to ischemia the pathology of neurapraxia (Denny-Brown and Brenner 1944b).

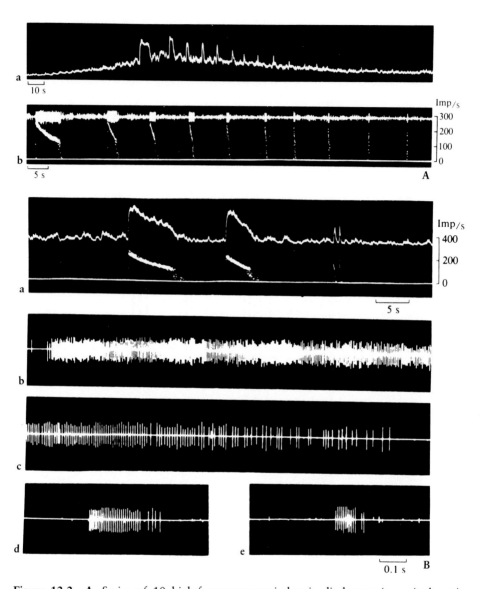

Figure 12.2 **A,** Series of 10 high-frequency postischemic discharges in a single unit recorded from the ulnar nerve at elbow level. **a,** Integrated neurogram, dominated by single unit bursts. Recording started on release of cuff in upper arm after 15 minutes of ischemia. **b,** Discriminated neurogram of part of the sequence shown in **a,** displayed at an extended time scale. *Upper trace* is original neurogram; *lower trace* displays "instantaneous" firing frequency of the unit. Note the fairly regular repeat of bursts and their decreasing duration. Note also the uniform impulse frequency at the onset of bursts and the progressive steepness of the frequency decay in subsequent bursts. There seems to be a critical firing frequency of about 130 Hz, below which the impulse frequency claudicates abruptly. **B,** Prolonged, high-frequency postischemic discharges in a single unit recorded from the median nerve at elbow level. Unitary bursts appeared during the second minute after release of cuff compression around forearm, maintained for 25 minutes. **a,** Integrated neurogram *(upper trace)* shows four abrupt deflections, representing single unit discharges,

200

Postischemic paresthesias typically occur after ischemia is released and motor and sensory deficit have resolved. In a classic study, Merrington and Nathan (1949) offered indirect evidence that postischemic paresthesias are caused by ectopic generation of nerve impulses. Microneurography directly confirms Merrington and Nathan's conclusion. Figure 12.2 shows recordings of paroxysmal ectopic nerve discharges from single sensory fibers in one of the authors (JO); these occurred at the same time as the abnormal postischemic sensations (Ochoa and Torebjörk 1980).

Nocturnal acroparesthesias in patients with chronic nerve entrapment may be induced by ischemia developed during transient local compression in sleep (presumably of positional origin). Alternatively, those paresthesias might be caused by increased mechanical deformation of nodes of Ranvier, possibly by sustained abnormal posture and further pressure during sleep.

Remarkably, nocturnal acroparesthesias largely involve tingling and buzzing. These are sensations that correspond to afferent activity in tactile, large-caliber mechanoreceptors (Ochoa and Torebjörk 1983). Patients with carpal tunnel syndrome are less likely to experience pains or thermal sensations, which are mediated by small-caliber nerve fibers (Ochoa and Torebjörk 1989). Small-caliber fibers tend not to engage in ectopic discharge during postischemic paresthesias (Ochoa and Torebjörk 1980).

PATHOPHYSIOLOGY OF VASA NERVORUM

Key aspects of the structure and pathophysiology of the delicate intraneural microcirculatory apparatus have been elucidated over the past two decades (Lundborg 1970, 1975, 1979, 1980; Olsson and Reese 1971; Olsson 1972; Lundborg and Rydevik 1973; Lundborg et al. 1973, 1983; Olsson and Kristensson 1973; Rydevik 1979; Myers et al. 1986; Powell and Myers 1986).

A vascular plexus of small vessels courses longitudinally at various depths in the epineurium, feeding smaller vessels running on the perineurial surface of nerve fascicles. These obliquely pierce the multicellular and collagenous layers of perineurium, to connect with endoneurial vessels of even smaller caliber. The anastomotic system supplying the endoneurial surface is relatively independent of the blood supply of the fascicular core. Thus, transperineurial vascular occlusion during nerve compression causes subperineurial nerve fiber pathology, whereas

also displayed in **b–e**. "Instantaneous" frequency plot *(lower trace)* shows initial frequency of about 220 Hz with exponential fall to about 150 Hz and subsequent breakdown. Duration of consecutive bursts diminished from an initial maximum of seven seconds. **b** displays the beginning and **c** the end of first unitary burst shown in **a**. Note regular firing frequency at the beginning and missing beats toward the end. Last two bursts in **a** are displayed in **d** and **e**. (Reproduced with permission of the authors and Oxford University Press from Ochoa JL, Torebjörk HE. Paresthesiae from ectopic impulse generation in human sensory nerves. Brain 1980;103:835–53.)

thrombosis of microcirculation causes necrosis of the central core of the fascicles (Parry and Brown 1981, Powell and Myers 1986) (Figure 12.3).

Once it reaches critical levels, ischemia sets off a serious pathophysiologic sequence. The resulting increased microvascular permeability leads to endoneurial edema and increased intrafascicular fluid pressure. The perineurium, relatively resistant to anoxia, remains comparatively stiff and impermeable. The resulting "microcompartment" state restricts endoneurial blood flow and is believed to promote nerve fiber pathology and endoneurial fibrosis (Lundborg 1988).

While disruption of intraneural circulation by nerve compression may cause local demyelinating nerve fiber damage, acute compression of nerve may additionally induce blockage of axoplasmic transport (Rydevik et al. 1980). Impaired axoplasmic transport conceivably may result in anterograde axonal atrophy or degeneration.

To supplement a warning given elsewhere in this chapter: It is as naive to blame the pathophysiology of nerve compression solely on ischemia as it is to do so just on primary mechanical damage.

ACUTE ISCHEMIA AND NERVE INFARCTION

Acute prolonged suppression of arterial blood supply to a limb leads to cell death. The characteristics of ischemic nerve infarctions have been well defined in animals and vary depending on the experimental approach (Korthals and Wisniewski 1975; Hess et al. 1979; Parry and Brown 1981; Nukada and Dyck 1984). Detailed neuropathologic examination of selected human cases has allowed definition of typical patterns of distribution of the pathology in naturally occurring nerve infarctions and of the kind and degree of pathologic reactions involving subtypes of nerve fibers (Raff et al. 1968, Asbury 1970; Asbury and Johnson 1978).

The subject of nerve infarction is relatively tangential to the pathology of carpal tunnel syndrome. However, even in infarction following severe acute nerve ischemia, unmyelinated fibers tend to be spared, while myelinated fibers are degenerating (Fujimura et al. 1991).

CHRONIC ISCHEMIA AND NERVE PATHOLOGY

Chronic nerve ischemia may also lead to pathologic changes in nerve trunks and clinical nerve fiber dysfunction. Early reports on pathology of human nerves in chronic ischemic conditions described concrete dropout of nerve fibers (Joffroy and Achard 1889; Gairns et al. 1960; Garven et al. 1962). Later, longitudinal microdissection of nerve fibers revealed that demyelination, not highlighted on nerve trunk cross sections, is commonplace in chronic ischemia (Eames and Lange 1967). Electron microscopy of these nerves has shown that—just as for acute nerve infarction—chronic ischemia tends to spare unmyelinated fibers in human

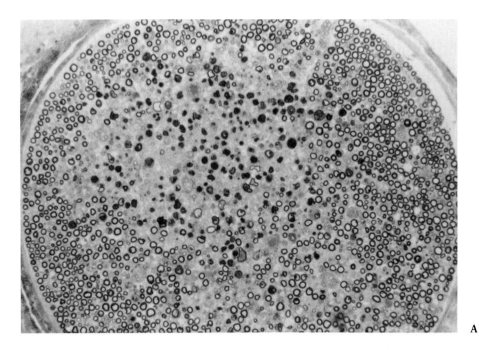

A

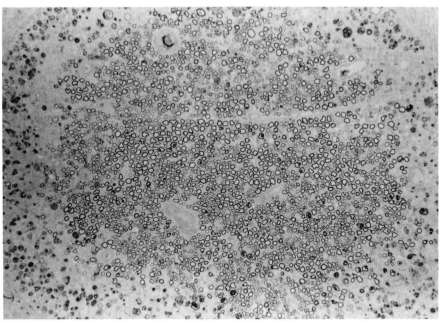

B

Figure 12.3 **A,** Light micrograph of cross section of tibial nerve of rat showing striking centrofascicular degeneration of nerve fibers due to experimentally induced partial nerve infarction. (Reproduced with permission of the author, Gareth J. Parry, M.D., unpublished material from Parry GJ, Brown MJ. See: J Neurol Sci 1980; 50:123). **B,** Light micrograph of cross section of tibial nerve of rat showing striking subperineurial demyelination due to interference with transperineurial blood supply caused by local external compression. (Reproduced with permission of the author, Henry Powell, Ph.D., unpublished material from Powell HC, Myers RR. See: Lab Invest 1986;55:91.)

nerves (Asbury and Johnson 1978; Ochoa, unreported). Development of animal experimental models of chronic nerve ischemia is still needed.

ACUTE, SEVERE LOCAL MECHANICAL TRAUMA TO NERVE

Cajal (1928) described the pathologic events that follow acute axonal transection ("axonotmesis" and "neurotmesis"; Seddon 1943) through the degenerative and regenerative stages. An acute mechanical injury to the median nerve leading to interruption of a population of axons might be delayed in its regenerative progress if the new axons must grow through an area of preexisting nerve pathology at the carpal tunnel. At usual sites of entrapment, common pathologic changes are endoneurial fibrosis, thickening of the perineurium and epineurium, formation of space-occupying Renaut bodies, and probably local disruption of microcirculation.

Severe acute mechanical trauma to median nerve at the wrist may cause ill-repaired pathologic changes such as formation of a posttraumatic neuroma. The acute injury may thus result in chronic symptoms. The clinical picture might be misinterpreted as reflecting chronic nerve entrapment deserving surgical decompression at the carpal tunnel. However, the pathology of chronic entrapment, featuring current damage, concurrent attempts at repair, and recurrent damage of old and new structures, is different from the stable pathology that may persist after an isolated traumatic episode. Appropriate therapy varies with the pathology; chronic compression does benefit from carpal tunnel decompression, but direct mechanical nerve trauma does not and may require microneurosurgery (Figure 12.4).

PERCUSSION INJURY

Like acute compression injury, a single percussive episode to peripheral nerve will cause different types of histopathologic consequences, depending on the force applied. S. Weir Mitchell is quoted by Richardson and Thomas (1979): "In some cases where I struck the nerve sharply with a smooth broad whalebone slip, allowing a thin layer of muscle to intervene, the paralysis which ensued, although temporary, was in degree complete. Within a few days, the rabbit showed no discernible paralysis." In turn, Denny-Brown and Brenner (1944a) state that after percussion injury to cat sciatic nerve, paralysis completely recovered within one week. The histopathologic correlate was focal demyelination with distal axonal degeneration in less than 2% of the fibers. More forceful blows by Richardson and Thomas (1979) caused increasing incidence of axonal degeneration.

The woodwind musician in Figure 12.4 violently percussed his median nerve at wrist level when he spanked a protruding piece of metal decorating his son's belt. Clinical and electrophysiologic evaluation showed definite axonal

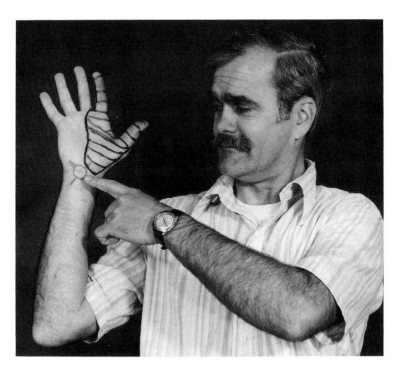

Figure 12.4 Patient points at site of previous mechanical injury that coincides with stationed point of Tinel's sign. Note involvement of palmar cutaneous branch. Following fascicular repair, there was additional early postoperative numbness of digits III and IV before eventual progressive recovery.

degeneration. Arrested recovery suggested neuroma formation, which was confirmed and treated microsurgically by fascicular repair.

NEURAPRAXIA

The median nerve, like any other, may develop an acute primary pathologic deformation of nerve fibers that leads to the clinical-electrophysiologic state of "neurapraxia" (Seddon 1943). While clinical neurapraxia is best exemplified by injury to the radial nerve in "Saturday night paralysis," it may also affect the median nerve at the carpal tunnel under unusual circumstances. Figure 12.5 illustrates a rare microscopic example of the primary neurapraxic lesion of myelinated fibers caused by acute local compression of the median nerve in the carpal canal (Neary et al. 1975).

In terms of duration of the clinical abnormalities, severity of the structural changes, and nature of the electrophysiologic correlates, neurapraxia represents an intermediate state between rapidly reversible ischemic nerve block and the

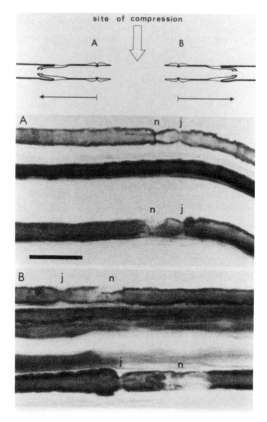

Figure 12.5 Fresh postmortem median nerve specimen obtained from the carpal tunnel of a 30-year-old man. He died after being for several hours in a state of decorticate rigidity with marked flexion of the wrists, maintained after death. This caused pressure on the nerve under the distal part of the flexor retinaculum. Microscopic abnormalities indicative of mechanical distortion of axons and myelin were found over a distance of ±7 mm. The figure reproduces single fibers to show displacement of the nodes of Ranvier in opposite directions: **A** = proximal, **B** = distal. *j*, Schwann cell junction; *n*, new position of node. Bar = 30 μm. (Reproduced with permission of the authors and publisher from Neary D, Ochoa JL, Gilliatt RW. Subclinical entrapment neuropathy in man. J Neurol Sci 1975; 24:283–98.)

devastating local lesion caused by severe mechanical trauma leading to interruption of nerve fibers (axonotmesis) or whole nerve trunks (neurotmesis) (Seddon 1943).

Clinically, in both neurapraxia and acute reversible ischemia there is a deficit of motor nerve function and of those sensory nerve functions served by large-caliber myelinated fibers, with sparing of sensory and autonomic functions served by small-caliber nerve fibers (Moldaver 1954; Bolton and McFarlane 1978). Thus, neurapraxic sensory loss differs from the multimodality sensory loss that correlates with gross interruption of axons. While functional recovery after transection of axons may take many months or years, recovery of neurapraxia usually takes weeks or a few months at most. Distal to a site of neurapraxic injury, a nerve remains electrically excitable (Erb 1876). In contrast, within days of axonal interruption, the fibers distal to the injury are no longer electrically excitable. Nerve conduction studies can often use this difference in physiology to distinguish neurapraxia from axonotmesis early after nerve injury, before muscle atrophy or electromyographic signs of denervation are evident.

The pathology of neurapraxia varies, depending on the time after injury at which the nerve is examined. The pathologic characteristics of the lesion underlying neurapraxia also differ, depending on the power of the examiner's microscope. The pioneering study by Denny-Brown and Brenner (1944b) emphasized late observations, by which time demyelination was present. Furthermore, the observations were limited to optic microscopy, preventing recognition of telltale fine structural changes that are a signature of their mechanical origin. Over and above the optical resolution handicap, Denny-Brown and Brenner were further handicapped by the limitations of contemporary knowledge. Indeed, local constriction of a limb by cuff leads to immediately reversible sensorimotor dysfunction caused by ischemia and not by direct mechanical pressure (Lewis et al. 1931). Since simple prolongation of local constriction time may lead to neurapraxia, neurapraxic demyelination logically seemed to result from sustained ischemia. However, as illustrated in Figures 12.6 and 12.7, finer methods for nerve histology show an early lesion of myelinated fibers in experimental neurapraxia.

Critical supporting evidence for the mechanical origin of the primary lesion underlying neurapraxia came from analysis of the ultrastructural features of single abnormal myelinated fibers. The fibers were selected by light microscopy and then subjected to ultrathin longitudinal sections for electron microscopy (Ochoa 1972). The technical demands for this kind of study have not been replicated over the past two decades.

This lesion is unquestionably mechanical in origin, as it involves displacement of structures in the direction of, and proportional to, abnormally operant forces (Ochoa et al. 1971, 1972). Demyelination is a secondary event after this lesion. Further evidence for the mechanical origin of this lesion is that it occurs in duplicate at either edge of the site of compression rather than under the whole area of compression (Figure 12.8). Moreover, the direction of displacement of structures is reversed at either edge, in keeping with the development of extruding forces generated from pressure gradients between compressed and uncompressed tissue. This occurrence, which establishes the mechanical nature of the lesion, also explains the lack of pertinence of another experiment that Denny-Brown and Brenner (1944b) cited in support of the ischemic hypothesis. This was a striking experiment by Grundfest (1936) that had shown that nerve segments, contained within pressure chambers, may continue to conduct nerve impulses even under huge pressures, provided oxygen is present in the chamber. This observation was misconstrued as indicating that nerve fibers are relatively indifferent to the effects of pressure; instead, in the lesion shown in Figures 12.6 through 12.8 at the edges of local compression of nerves in limbs, dependence on pressure gradients is self

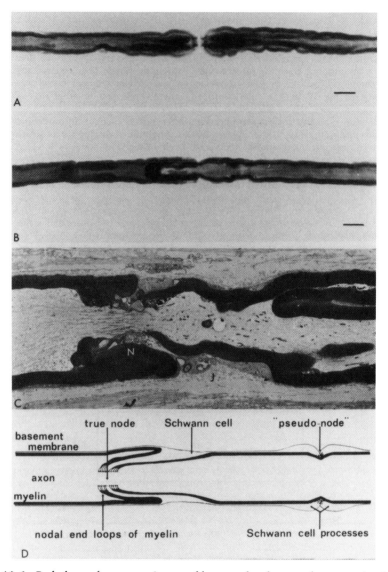

Figure 12.6   Pathology of neurapraxia caused by acute local external compression in limb of a baboon. **A,** Normal microdissected myelinated fiber showing node of Ranvier. Baboon tibial nerve. Bar = 10 μm. **B,** Abnormal fiber, early after acute compression. The nodal gap is occluded due to intussusception from right to left. An indentation (pseudonode) marks the original site of the node. Bar = 10 μm. **C,** Low-power electron micrograph of abnormal myelinated fiber, cut longitudinally after microdissection. Note indentation at Schwann cell junction *(J)* and new position of the node *(N)* under infolded myelin. (Reproduced with permission of the authors and publisher from Rudge P, Ochoa JL, Gilliatt RW. Acute peripheral nerve compression in the baboon. Anatomical and physiological findings. J Neurol Sci 1974;23:403–20.) **D,** Diagram of affected fiber showing invagination of one paranode by the adjacent one, movement occurring from right to left. (Reproduced with permission of the authors and publisher from Ochoa JL, Fowler TJ, Gilliatt RW. Changes produced by a pneumatic tourniquet. In: Desmedt JE, ed. New developments in electromyography and clinical neurophysiology. Basel: Karger, 1973; 2:166–73.)

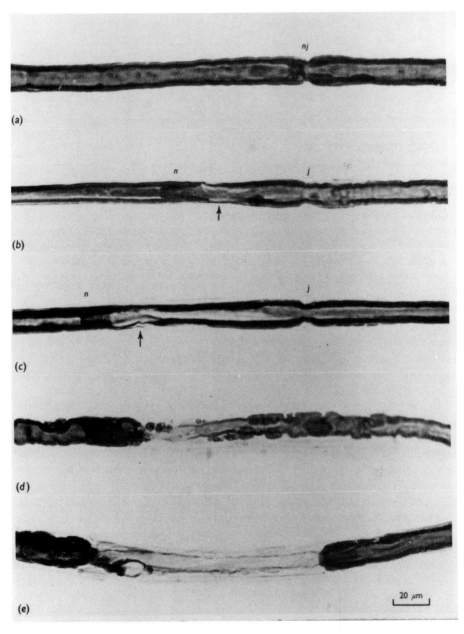

Figure 12.7 Pathology of neurapraxia caused by acute local external compression in limb of a baboon. **A–C,** Abnormal fibers, four days after compression, showing different degrees of nodal displacement (reaching 120 μm in **C**). *j,* Schwann cell junction; *n,* new position of node. Note thinning of myelin at *arrows.* **D,** A fiber, 15 days after compression, undergoing demyelination of the paranodal region. There is tapering of the myelin of the paranode on the *right.* **E,** A thinly myelinated intercalated segment, 61 days after compression. (Reproduced with permission of the authors and publisher from Ochoa JL, Fowler TJ, Gilliatt RW. Anatomical changes in peripheral nerves compressed by a pneumatic tourniquet. J Anat 1972;113:433–55.)

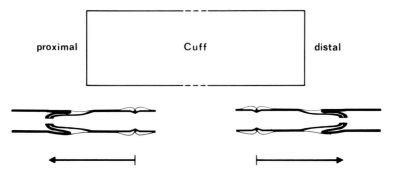

Figure 12.8 Pathology of neurapraxia caused by acute local external compression in limb of a baboon. Diagram describing the direction of displacement of the nodes of Ranvier in relation to the compressed zone. (Reproduced with permission of the authors and publisher from Ochoa JL, Fowler TJ, Gilliatt RW. Anatomical changes in peripheral nerves compressed by a pneumatic tourniquet. J Anat 1972;113:433–55.)

evident. In Grundfest's chamber, the nerve segments were subjected to uniform pressures; no pressure gradients could develop there. This primary mechanical lesion affecting myelinated fibers was also shown to develop under conditions of much more focal compression, as caused by a weighted string in baboons (Rudge et al. 1974) (Figures 12.9 through 12.11) or by 5-mm wide rubber bands applied to the thinner limbs of rodents (Ochoa, unpublished).

Unmyelinated fibers, and even small-caliber myelinated fibers, escape damage in neurapraxia. While functional sparing of small-caliber fibers during *acute* ischemia is explainable by differential susceptibility to anoxia; sparing of structure of small fibers in the mechanical lesion underlying neurapraxia has a different mechanism (Ochoa et al. 1972). However, the common feature was another reason why Denny-Brown and Brenner (1944b) mistakenly concluded that ischemia was the cause of the late demyelinating nerve lesion underlying neurapraxia.

In man, local mechanical nerve lesions often combine elements of neurapraxia and axonotmesis. This admixture is not at all surprising, as the experimental requirements to achieve relatively pure neurapraxia are stringent and demand rigorous titration of severity of the mechanical insult (Fowler et al. 1972; Fowler 1975). Naturally, less controlled experiments on acute nerve compression tend to yield a mixed pathology of axons and myelin sheaths (as they do in nerve percussion injury).

Clinical and electrophysiologic recovery from genuine neurapraxia may be substantially delayed in instances of particularly severe nerve compression (Rudge 1974; Harrison 1976). This protracted course correlates with the development of a component of edema of nerve fibers and necrosis of Schwann cells, affecting particularly the ad-axonal loops of Schwann cell cytoplasm. Such pathology is almost certainly a consequence of anoxia. Somehow, these aberrant structures that interfere with transmission of nerve impulses are tolerated by the organism; their scavenging and repair through remyelination being delayed (Ochoa et al. 1972; Ochoa 1981) (Figures 12.12 and 12.13).

In addition to this well-defined and electrophysiologically matched mechanical lesion underlying neurapraxia, acute or chronic local nerve compression may, under special circumstances, cause demyelination that is strikingly confined to subperineurial nerve fibers (Aguayo et al. 1971). The distinctive, strictly subperineurial localization of the demyelination suggests that impaired flow in transperineurial vessels causes the lesion through ischemia (Powell and Myers 1986). As discussed earlier, a separate microvascular system supplies nerve fibers in the core of the fascicles; these core fibers may be selectively infarcted in certain conditions (Parry and Brown 1981) but are spared in sub-perineural demyelination (Hess et al. 1979; Powell and Myers 1986) (see Figure 12.3A and B).

The application of constricting devices directly on the surface of nerve trunks may also lead to acute nerve pathology (Dyck 1969). More recently, Bennett and Xie (1988) have standardized a nerve constriction lesion caused by snug application of a series of ligatures along the sciatic nerve in rats. The ligatures lead predominantly to axonal degeneration of myelinated fibers and a remarkably well characterized set of physiologic and clinical consequences dominated by irritative sensory phenomena overshadowing sensorimotor deficit.

CHRONIC NERVE ENTRAPMENT

Chronic nerve entrapment causes distinct pathologic changes. These have been described in animal models of natural local nerve entrapment and also in archetypical syndromes of chronic nerve entrapment in humans. However, these pathologic lesions have not been reproduced through experimental local nerve constriction. The pathogenesis of the natural lesions is more complex than simple, steady constriction. For example, at the carpal tunnel the pressure on the median nerve varies during the day, and compression may be accompanied by intermittent ischemia, local nerve stretching, and friction from movement of adjacent structures. Marie and Foix (1913) provided a notable early description of the histopathologic correlates of local nerve entrapment. They documented that some forms of chronic thenar atrophy were caused by a lesion of the median nerve in the region of the carpal tunnel. Using classic myelin stains, they showed that myelinated fibers, traced from the forearm, disappeared at wrist level. Some 50 years later, in a clinical, electrophysiologic, and autopsy human study of proven carpal tunnel syndrome at Queen Square, Thomas and Fullerton (1963) confirmed the presence of local pathology in median nerve at the wrist. They found in nerve cross sections that density of myelinated fibers was partially preserved distal to the wrist, indicating that the demyelination at the wrist was not invariably accompanied by axonal interruption. At that time, demonstration of local demyelinating pathology carried no challenge to the prevailing assumption that local nerve demyelination associated with mechanical trauma must be ischemic in origin. Later, animals with chronic nerve entrapment were shown to exhibit similar changes (Fullerton and Gilliatt 1967) (Figure 12.14), and shortly after, a distinctive morphologic change was described in microdissected myelinated fibers: peculiar deformities of the myelin sheaths with thickening of proximal

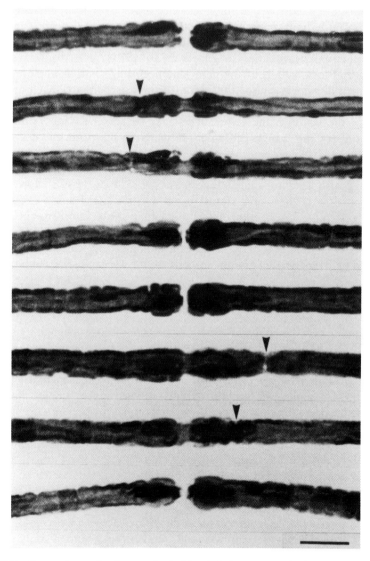

Figure 12.9 Successive nodes from a single fiber in left anterior tibial nerve 24 hours after compression (externally with string) (750 g for 90 minutes) to show extent of the lesion. The proximal end of the fiber is at the *top*. Note two normal nodes in center of lesion and nodal displacement in opposite directions on either side (new positions of nodes marked by *arrows*). Beyond these the nodes are again normal. Bar = 20 µm. (Reproduced with permission of the authors and publisher from Rudge P, Ochoa JL, Gilliatt RW. Acute peripheral nerve compression in the baboon. Anatomical and physiological findings. J Neurol Sci 1974;23:403–20.)

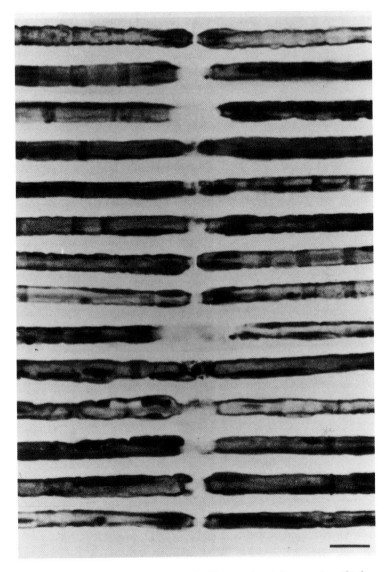

Figure 12.10 Successive nodes from a single fiber in the right anterior tibial nerve eight days after compression (with string) to show extent of lesion. Early demyelination is present. Note normal nodes at center (retouched) and at each edge of lesion. Bar = 20 μm. (Reproduced with permission of the authors and publisher from Rudge P, Ochoa JL, Gilliatt RW. Acute peripheral nerve compression in the baboon. Anatomical and physiological findings. J Neurol Sci 1974;23:403–20.)

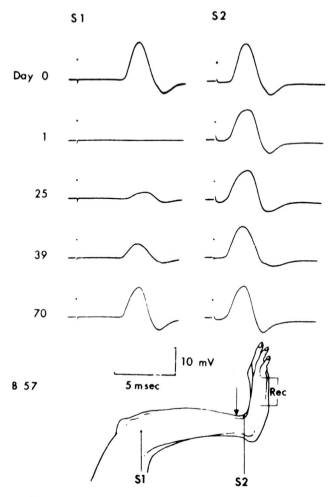

Figure 12.11 Evoked muscle action potentials from extensor digitorum brevis at different intervals after compression of the right anterior tibial nerve (externally with string at arrow) (1.5 kg for 90 minutes). Sites of stimulating and recording electrodes shown *below*. (Reproduced with permission of the authors and publisher from Rudge P, Ochoa JL, Gilliatt RW. Acute peripheral nerve compression in the baboon. Anatomical and physiological findings. J Neurol Sci 1974;23:403–20.)

paranodal myelin and thinning of distal paranodal myelin. The deformities were consistently polarized in consecutive myelin segments (Anderson et al. 1970) (Figure 12.15). This finding was not understood until the same polarized deformity was shown to be present in reverse, distal to the wrist (Ochoa and Marotte 1973) (Figure 12.16). The symmetry of the myelin changes suggested a mechanical origin in analogy to the distinct mechanical deformity, also polarized symmetrically around the compression, that had been described as a correlate of acute neurapraxia in experimentally compressed nerves (Ochoa et al. 1972). Certainly,

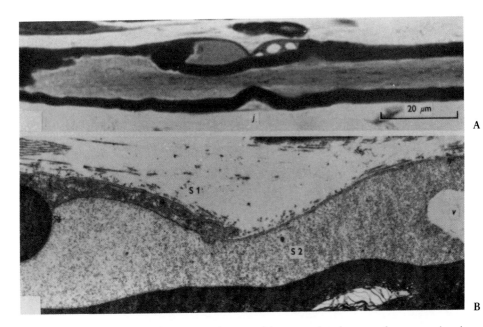

Figure 12.12 Pathology of neurapraxia caused by acute local external compression in limb of a baboon. **A,** Longitudinal section of fiber four days after compression, showing indented myelin at the Schwann cell junction (*j*) and swollen Schwann cell cytoplasm containing vacuoles. Epon-toluidine blue. **B,** Electron micrograph showing detail of the fiber shown *above*. The thin tongue of paranodal Schwann cell cytoplasm on the *left (S1)* has been dissected from the myelin by a swollen cell process intruding from the Schwann cell on the *right (S2)*. In the latter, cytoplasmic differentiation is lost, and there is a vacuole (*v*). ×8,700. (Reproduced with permission of the authors and publisher from Ochoa JL, Fowler TJ, Gilliatt RW. Anatomical changes in peripheral nerves compressed by a pneumatic tourniquet. J Anat 1972;113:433–55.)

the tapered paranodes of myelin segments and the buckled paranodes on the opposite ends result from displacement of inner myelin lamellae away from the entrapped site (Figure 12.17). Such pathologic profile of myelinated fibers in entrapped nerves disproves the hypothesis that local nerve anoxia is its cause. Local anoxia explains neither the tapering of myelin sheaths nor the focal demyelination which is so capriciously localized to the distal ends of internodes proximal to the entrapment and to the proximal end of internodes distal to the entrapment. Rather, compression causes myelin lamellae to slip because of mechanical stresses operating in opposite directions at the sites of nerve entrapment.

The dynamics of development of distortion of myelin segments in chronically entrapped nerve fibers, in a polarized and mirror-image fashion, are not precisely known. Our explanation of why the myelin lamellae closest to the axon are most affected has been speculative: Mechanical friction or stretching of the entrapped fibers may strain the specialized subcellular attachments of myelin to

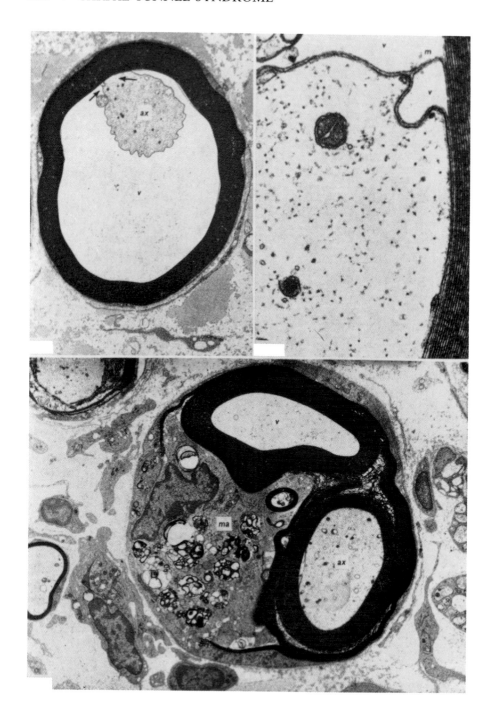

←

Figure 12.13 Pathology of neurapraxia caused by acute local external compression in limb of a baboon. **A,** Low-power electron micrograph of a nerve fiber swelling six weeks after compression. The swollen inner tongue of Schwann cell cytoplasm (*v*) separates most of the surface of the axon (*ax*) from the myelin sheath. A sector remains attached to the sheath. ×3,000. **B,** Enlargement of area *arrowed* in **A.** The mesaxon (*m*) is seen with swollen Schwann cell cytoplasm (*v*) on either side of it. ×44,000. **C,** A myelinated fiber from the same nerve as *above*, showing axon (*ax*) and a pocket of edema (*v*). A macrophage (*ma*) has penetrated the basement membrane and broken into the myelin sheath. ×4,600. (Reproduced with permission of the authors and publisher from Ochoa JL, Fowler TJ, Gilliatt RW. Anatomical changes in peripheral nerves compressed by a pneumatic tourniquet. J Anat 1972;113:433–55.)

axon; eventually, detached inner portions of myelin spiral may suffer progressive slippage following mechanical pressure waves propagated away from the site of entrapment; redundant inner myelin lamellae may be pushed into the envelope of outer myelin lamellae attached to the downstream paranode (Ochoa 1980) (Figure 12.18). When all myelin lamellae drift away, paranodal axons become obviously exposed—demyelinated. Redundant myelin lamellae at the distended paranodes may progressively compress the axon. This should alter electrical

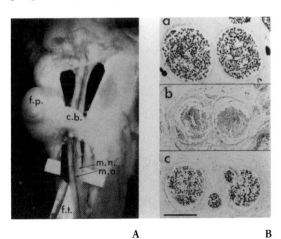

A   B

Figure 12.14 **A,** Chronic nerve entrapment in the guinea pig. A dissection of the palmar surface of the right wrist and forefoot of a young guinea pig. A piece of black card has been placed behind the median nerve (*m.n.*) and its accompanying artery (*m.a.*). The transverse cartilaginous bar (*c.b.*), which supports the footpad (*f.p.*), can be seen. Proximal to the wrist, a card marked with 1-mm squares has been inserted in front of the flexor tendons (*f.t.*). (Courtesy of Dr. J.E.C. Hern.) **B,** Two fascicles of the median nerve from transverse sections taken (*a*) above, (*b*) at, and (*c*) below the wrist. The distance between *a* and *b* was 2 mm and between *b* and *c* 3 mm. Sections fixed in Flemming's solution and stained by modified Weigert method to show myelin sheaths. Bar = 200 μm. (Reproduced with permission of the authors and publisher from Fullerton PM, Gilliatt RW. Median and ulnar neuropathy in the guinea-pig. J Neurol Neurosurg Psychiatry 1967;30:393–402.)

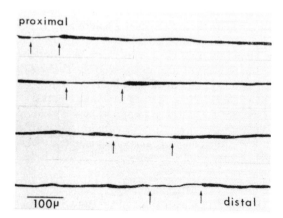

Figure 12.15 Pathology of chronic nerve entrapment in the guinea pig. Consecutive lengths of a single fiber from the median nerve in the midforearm to show intercalated segments occurring at regular intervals along the fiber. 1% osmium tetroxide. (Reproduced with permission of the authors and publisher from Anderson MH, Fullerton PM, Gilliatt RW, Hern JEC. Changes in the forearm associated with median nerve compression at the wrist in the guinea-pig. J Neurol Neurosurg Psychiatry 1970;33:70–79.)

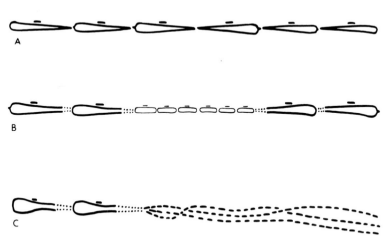

Figure 12.16 Pathology of chronic nerve entrapment in the guinea pig. **A,** Diagram showing distorted myelin segments from median nerve of young guinea pig. Note reversal of polarity at the wrist. **B,** Further distortion and exposure of the axon proximal and distal to the site of entrapment. The median nerve under the carpal tunnel has lost its original myelin segments: multiple, short remyelinated internodes repair the lesion. **C,** Advanced lesion with massive bulbs and axonal Wallerian degeneration and regeneration. (Reproduced with permission of the author and publisher from Ochoa JL. Nerve fiber pathology in acute and chronic compression. In: Omer GE Jr, Spinner M, eds. Management of peripheral nerve problems. Philadelphia: WB Saunders, 1980;495.)

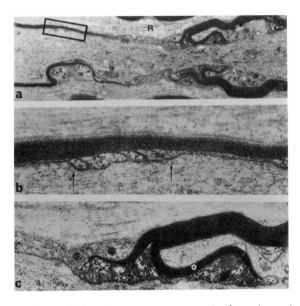

Figure 12.17 Pathology of chronic nerve entrapment in the guinea pig. **A,** Low-power electron micrograph of a moderately abnormal fiber taken from the median nerve of a guinea pig above the wrist. The paranode on the *left* is tapered. The bulbous paranode on the *right* shows inturning of a group of inner lamellae. R, node of Ranvier. ×7000. **B,** Enlargement of the area enclosed; in the *rectangle* in **A.** Six myelin lamellae end in cytoplasmic loops between the *arrows.* ×48,000. **C,** Detail of the bulbous paranode. ×20,000. (Reproduced with permission of the authors and publisher from Ochoa JL, Marotte L. The nature of the nerve lesion underlying chronic entrapment. J Neurol Sci 1973;19:491–95.)

axonal resistance and axoplasmic flow and eventually lead to axonal degeneration. Probably, critically narrowed axons distal to the site of entrapment undergo reversible partial atrophy before they degenerate. This "axon cachexia" explains subtle dysfunctions detectable electrophysiologically distal to sites of entrapment.

This distinctive pathology in chronic entrapment of animal nerves has been confirmed as a subclinical finding in human nerve trunks at common sites of entrapment (Neary and Eames 1975; Neary et al. 1975; Jefferson and Eames 1979) (Figures 12.19 and 12.20).

The myelin distortions that support a mechanical origin for the pathologic changes observed in local nerve entrapment cannot be naively taken to indicate that primary mechanical phenomena alone participate in the genesis of structural and physiologic abnormalities related to local nerve entrapment. As mentioned earlier, transient positive sensory phenomena related to local nerve entrapment probably reflect nerve fiber hyperexcitability caused by ischemia. Prolonged ischemia might cause nerve fiber hypoexcitability even in the absence of substantial morphologic changes (Sladky et al. 1991). Furthermore, subperineurial demyelination, if eventually demonstrated in human nerve fascicles at sites of

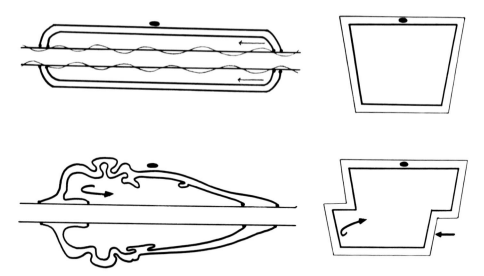

Figure 12.18 Pathology of chronic nerve entrapment in the guinea pig. *Top,* Normal myelin segment and unrolled myelin sheath *(right),* which is trapezoid shaped. Hypothetical pressure waves in the direction of the *arrows* along the axon. *Bottom,* Distorted segment with tapered end caused by myelin slippage, and bulbous end containing inturned redundant myelin lamellae. If the myelin were unrolled, it would be altered as indicated *(right).* (Reproduced with permission of the author and publisher from Ochoa JL. Nerve fiber pathology in acute and chronic compression. In: Omer GE Jr, Spinner M, eds. Management of peripheral nerve problems. Philadelphia: WB Saunders, 1980;497.)

chronic entrapment, might well be the consequence of ischemia due to impaired transperineurial circulation (Powell and Myers 1986). Finally, chronic endoneurial edema in entrapped nerves is a likely consequence of hemodynamic derangement (Sunderland 1976). Thus, both primarily mechanical and primarily ischemic events probably contribute to the development of structural abnormalities of nerve fibers, particularly of myelinated fibers, and to biophysical abnormalities leading to ectopic impulse generation, conduction block, and their clinical correlates.

SIGN OF TINEL IN CARPAL TUNNEL SYNDROME

Tinel's sign highlights a possible role of primary mechanical factors underlying the development of paresthesias in carpal tunnel. For this sign, a gentle mechanical force—tapping on the nerve—generates ectopic discharges (see Ochoa et al. 1982 for electrophysiologic evidence). The presence of hyperexcitable nerve sprouts or hyperexcitable dysmyelinated stretches of nerve fibers predisposes to the ectopic discharges (Konorski and Lubinska 1946; Brown and Iggo 1963; Smith and McDonald 1980, 1982). Therefore, conceivably, over and

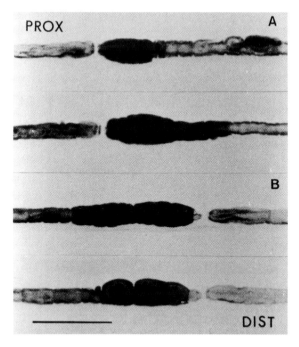

Figure 12.19 Pathology of chronic entrapment of human median nerve. **A,** two consecutive nodes from a single fiber proximal to the flexor retinaculum. **B,** Two consecutive nodes from a (different) single fiber distal to the upper border of the retinaculum. In each case, the fibers are mounted with their proximal portions to the left. Bar = 50 μm. (Reproduced with permission of the authors and publisher from Neary D, Ochoa JL, Gilliatt RW. Subclinical entrapment neuropathy in man. J Neurol Sci 1975;24:283–98.)

above ischemic and postischemic ionic phenomena, mechanical factors might operate on abnormal nerve fibers at sites of chronic entrapment to generate intermittent paresthesias, since the physiologic basis of Tinel's sign and of paresthesias is basically equivalent (Diamond et al. 1982).

RENAUT BODIES

After an original description by Renaut (1881), the peculiar bodies shown in Figure 12.21 became "forgotten endoneurial structures" (Asbury 1973). These Renaut bodies are conspicuous at sites of chronic nerve entrapment but are not exclusive to that pathologic state. We have found them in many locally entrapped nerve segments, particularly in the median and ulnar nerves at wrist and elbow, respectively. Jefferson et al. (1981) demonstrated that more than half of their 74 autopsied nerves showed these structures at sites of common entrapment but not in adjacent segments of the same nerves. They concluded that these bodies are pathologic formations without protective function.

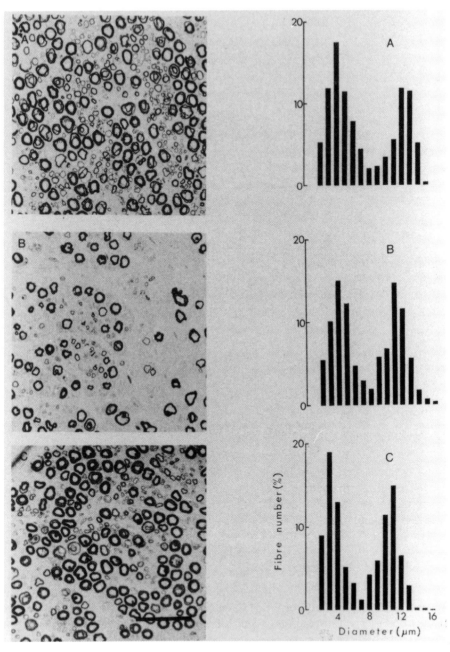

Figure 12.20 Pathology of chronic entrapment of human nerve. On the *left*, enlarged portions of transverse sections of ulnar nerve. On the *right*, histograms of fiber diameter from the same sections. **A,** Proximal to the elbow. **B,** In the ulnar groove. **C,** Distal to the elbow. Bar = 50 μm. (Reproduced with permission of the authors and publisher from Neary D, Ochoa JL, Gilliatt RW. Subclinical entrapment neuropathy in man. J Neurol Sci 1975;24:283–98.)

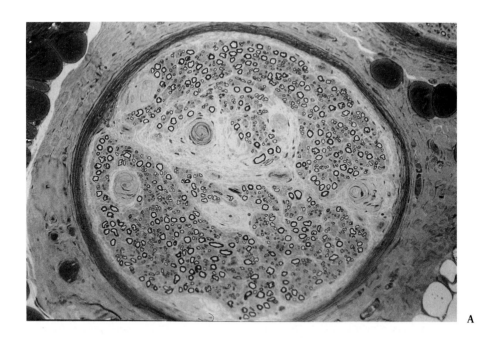

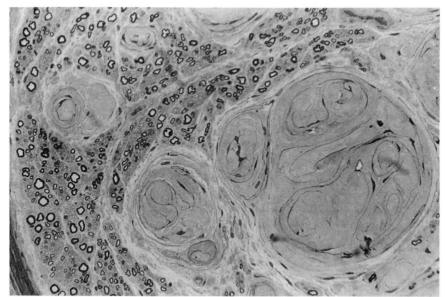

Figure 12.21 Chronic entrapment of human nerve. **A,** Cross section of fascicle obtained from the lateral femerocutaneous nerve of the thigh at the site of entrapment in a patient with meralgia paresthetica. Half a dozen Renaut bodies occur. **B,** Higher-power view of cross section of Renaut bodies from an adjacent level in the same nerve as **A.**

Renaut bodies can be microdissected out of entrapped nerves. They are spindle-shaped structures measuring up to 2 mm or more in length. While they do occupy endoneurial space, their pathophysiologic significance is unknown. Some of us have believed that they are organized remnants of endoneurial vessels. Their formation, featuring an early stage of endoneurial clefting, has been followed sequentially in experimental animals subjected to repeated mechanical trauma of plantar nerves (Ortman et al. 1983).

SOME PATHOLOGIC-PHYSIOLOGIC-CLINICAL CORRELATIONS IN CHRONIC NERVE ENTRAPMENT

The pathology of local nerve entrapment ranges from microscopically undetectable molecular disruption of the excitable biophysical apparatus, through demyelination and remyelination, to axonal degeneration and regeneration. Understandably, the clinical expression of nerve entrapment pathology include positive and negative motor and sensory and sympathetic phenomena. Regardless of whether mechanical or ischemic in origin, and regardless of whether stable or intermittent, derangements in nerve membrane excitability in local entrapment underlie the development of paresthesias and occasional myokymia and other positive phenomena traceable to motor nerve fibers. Muscle weakness associated with atrophy is obviously due to axonal interruption. Weakness may also occur when fibers with pathologic myelin sheaths develop conduction block. Moreover, weakness and muscle fatigue develop when those fibers are unable to sustain high rates of impulse discharge (McDonald 1982). Sensory deficit, when present, most commonly consists of diminished tactile acuity. Subtle sensory deficits may be expressed as clumsiness of manipulation and may be misconstrued as muscle weakness. Tactile proprioceptive deficits may interfere with performance of highly refined finger movements, such as those of skilled musicians (Johansson and Westling 1987).

Deficits in cold and warm perception and pain are inconspicuous manifestations of nerve entrapment partly because these pain and temperature modalities are served by small-caliber fibers that are affected late by pathology in local entrapment. Furthermore, patients are likely to be aware of deficits of tactile, discriminative ability of the hand, while overlooking mild deficits in protective nociception.

Similarly, sympathetic dysfunction tends not to be a prominent aspect of the clinical expression of chronic nerve entrapment (Aminoff 1979). However, in severe nerve pathology there may be clear signs of sympathetic deficit, in the form of anhydrosis and vasomotor denervation. Signs of irritation of sympathetic efferent nerve fibers in the form of excessive sweating and vasospasm are decidedly uncommon in chronic nerve entrapment and rarely reported in acute neurapraxia (Bolton and McFarlane 1978). The hypothermia related to vasospasm commonly observed in "causalgiform syndromes" usually represents a somatosympathetic reflex response rather than ectopic discharge in sympathetic fibers. Alternatively, a chronically vasoconstricted limb, a common consequence of local nerve injury, results from sympathetic denervation supersensitivity rather than from increased sympathetic neural activity.

The pathophysiology of pain in nerve injury and entrapment is treated in Chapter 16.

PRESSURE STUDIES

Measurement of physical pressure within body compartments, and even within a microenvironment such as the endoneurium, has helped understanding of the pathogenesis and mechanisms of acute nerve compression and chronic entrapment. In the mid-1970s, wick catheters became a new research and clinical tool (Whitesides et al. 1975; Mubarak et al. 1976). Measurements with these fine catheters inserted into limb compartments yield a range of normal interstitial intramuscular fluid pressures about 7 to 8 mm Hg in man. Pressures greater than 30 mm Hg presage complications such as neural deficit, Volkmann's contracture, or in extreme cases, gangrene (Mubarak et al. 1978). At pressures above 30 mm Hg, pain and paresthesias first appear (Mubarak et al. 1976; Lundborg et al. 1982; Gelberman et al. 1983). Normal capillary pressure in muscle is 20 to 30 mm Hg in cats (Fronek and Zweifach 1975) and dogs (Hargens et al. 1978). The need for dermotomy, fasciotomy, and epimysiotomy can be monitored by measuring intracompartmental fluid pressure. The most reliable physical indication of increased tissue pressure within a closed fascial space is sensory dysfunction, since all compartments in forearm and leg contain a nerve and since under the circumstances of pain and muscle swelling, motor performance is not a reliable measure. Compartment pressure sufficient to damage nerves and muscles is seldom sufficient to occlude a major artery, and thus common clinical signs of vascular dysfunction are late manifestation.

The micropipette method allows direct measurement of endoneurial fluid pressure (Low and Dyck 1977; Myers et al. 1978). Exposed rat sciatic nerves directly compressed within a special chamber for two to eight hours, at 30 mm Hg to interfere with venular flow, or at 80 mm Hg to cause circulatory arrest in the nerve, were found to have developed a three- to fourfold increase in endoneurial fluid pressure and endoneurial edema (Lundborg et al. 1983). Endoneurial edema becomes associated with progressive deposition of endoneurial collagen and may close a vicious cycle of nerve ischemia by interfering with nerve blood flow (Myers et al. 1982; Lundborg 1988). The hypertonic quality of endoneurial edema fluid may impair ionic equilibrium and interfere with excitable membrane function (Myers et al. 1978). As predicted from the distribution of nerve fiber damage in acute compression with tourniquet (Ochoa et al. 1972), the distribution of edema is at the edges of the microcuff used by Lundborg, Myers, and Powell, as strikingly illustrated to the naked eye by Evans blue extravasation (Lundborg 1988).

Findings and mechanisms analogous to those documented for nerve seem to apply to compression of dorsal root ganglia (Rydevik et al. 1989).

Pressure studies in the carpal tunnel have revealed striking correlations with clinical and electrophysiologic parameters in symptomatic patients with carpal tunnel syndrome. Increased canal pressures have been recorded in several independent studies (Gelberman et al. 1981; Lundborg et al. 1982; Werner et al. 1983; Chaise and Witvoet 1984; Szabo and Chidgey 1989). Patients often have pressures around 30 mm Hg with the wrist in the neutral position. This is just below the level needed to induce symptoms of nerve compression. The canal pressure in both normals and patients with carpal tunnel syndrome increases significantly with wrist flexion and extension so that pressure in the carpal tunnel fluctuates continually during normal daily activities (Smith et al. 1977; Werner et al. 1983). Increase in pressure with wrist flexion explains the effect of Phalen's wrist flexion test. Therapeutic wrist splinting prevents some of these recurring daily increases in canal pressure.

In patients with carpal tunnel syndrome, the pressure is usually highest in the distal third of the tunnel (Luchetti et al. 1989, 1990). Intraoperative sensory nerve conduction studies show the greatest slowing of nerve conduction and decrement of sensory nerve action potential (SNAP) amplitude along the nerve in this distal portion of the canal (Luchetti et al. 1990).

Carpal tunnel pressure measurements are not useful as a routine diagnostic test for carpal tunnel syndrome. In addition to their invasive nature, they do not reliably distinguish symptomatic from asymptomatic patients.

REFERENCES

Aguayo AJ, Nair CPV, Midgley R. Experimental progressive compression neuropathy in the rabbit. Histologic and electrophysiologic studies. Arch Neurol 1971;24:358–64.

Aminoff MJ. Involvement of peripheral vasomotor fibres in carpal tunnel syndrome. J Neurol Neurosurg Psychiatry 1979;42:649–55.

Anderson MH, Fullerton PM, Gilliatt RW, Hern JEC. Changes in the forearm associated with median nerve compression at the wrist in the guinea-pig. J Neurol Neurosurg Psychiatry 1970;33:70–79.

Asbury AK. Ischemic disorders of peripheral nerve. In: Vinken PJ, Bruyn GW, eds. Handbook of clinical neurology. Amsterdam: North-Holland, 1970;8:154–164.

Asbury AK. Renaut bodies: a forgotten endoneurial structure. J Neuropathol Exp Neurol 1973;32:334–43.

Asbury AK, Johnson PC. Pathology of peripheral nerve. Philadelphia: WB Saunders, 1978.

Bennett GJ, Xie Y-K. A peripheral mononeuropathy in rat that produces disorders of pain sensation like those seen in man. Pain 1988;33:87–107.

Bergmans J. Physiological observations on single human nerve fibres. In: Desmedt JE, ed. New developments in electromyography and clinical neurophysiology. Basel: S Karger, 1973;2:89–127.

Bergmans J. Modifications induced by ischemia in the recovery of human motor axons from activity. In: Culp WJ, Ochoa JL, eds. Abnormal nerves and muscles as impulse generators. New York: Oxford University Press, 1982a;419–42.

Bergmans J. Repetitive activity induced in single human motor axons: a model for pathological repetitive activity. In: Culp WJ, Ochoa JL, eds. Abnormal nerves and muscles as impulse generators. New York: Oxford University Press, 1982b;393–418.

Bolton FB, McFarlane RM. Human pneumatic tourniquet paralysis. Neurology (Minneap) 1978;28:787–93.

Brown AG, Iggo A. The structure and function of cutaneous "touch corpuscles" after nerve crush. J Physiol (Lond) 1963;165:28–29P.

Cajal SR. Degeneration and regeneration of the nervous system. Vols 1–2. London: Oxford University Press, 1928.

Chaise F, Witvoet J. Mesures des pressions intracanalaires dans le syndrome du canal carpien idiopathique non déficitaire. Rev. Chir. Orthop., 1984;70:75–78.

Culp WJ, Ochoa JL, eds. Abnormal nerves and muscles as impulse generators. New York: Oxford University Press, 1982.

Denny-Brown D, Brenner C. The effect of percussion of nerve. J Neurol Neurosurg Psychiatry 1944a;7:76–95.

Denny-Brown D, Brenner C. Paralysis of nerve induced by direct pressure and by tourniquet. Arch Neurol Psychiatry 1944b;51:1–26.

Diamond J, Ochoa JL, Culp WJ. An introduction to abnormal nerves and muscles as impulse generators. In: Culp WJ, Ochoa JL, eds. Abnormal nerves and muscles as impulse generators. New York: Oxford University Press, 1982;3–24.

Dyck PJ. Experimental hypertrophic neuropathy: pathogenesis of onion bulb formations produced by repeated tourniquet applications. Arch Neurol 1969;21:73–95.

Eames RA, Lange LS. Clinical and pathological study of ischaemic neuropathy. J Neurol Neurosurg Psychiatry 1967;30:215–26.

Erb W. Diseases of the peripheral cerebrospinal nerves. In: Ziemssen H von, ed. Cyclopedia of the practice of medicine. Vol 11. London: Samson Low, Marston, Searle and Rivington, 1876.

Erlanger J, Blair EA. Comparative observations on motor and sensory fibers with special reference to repetitiousness. Am J Physiol 1938;121: 431–453.

Fowler TJ. Tourniquet paralysis in the baboon. DM thesis, University of Oxford, 1975.

Fowler TJ, Danta G, Gilliatt RW. Recovery of nerve conduction after a pneumatic tourniquet: observations on the hind-limb of the baboon. J Neurol Neurosurg Psychiatry 1972;35:638–47.

Fowler TJ, Ochoa JL. Unmyelinated fibres in normal and compressed peripheral nerves of the baboon: a quantitative electron microscopic study. Neuropathol Appl Neurobiol 1975;1:247–65.

Fronek K, Zweifach BW. Microvascular pressure distribution in skeletal muscle and the effect of vasodilatation. Am J Physiol 1975;228:791–96.

Fujimura H, Lacroix C, Said G. Vulnerability of nerve fibres to ischaemia. A quantitative light and electron microscope study. Brain 1991;114:1929–42.

Fullerton PM, Gilliatt RW. Median and ulnar neuropathy in the guinea-pig. J Neurol Neurosurg Psychiatry 1967;30:393–402.

Gairns FW, Garven HSD, Smith G. The digital nerves and the nerve endings in progressive obliterative vascular disease of the leg. Scott Med J 1960;5:382–91.

Garven HSD, Gairns FW, Smith G. The nerve fibre populations of the nerves of the leg in chronic occlusive arterial disease in man. Scott Med J 1962;7:250–65.

Gasser HS. Conduction in nerves in relation to fiber types. Association for Research in Nervous and Mental Disease, 1935;15:35–59.

Gasser HS, Grundfest H. Action and excitability in mammalian A fibers. Am J Physiol 1936;117: 113–133.

Gelberman R, Hergenroeder P, Hargens A, Lundborg G, Akeson W. The carpal tunnel syndrome. A study of carpal tunnel pressures. J Bone Joint Surg 1981;61A:380–83.

Gelberman R, Szabo RM, Williamson RV, Dimick MP. Sensibility testing in peripheral nerve compression syndromes. An experimental study in humans. J Bone Joint Surg 1983;65A:632–38.

Grundfest H. Effects of hydrostatic pressures upon the excitability, the recovery, and the potential sequence of frog nerve. Cold Spring Harbor Symp Quant Biol 1936;4:179–87.

Hargens AR, Akeson WH, Mubarak SJ, Owen CA, Evans KL, Garetto LP, Schmidt DA.

Fluid balance within the canine anterolateral compartment and its relationship to compartment syndromes. J Bone Joint Surg 1978;60A:499–505.

Harrison MJG. Pressure palsy of the ulnar nerve with prolonged conduction block. J Neurol Neurosurg Psychiatry 1976;39:96–99.

Hess K, Eames RA, Darveniza P, Gilliatt RW. Acute ischaemic neuropathy in the rabbit. J Neurol Sci 1979;44:19–43.

Jefferson D, Eames RA. Subclinical entrapment of the lateral femoral cutaneous nerve: an autopsy study. Muscle Nerve 1979;2:145–54.

Jefferson D, Neary D, Eames RA. Renaut body distribution at sites of human peripheral nerve entrapment. J Neurol Sci 1981;49:19–29.

Joffroy A, Achard C. Nevrite périphérique d'origine vasculaire. Arch Med Exp 1889;1:229–40.

Johansson RS, Westling G. Significance of cutaneous input for precise hand movements. Electroencephalogr Clin Neurophysiol Suppl 1987;39:53–57.

Konorski J, Lubinska L. Mechanical excitability of regenerating nerve fibers. Lancet 1946;1:609–10.

Korthals JK, Wisniewski HM. Peripheral nerve ischemia. Part 1. Experimental model. J Neurol Sci 1975;24:65–76.

Kugelberg E. Accommodation in human nerves and its significance for the symptoms in circulatory disturbances and tetany. Acta Physiol Scand 1944;8: Suppl. XXIV, 1–105.

Lewis T, Pickering GW, Rothschild P. Centripetal paralysis arising out of arrested blood flow to the limb, including notes on a form of tingling. Heart 1931;16:1–32.

Low PA, Dyck PJ. Increased endoneurial fluid pressure in experimental lead neuropathy. Nature 1977;269:427–28.

Luchetti R, Schoenhuber R, Alfarano M, Deluca S, De Cicco G, Landi A. Carpal tunnel syndrome: correlations between pressure measurement and intraoperative electrophysiological nerve study. Muscle Nerve 1990;13:1164–68.

Luchetti R, Schoenhuber R, De Cicco G, Alfarano M, Deluca S, Landi A. Carpal-tunnel pressure. Acta Orthop Scand 1989;60:396–99.

Lundborg G. Ischemic nerve injury. Experimental studies on intraneural microvascular pathophysiology and nerve function in a limb, subjected to temporary circulatory arrest. Scand J Plastic Reconstr Surg Supplement 6 1970; pages 1–113.

Lundborg G. Structure and function of the intraneural microvessels as related to trauma, edema formation and nerve function. J Bone Joint Surg 1975;57A:938–48.

Lundborg G. The intrinsic vascularization of human peripheral nerves. Structural and functional aspects. J Hand Surg 1979;4:34–41.

Lundborg G. Intraneural microcirculation and peripheral nerve barriers. In: Omer G, Spinner M, eds. Management of peripheral nerve problems. Philadelphia: WB Saunders, 1980;903–16.

Lundborg G. Nerve injury and repair. New York, Edinburgh: Churchill Livingstone, 1988.

Lundborg G, Gelberman R, Minteer-Convery M, Lee VF, Hargens A. Median nerve compression in the carpal tunnel: the functional response to experimentally induced controlled pressure. J Hand Surg 1982;7:252–59.

Lundborg G, Myers R, Powell H. Nerve compression injury and increase in endoneurial fluid pressure: "miniature compartment syndrome." J Neurol Neurosurg Psychiatry 1983;46:1119–24.

Lundborg G, Nordborg C, Rydevik B, Olsson Y. The effect of ischemia on the permeability of the perineurium to protein tracers in rabbit tibial nerve. Acta Neurol Scand 1973;49:287–94.

Lundborg G, Rydevik B. Effects of stretching the tibial nerve of the rabbit. A preliminary study of the intraneural circulation and the barrier function of the perineurium. J Bone Joint Surg 1973;55B:390–401.

Marie P, Foix C. Atrophic isolée de l'éminence thénar d'origine névritique. Rôle du ligament annulaire antérieur du carpal dans la pathogénie de la lésion. Rev Neurol (Paris) 1913;26:647.

McDonald WI. Clinical consequences of conduction defects produced by demyelination. In: Culp WJ, Ochoa JL, eds. Abnormal nerves and muscles as impulse generators. New York: Oxford University Press, 1982;253–70.

Merrington WR, Nathan PW. A study of post-ischaemic paresthesiae. J Neurol Neurosurg Psychiatry 1949;12:1–18.

Moldaver J. Tourniquet paralysis syndrome. Arch Surg 1954;68:136–44.

Mubarak SJ, Hargens AR, Owen CA, Garetto LP, Akeson WH. The wick catheter technique for measurement of intramuscular pressure. A new research and clinical tool. J Bone Joint Surg 1976;58A:1016–20.

Mubarak SJ, Owen CA, Hargens AR, Garetto LP, Akeson WH. Acute compartment syndromes: diagnosis and treatment with the aid of the Wick catheter. J Bone Joint Surg 1978;60A:1091–95.

Myers RR, Mizisin AP, Powell HC, Lampert PW. Reduced nerve blood flow in hexachlorophene neuropathy. Relationship to elevated endoneurial fluid pressure. J Neuropathol Exp Neurol 1982;41:391–99.

Myers RR, Powell HC, Costello ML, Lambert PW, Zweifach BW. Endoneurial fluid pressure: direct measurement with micropipettes. Brain Res 1978;148:510–15.

Myers RR, Murakami H, Powell HC. Reduced nerve blood flow in edematous neuropathies—a biochemical mechanism. Microvasc Res 1986;32:145–51.

Nathan PW. Ischaemic and post-ischaemic numbness and paraesthesiae. J Neurol Neurosurg Psychiatry 1958;21:12–23.

Neary D, Eames RA. The pathology of ulnar nerve compression in man. Neuropathol Appl Neurobiol 1975;1:69–88.

Neary D, Ochoa JL, Gilliatt RW. Subclinical entrapment neuropathy in man. J Neurol Sci 1975;24:283–98.

Nukada H, Dyck PJ. Microsphere embolization of nerve capillaries and fiber degeneration. Am J Pathol 1984;115:275–87.

Ochoa JL. Ultrathin longitudinal sections of single myelinated fibres for electron microscopy. J Neurol Sci 1972;17:103–6.

Ochoa JL. Nerve fiber pathology in acute and chronic compression. In: Omer GE Jr and Spinner M, eds. Management of peripheral nerve problems. Philadelphia: WB Saunders, 1980;487–501.

Ochoa JL. Some aberrations of nerve repair. In: Gorio A, Millesi H, Mingrino S, eds. Post traumatic peripheral nerve regeneration: experimental basis and clinical implications. New York: Raven Press, 1981;147–55.

Ochoa JL, Danta G, Fowler TJ, Gilliatt RW. Nature of the nerve lesion caused by a pneumatic tourniquet. Nature 1971;233:265–66.

Ochoa JL, Fowler TJ, Gilliatt RW. Anatomical changes in peripheral nerves compressed by a pneumatic tourniquet. J Anat 1972;113:433–55.

Ochoa JL, Fowler TJ, Gilliatt RW. Changes produced by a pneumatic tourniquet. In: Desmedt JE, ed. New developments in electromyography and clinical neurophysiology. Basel: Karger, 1973;2:166–73.

Ochoa JL, Marotte L. The nature of the nerve lesion underlying chronic entrapment. J Neurol Sci 1973;19:491–95.

Ochoa JL, Torebjörk HE. Paresthesiae from ectopic impulse generation in human sensory nerves. Brain 1980;103:835–53.

Ochoa JL, Torebjörk HE. Sensations evoked by intraneural microstimulation of single mechanoreceptor units innervating the human hand. J Physiol, 1983;342:633–654.

Ochoa JL, Torebjörk HE. Sensations evoked by intraneural microstimulation of C nociceptor fibres in human skin nerves. J Physiol (London) 1989;415:583–99.

Ochoa JL, Torebjörk HE, Culp WJ, Schady W. Abnormal spontaneous activity in single sensory nerve fibers in humans. Muscle Nerve 1982;5:S74–S77.

Olsson Y. The involvement of vasa nervorum in diseases of peripheral nerves. In: Vimkem, PJ and Bruyn V, eds. Handbook of clinical neurology, part II. Vol 12. Vascular diseases of the nervous system. Amsterdam, North Holland Publishing Co., 1972;641–64.

Olsson Y, Kristensson K. The perineurium as a diffusion barrier to protein tracers following trauma to nerves. Acta Neuropathol (Berl) 1973;23:105–11.

Olsson Y, Reese TS. Permeability of vasa nervorum and perineurium in mouse sciatic nerve studied by fluorescence and electron microscopy. J Neuropathol Exp Neurol 1971;30:105–19.

Ortman JA, Sahenk Z, Mendell JR. The experimental production of Renaut bodies. J Neurol Sci 1983;62:233–41.

Parry GJ, Brown MJ. Arachidonate-induced experimental nerve infarction. J Neurol Sci 1981;50:123–33.

Powell HC, Myers RR. Pathology of experimental nerve compression. Lab Invest 1986;55:91–100.

Raff MC, Sangalang V, Asbury AK. Ischemic mononeuropathy multiplex associated with diabetes mellitus. Arch Neurol 1968;18:487–499.

Renaut J. Système hyalin de soutènement des centres nerveux et de quelques organes des sense. Arch Physiol Norm Pathol 1881;8:846–859.

Richardson PM, Thomas PK. Percussive injury to peripheral nerve in rats. J Neurosurg 1979;51:178–87.

Rudge P. Tourniquet paralysis with prolonged conduction block: electrophysiological study. J Bone Joint Surg 1974;56B:716–20.

Rudge P, Ochoa JL, Gilliatt RW. Acute peripheral nerve compression in the baboon. Anatomical and physiological findings. J Neurol Sci 1974;23:403–20.

Rydevik B. Compression injury of peripheral nerve. Experimental studies on microcirculation, oedema formation, axonal transport, fibre structure and function in nerves subjected to acute, graded compression. Thesis, University of Göteborg. Göteborg, 1979.

Rydevik B, McLean WG, Sjöstrand J, Lundborg G. Blockage of axonal transport induced by acute graded compression of the rabbit vagus nerve. J Neurol Neurosurg Psychiatry 1980;43:690–98.

Rydevik BL, Myers RR, Powell HC. Pressure increase in the dorsal root ganglion following mechanical compression. Closed compartment syndrome in nerve roots. Spine 1989;14:574–76.

Seddon HJ. Three types of nerve injury. Brain 1943;66:237–88.

Sinclair DC, Hinshaw JR. A comparison of the dissociation produced by procaine and by limb ischaemia. Brain 1950;73:480–98.

Sivak M, Ochoa JL. Positive manifestations of nerve fiber dysfunction: clinical, electrophysiologic, and pathologic correlates. In: Brown WF, Bolton CF, eds. Clinical electromyography: Boston: Butterworths, 1987;1–30.

Sladsky JT, Tschoepe RL, Greenberg JH, Brown MJ. Peripheral neuropathy after chronic endoneurial ischemia. Ann Neurol 1991;29:272–78.

Smith EM, Sonstegard DA, Anderson WH Jr. Carpal tunnel syndrome: contribution of flexor tendons. Arch Phys Med Rehabil 1977;58:379–85.

Smith KJ, McDonald WI. Spontaneous and mechanically evoked activity due to central demyelinating lesion. Nature 1980;286:154–55.

Smith KJ, McDonald WI. Spontaneous and evoked electrical discharges from a central demyelinating lesion. J Neurol Sci 1982;55:39–47.

Sunderland S. The nerve lesion in the carpal tunnel syndrome. J Neurol Neurosurg Psychiatry 1976;39:615–626.

Szabo RM, Chidgey LK. Stress carpal tunnel pressure in patients with carpal tunnel syndrome and normal patients. J Hand Surg 1989;14A:624–27.

Thomas PK, Fullerton PM. Nerve fiber size in the carpal tunnel syndrome. J Neurol Neurosurg Psychiatry 1963;26:520–27.

Werner CO, Elmquist D, Ohlin P. Pressure and nerve lesion in the carpal tunnel. Acta Orthop Scand 1983;54:312–16.

Whitesides TE Jr, Haney TC, Morimoto K, Harada H. Tissue pressure measurements as a determinant for the need of fasciotomy. Clin Orthop 1975;113:43–51.

Yarnitsky D, Ochoa JL. Release of cold-induced burning pain by block of cold-specific afferent input. Brain 1990;113:893–902.

Yarnitsky D, Ochoa JL. Differential effect of compression-ischaemia block on warm sensation and heat-induced pain. Brain 1991;114:907–13.

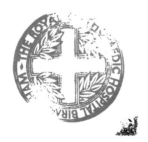

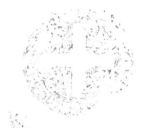

13

Activity, Occupation, and Carpal Tunnel Syndrome

Activities that can cause carpal tunnel syndrome include sustained wrist or palmar pressure, repetitive hand and wrist use, work with vibrating tools, and possibly hand use in the cold.

HISTORICAL BACKGROUND

Insight into the role of activities or occupations in causing median neuropathy has a long tradition. Before recognition of the pathogenic importance of the carpal tunnel, Oppenheim's *Textbook of Nervous Diseases* (1911) listed laundry women, joiners, locksmiths, milkers, cigar makers, carpet beaters, and dentists among those prone to occupational median nerve pareses. In their seminal report on carpal tunnel syndrome in six women, Brain et al. (1947) characterized median nerve compression in the carpal tunnel as "spontaneous" but thought that manual work was a contributing factor to development of the syndrome. Kendall (1950, 84) described five cases of carpal tunnel syndrome that he attributed to "unusually heavy household duties rather late in life." Tanzer (1959) stressed the role of increased hand use prior to onset of symptoms.

Over the years, numerous reports have associated carpal tunnel syndrome with various professions. Most of these reports have been based on single cases or clusters of cases, and skeptics have pointed to the high incidence of carpal tunnel syndrome in the general population as evidence that these associations may be fortuitous. For example, Phalen (1966, 219) emphasized that the largest group of his patients were housewives and wrote, "Common, typical, carpal-tunnel syndrome—spontaneous compression neuropathy of the median nerve in the carpal tunnel—is not an occupational disease." He thus evaded the issue of whether the activities of a housewife might be a contributing factor to pathogenesis. He did, however, concede that excessive hand use is a contributing factor in some cases.

Birkbeck and Beer (1975) surveyed the activities of 588 patients who had both symptoms of carpal tunnel syndrome and abnormal median nerve conduction studies. Of the employed patients without medical conditions that might predispose to development of carpal tunnel syndrome, 79% worked in occupations requiring repetitive hand movements. Of the 72 housewives, 51% were knitters. The study made no attempt to quantify or better define "repetitive hand movement" and provided no control data on the activities or hobbies of a nonaffected peer group. Table 13.1 lists selected case reports and case clusters to illustrate the wide variety of activities and professions that have been purported to cause carpal syndrome.

CONTROVERSY

Despite widespread recognition of the relationship between hand and wrist use and symptoms of carpal tunnel syndrome, some authors still debate whether activities are a cause of the basic pathology underlying the syndrome. For instance, Hadler (1987), Nathan et al. (1988), and Schottland et al. (1991) have been dubious of a causal role for occupation in carpal tunnel syndrome patients.

Nathan et al. and Schottland et al. have shown that subtle abnormalities of median nerve conduction can frequently be detected in workers whether or not they use their hands for heavy or repetitive work. Since median nerve conduction

Table 13.1 Examples of occupations and conditions associated with carpal tunnel syndrome

Setting	Reference
Automotive worker	Gordon et al. 1987 Rothfleisch and Sherman 1976
Cardiologist	Stevens 1990
Cornhusker	Jones and Scheker 1988
Dental hygienist	Osborn et al. 1990 Bauer 1985
Dystonic-athetotic wrist posture	Alvarez et al. 1982
Electrician	Bleecker et al. 1985
Forester, logger	Farkkila et al. 1988
Grocery checker	Barnhart and Rosenstock 1987
Musician	Hochberg et al. 1983
Paraplegic	Gellman et al. 1988 Aljure et al. 1985
Polio victim	Werner et al. 1989 Waring and Werner 1989
Rock driller	Chatterjee et al. 1982
Sign language interpreter	Stedt 1989
Staple gun user	Hoffman and Hoffman 1985

abnormalities can be asymptomatic, these observations do not resolve the issue of whether certain activities can cause carpal tunnel syndrome.

Armstrong and Silverstein (1987) have urged use of a formal epidemiologic analysis to clarify the controversy. Epidemiologic evidence for a causal relationship starts with demonstration of a strong and consistent statistical correlation between activities and the occurrence of carpal tunnel syndrome. In addition to the statistical correlation, the dose-response relation between reputed cause and effect, the temporal relation between reputed cause and effect, and the biologic plausibility of the relation are needed to support the causal nature of the association (MacMahon and Pugh 1970; Fletcher et al. 1982; Mausner and Kramer 1985).

EPIDEMIOLOGY

There is little published data on the incidence of carpal tunnel syndrome among workers. The data available suggest that carpal tunnel syndrome among workers differs in incidence and in age and sex distribution compared with carpal tunnel syndrome in the general population.

For the 1.3 million workers covered by the Washington State workers' compensation system, the incidence of accepted claims for carpal tunnel syndrome was 1.7 cases per 1,000 workers per year from 1984 to 1988 (Franklin et al. 1990, 1991). Workers in some industries had yearly incidences of over 10 cases per 1,000 workers; oyster, crab, and clam packers had the highest yearly incidence, with 26 cases per 1,000 workers. Table 13.2 contrasts the epidemiology of carpal tunnel syndrome in Washington State workers and in the citizens of Rochester, Minnesota (Stevens et al. 1988). The incidence of carpal tunnel syndrome is higher among workers than in the general population. Carpal tunnel syndrome is likely to occur at a younger age in workers than in the general population. Male workers are more likely than males in the general population to develop carpal tunnel syndrome.

The workers' compensation claims for carpal tunnel syndrome in Oregon State for the year 1988 showed a different incidence of the syndrome (Oregon Department of Insurance and Finance 1990). There was 1 accepted carpal

Table 13.2 Epidemiology of carpal tunnel syndrome

	Washington State Workers, 1984–1988[a]	Rochester, Minnesota, General Population, 1976–80[b]
Cases per 1,000 person years	1.7	0.12
Peak age incidence	25–34 years	55–64 years
Female-to-male case ratio	1.2	2.8

[a]Data from Franklin et al. 1991. [b]Data from Stevens et al. 1988.

tunnel syndrome claim for disability for every 1,000 Oregon workers. The incidence was highest (2.1/1,000 workers) in manufacturing and lowest (0.3/1,000 workers) in finance, insurance, and real estate. Peak age incidence was 37 years. Female to male ratio was 1.1.

The Oregon and Washington state workers' compensation data may not be strictly comparable with the Rochester population study. The Rochester series took great care to confirm that the diagnosis was made uniformly and correctly. Matte et al. (1989) have proposed guidelines for detection of work-related carpal tunnel syndrome to improve case recognition and reporting. The recent media and lay attention to carpal tunnel syndrome may have lead to increased case recognition or even overdiagnosis in recent years compared with the 1970s. Nonetheless, the comparison supports the thesis that among manual workers, carpal tunnel syndrome may occur with higher incidence, at a younger age, and more often in males than carpal tunnel syndrome in a population unselected for occupation.

STATISTICAL STUDIES ON RELATION BETWEEN MANUAL ACTIVITY AND CARPAL TUNNEL SYNDROME

A correlation between manual activity and detection of cases of carpal tunnel syndrome has been shown most convincingly in meat and poultry processors, electronics assemblers, garment workers, aircraft workers, and frozen food processors.

Repetitive hand activities can cause hand and arm symptoms through mechanisms other than carpal tunnel syndrome. Some of the literature on occupational hand symptoms does not carefully separate patients with carpal tunnel syndrome from patients with other hand syndromes. Carpal tunnel syndrome in the workplace has received widespread public attention, and workers now often assume that their hand symptoms are due to carpal tunnel syndrome; however, a careful clinical assessment may establish a different diagnosis. The studies reviewed here are chosen for their care in defining carpal tunnel syndrome and, in most cases, for their comparison of affected workers to control populations.

Meat and Poultry Processors

Masear et al. (1986) described a meat packing plant in Illinois in which 15% of employees underwent carpal tunnel release over 12 years. Carpal tunnel syndrome, severe enough to require surgical therapy, occurred in 19% of workers doing boning activities that required bilateral repetitive wrist motions, including extreme flexion and ulnar deviation and work with meat cooled to 3° C. In comparison, workers on the loading dock and in sanitation had an incidence of carpal tunnel surgery of 4%. Of the 117 employees with carpal tunnel syndrome, 64 had bilateral surgery. Most of the patients with unilateral carpal tunnel syndrome had involvement of their dominant hand. The authors concluded that wrist motions during meat cutting contributed to the high incidence of carpal tunnel syndrome among the workers.

The study was retrospective and not formally controlled. The authors cited a meat packing plant in a different state with a much lower prevalence of carpal tunnel syndrome than in the plant they studied. They questioned what roles worker awareness of carpal tunnel syndrome and size of workers' compensation benefits played in explaining differences in prevalence.

Falck and Aarnio (1983) provided data from another group of butchers. They studied 17 butchers in two slaughterhouses in a Finnish town. In these plants the butchers usually used their knives or other tools in their dominant right hand, while using the left hand to grasp, lift, or tear the carcass. The incidence of symptomatic carpal tunnel syndrome was 4 of 17 in the right hand and 9 of 17 in the left hand. In cases with bilateral symptoms, the right hand was always less severely affected. Falck and Aarnio proposed that vigorous use of the nondominant hand explained the unusually high incidence of carpal tunnel syndrome in these workers.

Electronics Assemblers

Feldman et al. (1987) studied an electronics assembly plant with 700 employees. The plant came to their attention because 52 workers' compensation claims for carpal tunnel syndrome had been filed among its employees within five years. The authors divided the plant into high-risk and low-risk jobs. The high-risk jobs (shaker bar welding, radial welding, axial welding, and integrated line work) were reviewed and found to require highly repetitive "exertional flexion-extension-pinching motions." Workers from the high-risk jobs were more likely than workers from the low-risk jobs to have hand symptoms, positive Phalen's signs, or hand weakness.

Garment Workers

Punnett et al. (1985) surveyed women working in a garment sewing shop near Boston. Women working in a hospital (nurses, laboratory technicians, food and laundry workers, and administrative personnel but not typists) served as controls. The prevalence of carpal tunnel syndrome was 18% in the garment workers but only 6% in the hospital workers. Garment workers were three times more likely than hospital workers to have carpal tunnel syndrome diagnosed (95% confidence limits of relative risk were 1.2 to 7.6). Among the garment workers, incidence of carpal tunnel syndrome varied with task. The highest incidence, 5.6 times higher than hospital workers, was among linings stitchers. This job required repetitive low-force wrist and fine finger movements. Underpressers, who did hand ironing requiring arm pressure but less movement at the wrists and fingers, were only 1.5 times more likely than hospital workers to develop carpal tunnel syndrome.

Aircraft Builders

Cannon et al. (1981) studied carpal tunnel syndrome in four plants of the Pratt and Whitney Aircraft Company. They compared the manual activities of 30 patients with carpal tunnel syndrome to those of 90 matched control employees without carpal tunnel syndrome. Some 70% of patients but only 14% of controls worked with vibrating hand tools (surface grinders, polisher/buffers, and small hand tools), giving a statistically significant association between vibrating tool use and carpal tunnel syndrome ($p < 0.01$ by chi-square). A nonstatistically significant association was found with "performance of repetitive motion tasks." The results are illustrated in Figure 13.1.

Processors of Frozen Food

Among workers in a Taiwanese frozen food processing plant, those whose work required repetitive wrist movement were 14 times more likely than other workers to develop carpal tunnel syndrome (Chiang et al. 1990). Hand exposure to cold during work was also associated with an increased risk of developing carpal tunnel syndrome.

Surgical Patients

Wieslander et al. (1989) used hospital records to match patients who had had carpal tunnel surgery to randomly chosen controls. The patients who had carpal tunnel surgery were significantly more likely than controls to use vibrating

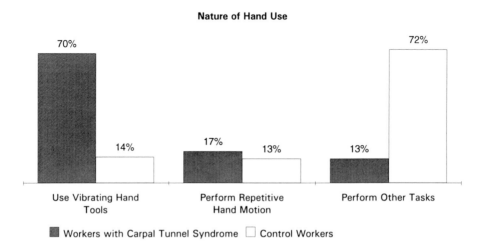

Figure 13.1 Development of carpal tunnel syndrome in aircraft builders. Use of vibrating tools was a statistically significant risk factor ($p < 0.01$) for developing carpal tunnel syndrome. The relationship between performing repetitive motion tasks and development of carpal tunnel syndrome was not statistically significant in this study. (Data from Cannon et al. 1981.)

hand tools, to do repetitive wrist movements, or to do work that placed a heavy load on their wrists.

TEMPORAL RELATIONSHIP—ACTIVITY AND CARPAL TUNNEL SYNDROME

Patients with carpal tunnel syndrome commonly observe that symptoms are closely related in time to certain hand activities. Symptoms routinely occur with rest or sleep following those activities. Frequently, workers with carpal tunnel syndrome can identify job tasks that are likely to make them symptomatic. They may note transient relief of symptoms on weekends or vacations. A job change may lead to complete resolution of symptoms (Gordon et al. 1987).

The connection between hand use and *symptoms* of carpal tunnel syndrome is unequivocal. However, whether hand use is the *cause* of the median neuropathy underlying the carpal tunnel syndrome is a more difficult question. For example, the occurrence of symptoms while driving is a common experience, but this no more proves that driving is a cause of pathology than does the prevalence of nocturnal symptoms implicate sleep as a causative factor. Nonetheless, the persuasive temporal patterns of certain activities convincingly preceding the appearance of symptoms, in many individuals, support the hypothesis that hand usage may cause median nerve pathology and trigger expression of carpal tunnel syndrome.

DOSE-RESPONSE RELATIONSHIP

Many carpal tunnel syndrome patients can clearly delineate a personal dose-response relationship, describing activities of specific nature or duration that induce their symptoms. For example, a questionnaire study of supermarket checkers showed an increased incidence of hand symptoms in workers with more years on the job, more hours worked weekly, and more use of laser scanners (Margolis and Kraus 1987). However, the differences were small, and statistical significance was not analyzed.

There are few studies that formally correlate "dose" of hand activity with development of symptoms of carpal tunnel syndrome. Silverstein et al. (1987) surveyed 652 workers in six industries (electronics assembly, major appliance manufacture, investment casing, apparel sewing, ductile iron foundry, and bearing manufacture). They inspected each job and classified it as high or low repetitiveness and high or low force. The classifications were carefully defined and confirmed by videotape and electromyographic analysis of the job activity. As shown in Figure 13.2, the prevalence of carpal tunnel syndrome was lowest among workers on "low-force, low-repetitiveness" jobs and highest among workers on "high-force, high-repetitiveness" jobs. Highly repetitive wrist movement was a greater risk factor for development of carpal tunnel syndrome than was forceful wrist use.

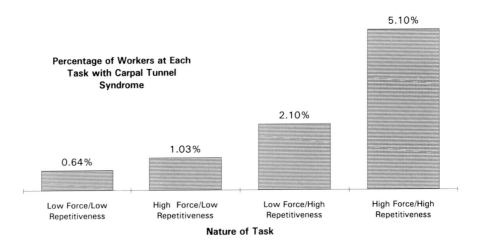

Figure 13.2 "Dose" of wrist activity and risk of developing carpal tunnel syndrome. (Data from Silverstein et al. 1987.)

BIOLOGIC PLAUSIBILITY

The causal relationship between mechanical activities of the hand and development of local median nerve pathology that is expressed as carpal tunnel syndrome is solidly supported by two facts:

1. Carpal tunnel syndrome results from chronic focal compressive neuropathy. Pathologically, the portion of the median nerve contained within the carpal tunnel shows physical slippage of myelin lamellae in opposite directions on either end of the site of entrapment (Ochoa and Marotte 1973; see Chapter 12 for detailed discussion). This localized nerve pathology documents the focal and mechanical nature of the pathogenetic process.

2. As a result of variations in wrist posture and activity, pressure increases intermittently within the carpal tunnel to levels high enough to cause nerve injury. Chapter 12 provides a review of studies of pressure in the carpal tunnel. Patients with carpal tunnel syndrome frequently have elevated resting pressures in the carpal canal. Pressures on the order of 30 mm Hg may not cause steady symptoms of nerve compression but do cause endoneurial edema and pathologic change in nerve (Lundborg et al. 1983).

The chronic increase in canal pressure in most patients with carpal tunnel syndrome is caused by synovial edema in the flexor tendons. In most patients with carpal tunnel syndrome, flexor synovium does typically show edema and fibrosis without evidence of a cellular inflammatory response (Faithfull et al. 1986; and others; see further discussion in Chapter 5).

The flexor tendon edema is probably caused in many cases by repetitive finger and wrist use. In rabbits, repetitive wrist and finger flexion induced by median nerve stimulation at 80/min for 10 hours led to edema within the carpal tunnel and to slowed median nerve conduction across the carpal tunnel (Andersson 1970). After one day of nerve stimulation, both edema and slowing of nerve conduction disappeared within 96 hours. If the flexor retinaculum was sectioned before the period of repetitive stimulation, the mechanical activity still elicited synovial edema, but median nerve conduction was not slowed. The tendency for repetitive tendon movement to induce tenosynovial edema may explain why high repetitiveness is more important than high force in causing carpal tunnel syndrome.

Individual Susceptibility

Any theory linking carpal tunnel syndrome to job activity needs to consider variations in individual susceptibility to development of carpal tunnel syndrome, the dissociation between the pathology of median nerve compression and the symptoms of carpal tunnel syndrome, and the amount of activity necessary to cause the syndrome.

The guinea pig model of plantar nerve compression, a parallel of median nerve compression in the carpal tunnel, illustrates the combined roles of individual susceptibility and exposure to trauma in development of carpal tunnel syndrome. Guinea pigs characteristically develop electrophysiologic and pathologic evidence of focal compression of the plantar nerves of the hindfoot after prolonged housing in cages with wire mesh floors but not after housing on solid floors (Fullerton and Gilliatt 1965). The animals become more susceptible if injected with an agent that causes demyelination, like diphtheria toxin, but even then the focal compressive neuropathy can be prevented by suspending the animals so that their hindlegs do not touch the floor (Hopkins and Morgan-Hughes 1969).

Among a group of workers performing a task, only a fraction will develop carpal tunnel syndrome. In a small percentage of patients, an underlying medical illness such as diabetes, rheumatoid arthritis, acromegaly, or hypothyroidism helps explain their susceptibility to median nerve compression. In most other patients the susceptibility is not as readily explained.

An attractive hypothesis posits that congenitally small carpal canals may predispose to median nerve compression and, with sufficient hand use, to symptomatic carpal tunnel syndrome. Some computed tomography (CT) scan measurements of the cross-sectional area of the carpal tunnel support this hypothesis, but there is contradictory data on the relationship between carpal canal size and risk of development of carpal tunnel syndrome (Bleecker 1987; Winn and Habes 1990).

Gordon et al. (1988) have suggested that at least some members of the susceptible subpopulation can be identified by the ratio of wrist anteroposterior diameter to mediolateral diameter measured at the distal wrist crease. New workers in whom this ratio was greater than or equal to 0.70 were more likely to develop carpal tunnel syndrome symptoms within the first year of employment.

The value of wrist ratio measurement in preemployment screening remains unconfirmed (Wyles and Rodriquez 1991).

The existence of a subpopulation of workers who are more susceptible to development of carpal tunnel syndrome may explain the finding in some series that the incidence of carpal tunnel syndrome is higher in workers with fewer years on the job (Falck and Aarnio 1983; not confirmed in all series, see Cannon et al. 1981; Margolis and Kraus 1987). In some settings, there may be a survivor effect whereby more susceptible workers become symptomatic and change jobs, whereas less susceptible workers remain asymptomatic and become veteran employees.

Pathology Versus Symptoms

Asymptomatic median nerve abnormalities at wrist level are common and can be demonstrated both pathologically and by nerve conduction studies (Neary et al. 1975; Nathan et al. 1988). Is it possible that those people who have mild nerve conduction abnormalities are the susceptible subpopulation and would inevitably develop carpal tunnel syndrome, and that work activities simply make their condition symptomatic? There is still relatively little long-term data on the natural history of these mild asymptomatic abnormalities, but an initial report of longitudinal nerve conduction studies suggests that these abnormalities are not rapidly progressive (Nathan 1991). The incidence of very mild abnormalities, more than 20% in Nathan et al.'s (1988) series and more than 40% in the study of pathology by Neary et al. (1975), far exceeds the incidence of carpal tunnel syndrome in epidemiologic studies; so many individuals with mild asymptomatic abnormalities remain asymptomatic for years. If they develop persistent symptoms of carpal tunnel syndrome, they usually have nerve injury or dysfunction in excess of the mild asymptomatic pathology.

Amount of Activity Needed to Cause
Carpal Tunnel Syndrome

Quantitatively, little is known about the degree and duration of wrist and hand activity needed to cause synovial changes in the carpal tunnel. For example, we do not know whether Andersson's (1970) experimental model in rabbits approximates industrial hand use or average quotidian hand use. Nor do we know exactly how repetitive hand use leads to chronic synovial thickening and chronic changes in nerve structure and function.

Nonetheless, the epidemiologic data discussed earlier clearly indicate that for many individuals specific work activities, rather than routine daily hand use, are the source of sufficient mechanical stress to cause median nerve pathology and its clinical expression as carpal tunnel syndrome.

VIBRATION EXPOSURE AND
CARPAL TUNNEL SYNDROME

Occupational exposure to vibration may cause carpal tunnel syndrome, but carpal tunnel syndrome accounts for only a fraction of the hand and arm symptoms experienced by workers who are exposed to vibration. Vibration can also cause both "vibration white finger" and a neuropathy predominantly affecting digital nerves.

In the study of aircraft builders by Cannon et al. (1981), the only job activity that was definitely identified as a risk factor for development of carpal tunnel syndrome was use of vibrating tools such as surface grinders, polishers, buffers, or small hand tools. Koskimies et al. (1990) found symptoms and nerve conduction abnormalities consistent with carpal tunnel syndrome in 20% of forestry workers who were exposed to the vibration of chain saws.

Exposure to vibration is also associated with mild asymptomatic abnormalities of nerve conduction across the carpal tunnel. Nathan et al. (1988) found that 61% of grinder workers but only 28% of administrative or clerical workers had focal median nerve sensory conduction slowing on the serial stimulation test. Chatterjee et al. (1982) found that 44% of rock drillers exposed to low-frequency vibration had decreased amplitude of median sensory nerve action potentials from the index finger compared with ulnar sensory nerve action potentials from the little finger, whereas only 7% of controls had this abnormality.

Prolonged occupational exposure to low-frequency vibration can also cause a more diffuse neuropathy in the hands, particularly affecting sensory function in digital branches of median and ulnar nerves (Brammer and Pyykko 1987). Patients may have impaired acuity for warm and cold sensation in the fingers, even with normal nerve conduction studies, suggesting dysfunction of unmyelinated and small myelinated fibers (Ekenvall et al. 1986). Individuals exposed to vibration may also display abnormalities of conduction in motor fibers, such as in the ulnar nerve in the forearm, but special techniques to measure conduction in slower motor fibers need to be applied to demonstrate an abnormality (Alaranta and Seppalainen 1977).

Vibration white finger, dead man's hand, and *traumatic vasospastic disease* are among the names given to another syndrome of hand and arm symptoms induced by vibration (Brammer and Taylor 1988; Taylor and Wasserman 1988). Symptoms include finger blanching, numbness, tingling, hand pain, grip weakness or fatigue, and joint stiffness. In individual patients, vasospasm, damage to Pacinian corpuscles, digital sensory neuropathy, carpal tunnel syndrome, and musculoskeletal changes are claimed to contribute to the symptom complex (Taylor 1988).

Among patients with symptoms of vibration-induced vasospasm, the presence of nocturnal hand paresthesias may be a clue to coexistence of carpal tunnel syndrome. Boyle et al. (1988) described 19 patients who had worked for years with vibrating tools and who had episodic finger blanching, usually associated with hand tingling or numbness. Table 13.3 shows the relationship in these patients between presence of hand tingling at night (unassociated with blanching) and occurrence of abnormal nerve conduction across the carpal tunnel.

Table 13.3 Symptoms versus nerve conduction in vibration white finger

Nerve Conduction Across the Carpal Tunnel	Nocturnal Hand Paresthesias	
	Yes	No
Abnormal	10	2
Normal	2	5

(Data from Boyle et al. 1988.)

PREVENTION OF OCCUPATIONAL CARPAL TUNNEL SYNDROME

The ergonomic method provides an approach to prevention of carpal tunnel syndrome (Armstrong 1983; Feldman et al. 1983). It starts with a thorough analysis of tasks and tools, looking for those aspects of a job that might contribute to tenosynovial or nerve irritation or lead to increases in carpal canal pressure.

Tichauer and Gage (1977) recommend paying attention to a number of features of hand tool design: optimization of tool forces with good sensory feedback from the tool, distribution of tool contact pressures, use of appropriate work gloves, promotion of optimal postures and motions, and matching tool size to the worker. These principles can translate to some clever adaptations such as angling the handle of a hammer so that the worker can use the tool with less ulnar wrist deviation (Schoenmarklin and Marras 1989). Changes in the work task and workstation can also minimize abnormal wrist postures or decrease the need for repetitive movements (Armstrong 1983). Table 13.4 summarizes some job modifications that might help prevent carpal tunnel syndrome.

The probable value of ergonomic intervention for prevention of carpal tunnel syndrome has not been rigorously proven. Armstrong et al. (1982) surveyed a poultry processing plant using both film and electromyographic data to provide detail on the hand and arm movements required for turkey boning. They then recommended changes in the workers' tools and techniques and in the design of the workstations to minimize hand stresses. They provide no data on the

Table 13.4 Prevention of carpal tunnel syndrome

The Task	The Tools
Match worker to job	Keep wrist straight
Improve workstations	Optimize center of gravity
Avoid pinching, wringing, grasping	Maximize mechanical advantage
Reduce task frequency	Avoid palmar pressure
Rotate tasks	Encourage ambidexterity
Schedule regular breaks	
Use appropriate gloves and padding	

(Modified from Feldman et al. 1983.)

effectiveness of their proposed changes. Feldman et al. (1987) proposed ergonomic improvements in an electronics assembly plant to prevent carpal tunnel syndrome but were unable to implement, let alone assess, the changes that they proposed.

Analysis of a telecommunications manufacturing facility led to modifications in a number of hand tool operations (McKenzie et al. 1985). The following year the number of workdays lost to reportable arm cumulative trauma disorders dropped precipitously. McKenzie et al. did not separate carpal tunnel syndrome from other causes of hand and arm symptoms. They emphasized that their study was not controlled and that the drop in incidence of disorders might not have been attributable to their intervention.

MEDICAL-LEGAL ISSUES

There have been hundreds of court decisions discussing the causal relationship between numerous occupations and carpal tunnel syndrome. This body of law will not be reviewed here, but we will discuss legal issues that arise for physicians who participate in the care and evaluation of workers with carpal tunnel syndrome.

When an individual worker develops carpal tunnel syndrome, the workers' compensation system often queries the physician as to the causal relation between the worker's job activities and the development of the syndrome. An informed and well-reasoned medical opinion is essential, because courts will usually rely heavily on medical experts to determine causation. Analysis of these questions can be challenging; for example, the worker may have had more than one employer, have vigorous avocational hand use, have worked on a job for only a brief period of time, or have an underlying medical condition that predisposes to development of carpal tunnel syndrome.

The analysis is also complicated because the pathologic processes, both in nerve and in synovial tissue, that underlie carpal tunnel syndrome usually have been present for an unknown amount of time before the symptoms of carpal tunnel syndrome appear. Furthermore, in some patients the symptoms are transient, easily reversible, and not necessarily indicative of irreversible pathologic damage to nerve or synovium. In other patients, the symptoms are recurrent or progressive and do reflect increasing nerve injury.

Before considering causation, the physician must ascertain that the diagnosis of carpal tunnel syndrome is correct. Epidemics of ill-defined hand complaints can occur in the workplace. Miller and Topliss (1988), studying an epidemic of hand symptoms among Australian workers, found that carpal tunnel syndrome was rarely the cause of their complaints, and many of the workers had no demonstrable clinical or electrophysiological derangements.

When rendering an opinion on causation, the physician should assess the worker's vocational and avocational activities with attention to the extent of repetitive hand and wrist use, wrist and grip force, palmar pressure, cold exposure, and vibration exposure. The existence of any medical condition predisposing to carpal tunnel syndrome should be considered. The prevalence of carpal tunnel syndrome in the worker's colleagues is of potential import, but usually this information is available only as rumor rather than as reliable statistics.

The temporal relationships between the suspect activities and symptoms of carpal tunnel syndrome often provides the best clues to answering the difficult question of causation. The occurrence of symptoms during work, at night, or at rest after work is important. Timing of symptoms in relation to changes in job tasks, vacations, days off, and changes in employment can be relevant.

At times, a careful occupational history may establish that the patient's occupation is the probable, major contributing cause of the carpal tunnel syndrome. In other patients, the carpal tunnel syndrome will have nonoccupational causes, or the role of occupation in genesis of the carpal tunnel syndrome will be equivocal.

QUESTIONS FOR THE FUTURE

Occupational hand use is one common cause of carpal tunnel syndrome. Controversy about the association persists, in part because of methodologic imperfections of available statistical studies and in part because of gaps in understanding the pathophysiology of carpal tunnel syndrome. Nonetheless, a temporal link between activities and development of symptoms of carpal tunnel syndrome, available statistical studies, and the known elements of pathophysiology provide evidence of a causal relationship in some patients.

A number of questions remain for future consideration:

- What is the natural history of chronic asymptomatic median nerve entrapment?
- What personal factors predispose to susceptibility to local median nerve pathology and its expression as carpal tunnel syndrome?
- Is there any role for preemployment screening in the prevention of carpal tunnel syndrome?
- What are the dose-response relationships between various types of hand use and development of carpal tunnel syndrome in susceptible individuals?
- How much synovial edema can occur before the synovium is irreversibly thickened?
- How much nerve compression can occur before the structure and function of the median nerve are chronically damaged?
- What is the efficacy of ergonomic interventions in the prevention of symptomatic carpal tunnel syndrome?

REFERENCES

Alaranta H, Seppalainen AM. Neuropathy and the automatic analysis of electromyographic signals from vibration exposed workers. Scand J Work Environ Health 1977;3:128–34.

Aljure J, Eltorai I, Bradley WE, Lin JE, Johnson B. Carpal tunnel syndrome in paraplegic patients. Paraplegia 1985;23:182–86.

Alvarez N, Larkin C, Roxborough J. Carpal tunnel syndrome in athetoid-dystonic cerebral palsy. Arch Neurol 1982;39:311–12.

Andersson A. Reaction in the tissues of the carpal tunnel after repeated contractions of the muscles innervated by the median nerve. An experimental investigation on the rabbit. Scand J Plast Reconstr Surg 1970;Sup. 5:3–67.

Armstrong TJ. An ergonomics guide to carpal tunnel syndrome. Akron: American Industrial Hygiene Association, 1983.

Armstrong TJ, Foulke JA, Joseph BS, Goldstein SA. Investigation of cumulative trauma disorders in a poultry processing plant. Am Ind Hyg Assoc J 1982;43:103–16.

Armstrong TJ, Silverstein BA. Upper-extremity pain in the workplace—role of usage in causality. In: Hadler NM, ed. Clinical concepts in regional musculoskeletal illness. Orlando: Grune & Stratton, 1987;333–54.

Barnhart S, Rosenstock L. Carpal tunnel syndrome in grocery checkers. A cluster of a work-related illness. West J Med 1987;147:37–40.

Bauer ME. Carpal tunnel syndrome. An occupational risk to the dental hygienist. Dent Hyg (Chic) 1985;59:218–21.

Birkbeck MQ, Beer TC. Occupation in relation to the carpal tunnel syndrome. Rheumatol Rehabil 1975;14:218–21.

Bleecker ML. Medical surveillance for carpal tunnel syndrome in workers. J Hand Surg 1987;12A:845–48.

Bleecker ML, Bohlman M, Moreland R, Tipton A. Carpal tunnel syndrome: role of carpal canal size. Neurology (Minneap) 1985;35:1599–1604.

Boyle JC, Smith NJ, Burke FD. Vibration white finger. J Hand Surg 1988;13B:171–76.

Brain WR, Wright AD, Wilkinson M. Spontaneous compression of both median nerves in the carpal tunnel. Lancet 1947;1:277–82.

Brammer AJ, Pyykko I. Vibration-induced neuropathy. Detection by nerve conduction measurements. Scand J Work Environ Health 1987;13:317–22.

Brammer AJ, Taylor W. Vibration effects on the hand and arm in industry. In: Brammer AJ, Taylor W, eds. Vibration effects on the hand and arm in industry. New York: John Wiley & Sons, 1988;1–11.

Cannon LJ, Bernacki EJ, Walter SD. Personal and occupational factors associated with carpal tunnel syndrome. JOM 1981;23:255–58.

Chatterjee DS, Barwick DD, Petrie A. Exploratory electromyography in the study of vibration-induced white finger in rock drillers. Br J Ind Med 1982;39:89–97.

Chiang HC, Chen SS, Yu HS, Ko YC. The occurrence of carpal tunnel syndrome in frozen food factory employees. Kaohsiung J Med Sci 1990;6:73–80.

Ekenvall L, Nilsson BY, Gustavsson P. Temperature and vibration thresholds in vibration syndrome. Br J Ind Med 1986;43:825–29.

Faithfull DK, Moir DH, Ireland J. The micropathology of the typical carpal tunnel syndrome. J Hand Surg 1986;11B:131–32.

Falck B, Aarnio P. Left-sided carpal tunnel syndrome in butchers. Scand J Work Environ Health 1983;9:291–97.

Farkkila M, Pyykko I, Jantti V, Aatola S, Starck J, Korhonen O. Forestry workers exposed to vibration: a neurological study. Br J Ind Med 1988;45:188–92.

Feldman RG, Goldman R, Keyserling WM. Classical syndromes in occupational medicine. Peripheral nerve entrapment syndromes and ergonomic factors. Am J Ind Med 1983;4:661–81.

Feldman RG, Travers PH, Chirico-Post J, Keyserling WM. Risk assessment in electronic assembly workers: carpal tunnel syndrome. J Hand Surg 1987;12A:849–55.

Fletcher RH, Fletcher SW, Wagner EH. Clinical epidemiology, the essentials. Baltimore: Williams & Wilkins, 1982.

Franklin GM, Haug J, Heyer N, Checkoway H, Peck N. Occupational carpal tunnel syndrome in Washington State, 1984–1988. Am J Public Health 1991;81:741–46.

Franklin GM, Haug JA, Peck NB, Heyer N, Checkoway H. Occupational carpal tunnel syndrome in Washington State, 1984–1987. Neurology (Minneap) 1990;40:420.

Fullerton PM, Gilliatt RW. Changes in nerve conduction in caged guinea-pigs. J Physiol (Lond) 1965;178:47–48.

Gellman H, Sie I, Waters RL. Late complications of the weight-bearing upper extremity in the paraplegic patient. Clin Orthop 1988;233:132–35.

Gordon C, Bowyer BL, Johnson EW. Electrodiagnostic characteristics of acute carpal tunnel syndrome. Arch Phys Med Rehabil 1987;68:545–48.

Gordon C, Johnson EW, Gatens PF, Ashton JJ. Wrist ratio correlation with carpal tunnel syndrome in industry. Am J Phys Med Rehabil 1988;67:270–72.

Hadler NM. Is carpal tunnel syndrome an injury that qualifies for workers' compensation insurance? In: Hadler NM, ed. Clinical concepts in regional musculoskeletal illness. Orlando: Grune & Stratton, 1987;355–60.

Hochberg FH, Leffert RD, Heller MD, Merriman L. Hand difficulties among musicians. JAMA 1983;249:1869–72.

Hoffman J, Hoffman PL. Staple gun carpal tunnel syndrome. JOM 1985;27:848–49.

Hopkins AP, Morgan-Hughes JA. The effect of local pressure in diphtheritic neuropathy. J Neurol Neurosurg Psychiatry 1969;32:614–23.

Jones WA, Scheker LR. Acute carpal tunnel syndrome: a case report. J Hand Surg 1988;13B:400–401.

Kendall D. Non-penetrating injuries of the median nerve at the wrist. Brain 1950;73:84–94.

Koskimies K, Farkkila M, Pyykko I, Jantti V, Aatola S, Starck J, Inaba R. Carpal tunnel syndrome in vibration disease. Br J Ind Med 1990;47:411–16.

Lundborg G, Myers R, Powell H. Nerve compression injury and increased endoneurial fluid pressure: a "miniature compartment syndrome." J Neurol Neurosurg Psychiatry 1983;46:1119–24.

MacMahon B, Pugh TF. Epidemiology principles and methods. Boston: Little, Brown, 1970.

Margolis W, Kraus JF. The prevalence of carpal tunnel syndrome symptoms in female supermarket checkers. JOM 1987;29:953–56.

Masear VR, Hayes JM, Hyde AG. An industrial cause of carpal tunnel syndrome. J Hand Surg 1986;11A:222–27.

Matte TD, Baker EL, Honchar PA. The selection and definition of targeted work-related conditions for surveillance under SENSOR. Am J Public Health Suppl 1989;79:21–25.

Mausner JS, Kramer K. Mausner and Bahn epidemiology—an introductory text. 2nd ed. Philadelphia: WB Saunders, 1985.

McKenzie F, Storment J, Van-Hook P, Armstrong TJ. A program for control of repetitive trauma disorders associated with hand tool operations in a telecommunications manufacturing facility. Am Ind Hyg Assoc J 1985;46:674–78.

Miller MH, Topliss DJ. Chronic upper limb pain syndrome (repetitive strain injury) in the Australian workforce: a systematic cross sectional rheumatological study of 229 patients. J Rheumatol 1988;15:1705–12.

Nathan PA. (Letter). J Hand Surg 1991;16B:231–32.

Nathan PA, Meadows KD, Doyle LS. Occupation as a risk factor for impaired sensory conduction of the median nerve at the carpal tunnel. J Hand Surg 1988;13B:167–70.

Neary D, Ochoa J, Gilliatt RW. Sub-clinical entrapment neuropathy in man. J Neurol Sci 1975;24:282–98.

Ochoa J, Marotte L. Nature of nerve lesion caused by chronic entrapment in guinea-pig. J Neurol Sci 1973;19:491–95.

Oppenheim H. Textbook of nervous diseases. 5th ed. Vol 1. London: TN Foulis, 1911.

Oregon Department of Insurance and Finance. Carpal tunnel syndrome in Oregon 1984–1988. Letter to physicians. April 1990.

Osborn JB, Newell KJ, Rudney JD, Stoltenberg JL. Carpal tunnel syndrome among Minnesota dental hygienists. J Dent Hyg 1990;64:79–85.

Phalen GS. The carpal-tunnel syndrome. Seventeen years' experience in diagnosis and treatment of six hundred fifty-four hands. J Bone Joint Surg 1966;48A:211–28.

Punnett L, Robins JM, Wegman DH, Keyserling WM. Soft tissue disorders in the upper limbs of female garment workers. Scand J Work Environ Health 1985;11:417–25.

Rothfleisch S, Sherman D. Carpal tunnel syndrome—biomechanical aspects of occupational occurrence and implications regarding surgical management. Orthop Rev 1976;7:107–9.

Schoenmarklin RW, Marras WS. Effects of handle angle and work orientation on hammering: I. Wrist motion and hammering performance. Hum Factors 1989;31:397–411.

Schottland JR, Kirschberg GJ, Fillingim R, Davis VP, Hogg F. Median nerve latencies in poultry processing workers: an approach to resolving the role of industrial "cumulative trauma" in the development of carpal tunnel syndrome. JOM 1991;33:627–31.

Silverstein BA, Fine LJ, Armstrong TJ. Occupational factors and carpal tunnel syndrome. Am J Ind Med 1987;11:343–58.

Stedt JD. Carpal tunnel syndrome: the risk to educational interpreters. Am Ann Deaf 1989;134:223–26.

Stevens JC, Sun S, Beard CM, O'Fallon WM, Kurland LT. Carpal tunnel syndrome in Rochester, Minnesota, 1961 to 1980. Neurology (Minneap) 1988;38:134–38.

Stevens K. The carpal tunnel syndrome in cardiologists (letter). Ann Intern Med 1990;112:796.

Tanzer RC. The carpal-tunnel syndrome. J Bone Joint Surg 1959;41A:626–34.

Taylor W. Biological effects of the hand-arm vibration syndrome: historical perspective and current research. J Acoust Soc Am 1988;83:415–22.

Taylor W, Wasserman DE. Occupational vibration. In: Zenz C, ed. Occupational medicine. 2nd ed. Chicago: Year Book Medical Publishers, 1988;324–33.

Tichauer ER, Gage H. Ergonomic principles basic to hand tool design. Am Ind Hyg Assoc J 1977;38:622–34.

Waring III WP, Werner RA. Clinical management of carpal tunnel syndrome in patients with long-term sequelae of poliomyelitis. J Hand Surg 1989;14A:865–69.

Werner R, Waring W, Davidoff G. Risk factors for median mononeuropathy of the wrist in postpoliomyelitis patients. Arch Phys Med Rehabil 1989;70:464–67.

Wieslander G, Norback D, Gothe CJ, Juhlin L. Carpal tunnel syndrome (CTS) and exposure to vibration, repetitive wrist movements, and heavy manual work: a case-referent study. Br J Ind Med 1989;46:43–47.

Winn FJ Jr, Habes DJ. Carpal tunnel area as a risk factor for carpal tunnel syndrome. Muscle Nerve 1990;13:254–58.

Wyles JM, Rodriquez AA. The predictive value of wrist dimension measurement in median sensory latencies in carpal tunnel syndrome. Muscle Nerve 1991;14:902.

14

Nonsurgical Treatment of Carpal Tunnel Syndrome

For most patients with carpal tunnel syndrome, the first therapeutic approaches should be nonsurgical. A variety of nonoperative therapies are available. Unfortunately, many patients who initially respond to nonoperative therapy have recurrence of symptoms.

CHOICE OF THERAPY

Many carpal tunnel syndrome patients with mild, intermittent symptoms appropriately choose no therapy. These patients should be alerted to watch for progression of symptoms. If pain and paresthesias become more frequent and particularly if weakness, sensory loss, or atrophy develops, they must seek reevaluation and be advised to reconsider their decision.

A survey of hand surgeons showed that they usually begin treatment with a few weeks of nonoperative therapy (Duncan et al. 1987). The most common therapies used were splinting (77% of surgeons), steroid injection into the carpal canal (60%), and nonsteroidal antiinflammatory drugs (47%). Oral steroids or diuretics were prescribed less frequently. Phalen (1966) reported that in his experience most patients with carpal tunnel syndrome do not require surgical therapy.

In some patients with acute carpal tunnel syndrome and associated neurologic deficit, surgical therapy should not be delayed. Patients with established neurologic deficit and neurologic signs of median neuropathy, such as loss of two-point discrimination or thenar atrophy, are unlikely to be cured by nonoperative therapy. Most surgeons will operate on these severe cases of carpal tunnel syndrome without delay (Duncan et al. 1987). An alternative approach is a brief trial of conservative modalities: If pain and paresthesia are relieved, and the neurologic deficit is not progressive during careful follow-up, a rare patient with severe carpal tunnel syndrome may show gradual improvement in neurologic deficit with nonoperative therapy.

INITIAL TREATMENT

Treatment should begin with attention to repetitive hand activities that are causing or exacerbating symptoms and, whenever possible, with treatment of any medical condition apparently contributing to the median nerve compression. In many patients, symptoms are closely related to repetitive hand activities. Often, the best treatment for these patients is stopping the offending activity. At times the activity can be redesigned or modified to protect against carpal tunnel syndrome. The section "Prevention of Occupational Carpal Tunnel Syndrome" in Chapter 13 discusses task modification in greater detail.

When carpal tunnel syndrome is caused or exacerbated by a medical condition, carpal tunnel symptoms will often resolve with successful treatment of the underlying problem. For example, the response of symptoms to treatment of hypothyroidism, acromegaly, or rheumatoid arthritis is discussed in Chapter 5.

When symptoms of carpal tunnel syndrome develop during pregnancy, they usually resolve following delivery (see Chapter 5 for more detailed data). Most pregnant patients with carpal tunnel syndrome need no specific therapy. If symptoms do require therapy, splinting or steroid injection of the carpal tunnel is often successful.

SPLINTING

Splinting is a mainstay of conservative therapy. It is simple, safe, relatively inexpensive, and often effective, at least initially.

Technique

A wide variety of splints are now available commercially. An example is shown in Figure 14.1. The splint should firmly immobilize the wrist in the neutral position or with extension up to 30° and with about 10° of ulnar deviation. The thumb should be free and able to flex to the index finger, but the splint should prevent thumb opposition to the little finger. Finger movement should be free. The fit, while firm, should not interfere with circulation or have focal sites that might cause skin irritation (Falkenburg 1987).

The splint should be worn during sleep and whenever possible during wakefulness. Some carpal tunnel syndrome patients note symptomatic benefit if they can use the splint during their daily activities. This is not always possible, either because the splint is too restrictive on finger movement for the task or because repetitive finger movement, even with the wrist splinted, can increase median nerve compression in the carpal tunnel.

Results

In response to the landmark description of carpal tunnel surgery by Brain et al. (1947), Roaf (1947) wrote that many patients with carpal tunnel syndrome did not require surgery and suggested three to four weeks of wrist immobilization

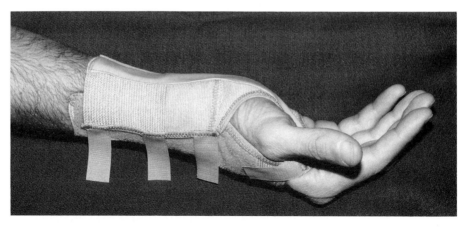

Figure 14.1 The splint used for treatment of carpal tunnel syndrome should maintain up to 30° of wrist extension and slight ulnar deviation.

as initial treatment of, and as a diagnostic test for, carpal tunnel syndrome. Heathfield (1957) prescribed wrist splinting in the neutral position for 51 patients with carpal syndrome. Patients used the splints for 6 to 12 weeks, at night if symptoms were nocturnal, or day and night if symptoms were continual; 48 patients had excellent relief of symptoms, and only 6 relapsed.

The success rate in subsequent series has been less impressive. Quin (1961) prescribed a wrist splint in the neutral position and obtained relief of symptoms in 28 of 47 patients. The results of Crow (1960) are shown in Figures 14.2 and 14.3. He splinted the wrists of 36 patients in the neutral position at night; about one half the patients noted immediate relief of nocturnal symptoms and gradual improvement in diurnal symptoms. One quarter of the patients did not note benefit until the splints had been in use for a week or two. An occasional patient benefited immediately from splinting and then had a recurrence of symptoms while still using the splint. One quarter of the patients did not benefit from the splints. Rarely, patients reported an increase in symptoms coincident with splint use.

In most patients in Crow's series, symptoms recurred after the splinting was stopped. Only one eighth of the patients had lasting relief of symptoms after splinting, and usually patients who had sustained improvement after splinting had also changed their hand activities or had been treated for an underlying causal condition.

In a group of patients with carpal tunnel syndrome, Goodman and Gilliatt (1961) performed serial nerve conduction studies during treatment by splinting. In patients with pretreatment median distal motor latencies between 5 and 10 msec, a few showed a 20% or better improvement in distal motor latency, but others showed no improvement or even had slight worsening of median distal motor latency.

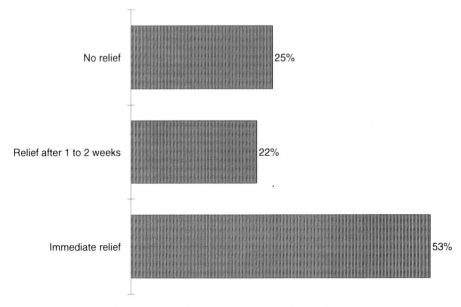

Figure 14.2 Early effects of splinting for treatment of carpal tunnel syndrome. (Data from Crow 1960.)

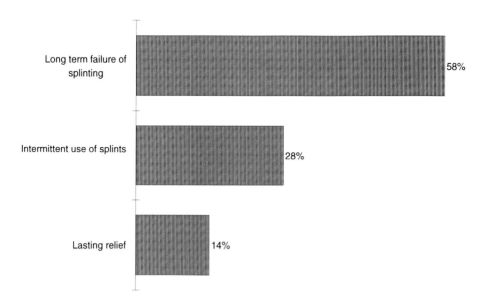

Figure 14.3 Late effects of splinting for treatment of carpal tunnel syndrome. (Data from Crow 1960.)

STEROID INJECTION INTO THE CARPAL TUNNEL

Injection of corticosteroids into the carpal tunnel often leads to excellent relief of symptoms. Unfortunately, the improvement is rarely permanent.

Technique

Steroid injection is typically done with a 25-gauge needle 1 cm proximal to the distal wrist crease. Positioning of the syringe is shown in Figure 14.4. The needle may be inserted between the palmaris longus and flexor carpi radialis tendons or on the ulnar side of the palmaris longus tendon (Gelberman et al. 1980; Green 1984). While the needle is advanced about 1 cm to enter the carpal tunnel through the flexor retinaculum, the patient is asked to report any paresthesias. If paresthesias do occur, the needle should be withdrawn and reinserted about 1 cm more proximally. When the steroid solution is successfully injected into the carpal tunnel, a slight bulge should be visible or palpable in the proximal palm (Green 1984).

Another approach is to inject along the flexor tendons just proximal to the carpal tunnel. Before injection, the patient flexes his or her fingers slightly; movement of the needle and syringe confirms that the needle is in contact with the flexor synovium (Dawson et al. 1990). Experiments with methylene blue in cadaver forearms show that injection of two ml solutions, three cm proximal to

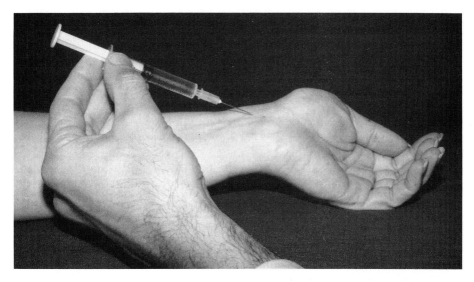

Figure 14.4 The needle is poised for injection of steroid into the carpal tunnel. The angle is about 30° with the needle tip 1 cm proximal to the distal wrist crease between the tendons of palmaris longus and flexor carpi radialis.

the distal wrist crease, followed by flexion and extension of the fingers, is another technique for introducing medication into the carpal tunnel (Minamikawa et al. 1992).

Results

Phalen and Kendrick (1957) reported treatment of carpal tunnel syndrome by injection of 1 ml of hydrocortisone into the carpal tunnel. Sixteen of 20 patients improved. Kopell (1958) added a case report of treatment by steroid injection into the canal. Van der Bracht (1958) was another early proponent of treatment with injection of hydrocortisone into the canal. Foster (1960) confirmed a similar response rate to this therapy but noted a high relapse rate at one-year follow-up. Quin (1961) found that improvement from hydrocortisone injection lasted less than a week in some patients.

Crow (1960) injected 25 to 50 mg of hydrocortisone acetate. He treated 31 hands and noted dramatic improvement in symptoms in 28 hands within 48 hours of injection. Symptomatic relief occurred rapidly, even in patients who had chronic symptoms and objective findings of median nerve dysfunction on examination. Unfortunately, 80% of patients noted recurrence of symptoms within one to eight months of the injection. On occasion, these patients received a second injection, but most of those who improved after the second injection had recurrence of symptoms within months.

Goodman and Foster (1962) injected 10 mg (1 ml) of prednisolone. They performed repeated median nerve motor conduction studies in their patients before and after injection of steroid into the carpal tunnel. Median distal motor latency often decreased at the initial follow-up, a few weeks after injection, and then again increased in subsequent months paralleling the clinical observation that symptomatic relief was usually transient.

Gelberman et al. (1980) injected 30 mg of triamcinolone (0.75 ml) and an equal volume of 1% lidocaine without epinephrine, then splinted the wrist continuously for three weeks in the neutral position. Three quarters of the patients were asymptomatic six weeks after injection, but less than one quarter remained asymptomatic after months of follow-up. Patients were more likely to have lasting benefit if symptoms were intermittent or had been present less than one year prior to treatment. Some 40% of patients with intermittent symptoms, normal strength, and normal two-point discrimination were asymptomatic 18 months following treatment.

Giannini et al. (1991) selected patients with mild carpal tunnel syndrome for treatment by canal injection with steroids. They found that six months after injection, 93% of their patients had good symptomatic improvement, and many had concomitant improvement in median nerve conduction studies.

Even an occasional patient with evidence of more severe median neuropathy was cured by the three-week treatment regimen (Gelberman et al. 1980). Criteria for severe median neuropathy included thenar weakness and atrophy, decreased median two-point discrimination, absent median sensory nerve action potential, median distal motor latency over 6 msec, or fibrillations on thenar electromyography. Table 14.1 compares the initial and late response rates to steroid injection into the carpal tunnel in various series.

The value of steroid injection is local rather than systemic. In a controlled series, women with idiopathic carpal tunnel syndrome received 1.5 mg of betamethasone injected into the deltoid or into the carpal tunnel. At follow-up after one month, the improvement rate was 50% following carpal tunnel injection but only 6% following deltoid injection (Ozdogan and Yazici 1984).

Complications

Some patients have transient increase in wrist discomfort at the time of injection. Increased pain may last one or two days (Phalen 1966). Experience with intraarticular injection of other joints suggests that some patients may develop a transient chemical synovitis in response to steroid crystals (Gray and Gottlieb 1983).

Crow (1960) noted one case of flexor tendon synovial infection introduced in the course of 65 injections. The patient recovered completely from the infection after antibiotic therapy. More severe infection may require acute exploration and drainage of the carpal tunnel (Gottlieb and Riskin 1980).

Bilateral digital flexor tendon ruptures occurred in a woman treated for bilateral idiopathic carpal tunnel syndrome with 29 injections of steroids into the carpal tunnel over seven years (Gottlieb and Riskin 1980).

Accidental steroid injection into the median nerve can worsen median neuropathy (Linskey and Segal 1990; McConnell and Bush 1990). When surgery is done after intraneural steroid injection, accumulated steroid may be visible in the nerve.

Local steroid injections may be complicated on rare occasions by local

Table 14.1 Efficacy of steroid injection in the carpal tunnel for patients with carpal tunnel syndrome

Reference	Hands with Initial Benefit (%)	Hands with Sustained Benefit (%)
Crow 1960	90	13
Goodman and Foster 1962	88	60
Foster 1960	92	24
Gelberman et al. 1980	76	22
Phalen 1966	92	19
Wood 1980	90	33
Green 1984	81	37

allergic dermatitis, acne, skin atrophy or depigmentation, or systemic flushing (Gottlieb and Riskin 1980).

PYRIDOXINE (VITAMIN B₆)
Therapeutic Controversy

Therapy of carpal tunnel syndrome with vitamin B_6 has strong advocates, but proof of its efficacy is still awaited. In a series of papers, Folkers, Ellis, et al. have proposed that many cases of carpal tunnel syndrome are caused by pyridoxine deficiency (Ellis et al. 1976, 1977, 1979, 1981; Folkers et al. 1978; Ellis and Folkers 1990). They measured erythrocyte glutamic-oxaloacetic transaminase (EGOT) activity in vitro before and after addition of pyridoxal phosphate. Patients with carpal tunnel syndrome had lower EGOT activity than controls. Addition of pyridoxal phosphate to the in vitro assay or addition of pyridoxine to the patients' diets led to correction of the EGOT activities of these patients, 2 mg of oral pyridoxine daily was less effective than 100 mg daily in correcting the results of the assay.

Fuhr et al. (1989) found low serum vitamin B_6 levels in some patients with carpal tunnel syndrome. Smith et al. (1984) found normal pyridoxal and pyridoxal phosphate levels in six patients with carpal tunnel syndrome.

Ellis et al. (1982) reported apparent clinical benefit of pyridoxine in seven patients in a crossover double-blind trial against placebo, but only two of the patients had nerve conduction abnormalities to the diagnosis of carpal tunnel syndrome, and the clinical descriptions suggest that many of the patients' symptoms were not those of carpal tunnel syndrome. Wolaniuk et al. (1983) reported serial nerve conduction studies in three patients treated with pyridoxine. One of these patients showed statistically significant improvement in right median distal motor latency and left median wrist-to-index finger sensory latency following treatment.

Folkers et al. (1984) described a patient in whom they attributed carpal tunnel syndrome to combined pyridoxine and riboflavin deficiency.

In one series, pyridoxine, 100 mg twice daily, was added to a conservative regimen of splinting, antiinflammatory drugs, job changes, or carpal tunnel steroid injections, and 68% of patients improved without surgery (Kasdan and Janes 1987). In previously treated patients given the same conservative regimen without pyridoxine supplements, 14% of patients with carpal tunnel syndrome responded well to conservative therapy. An accompanying discussion emphasized the inadequacy of control data in this paper and called for a well-designed prospective therapeutic trial.

Other small series have reported unimpressive responses to pyridoxine therapy (Amadio 1985; Scheyer and Haas 1985). One double-blind study found no benefit of pyridoxine over placebo, but small sample size (six patients treated with pyridoxine) and high response rate in control patients might have masked treatment benefit (Stransky et al. 1989).

Byers et al. (1984) criticized the Folkers and Ellis data for poorly separating symptoms of carpal tunnel syndrome from those of other conditions such as peripheral neuropathy. In patients studied by Byers et al., pyridoxine deficiency on the EGOT assay correlated better with evidence of generalized peripheral neuropathy than with evidence of carpal tunnel syndrome.

Toxicity

Neuropathy is now recognized as a complication of high-dose pyridoxine use (Schaumberg et al. 1983). A patient receiving 3 g of pyridoxine daily for treatment of carpal tunnel syndrome developed pyridoxine neuropathy (Vasile et al. 1984). Ellis and Folkers describe use of a dose of 200 mg daily in their patients. In patients without carpal tunnel syndrome, pyridoxine toxic neuropathy has been reported in patients on doses as low as 200 mg daily (Parry and Bredesen 1985).

DIURETICS, ANTIINFLAMMATORIES

Many physicians treat carpal tunnel syndrome with nonsteroidal anti-inflammatory drugs. When we do so, we use a two- to four-week trial unless limited by side effects such as gastrointestinal intolerance. An occasional patient reports an increase in carpal tunnel syndrome symptoms while on these drugs, possibly because of drug-induced fluid retention. There is no published controlled study on use of these drugs in carpal tunnel syndrome.

Use of a mild diuretic is another common, but poorly studied, treatment of carpal tunnel syndrome. There are a number of letters attesting to the value of diuretics in treatment of carpal tunnel syndrome in pregnancy (Donaldson 1959; McCallum 1959; Wood 1959). The theoretical rationale is to decrease synovial edema or vascular congestion in the carpal tunnel.

SUMMARY

Treatment of patients with carpal tunnel syndrome begins, whenever possible, with efforts to decrease recurrent wrist use and to treat causative medical illnesses. Many patients benefit from a simple wrist splint.

Injection of steroids into the carpal canal often gives impressive relief of symptoms. Some physicians use steroid injections frequently; others are un-enthusiastic about injections because benefit is rarely permanent, and complications may occur.

Diuretics or nonsteroidal antiinflammatory drugs are commonly used, but evidence for their value is only anecdotal. The value of pyridoxine therapy is unproven. If pyridoxine is prescribed, the dose should be kept under 200 mg daily.

Many patients with carpal tunnel syndrome can be treated successfully without surgery; however, surgical therapy is indicated for most patients with fixed or progressive neurologic deficit and also for those patients without neurologic deficit who have troublesome symptoms that have not been relieved by conservative therapy.

REFERENCES

Amadio PC. Pyridoxine as an adjunct in the treatment of carpal tunnel syndrome. J Hand Surg 1985;10A:237–41.

Brain WR, Wright AD, Wilkinson M. Spontaneous compression of both median nerves in the carpal tunnel. Lancet 1947;1:277–82.

Byers CM, DeLisa JA, Frankel DL, Kraft GH. Pyridoxine metabolism in carpal tunnel syndrome with and without peripheral neuropathy. Arch Phys Med Rehabil 1984;65:712–16.

Crow RS. Treatment of the carpal-tunnel syndrome. Br Med J 1960;1:1611–15.

Dawson DM, Hallett M, Millender LH. Carpal tunnel syndrome. In: Entrapment neuropathies. 2nd ed. Boston: Little, Brown, 1990;25–92.

Donaldson M. Carpal tunnel syndrome. Br Med J 1959;1:1184.

Duncan KH, Lewis RC Jr, Foreman KA, Nordyke MD. Treatment of carpal tunnel syndrome by members of the American Society for Surgery of the Hand: results of a questionnaire. J Hand Surg 1987;12A:384–91.

Ellis JM, Azuma J, Watanabe T, Fokers K, Lowell JR, Hurst GA, Ho-Ahn C, Shuford EH Jr, Ulrich RF. Survey and new data on treatment with pyridoxine of patients having a clinical syndrome including the carpal tunnel and other defects. Res Commun Chem Pathol Pharmacol 1977;17:165–77.

Ellis JM, Folkers K. Clinical aspects of treatment of carpal tunnel syndrome with vitamin B_6. Ann NY Acad Sci 1990;585:302–20.

Ellis JM, Folkers K, Levy M, Shizukuishi S, Lewandowski J, Nishii S, Schubert HA, Ulrich R. Response of vitamin B-6 deficiency and the carpal tunnel syndrome to pyridoxine. Proc Natl Acad Sci USA 1982;79:7494–98.

Ellis J, Folkers K, Levy M, Takemura K, Shizukuishi S, Ulrich R, Harrison P. Therapy with vitamin B_6 with and without surgery for treatment of patients having the idiopathic carpal tunnel syndrome. Res Commun Chem Pathol Pharmacol 1981;33:331–44.

Ellis J, Folkers K, Watanabe T, Kaji M, Saji S, Caldwell JW, Temple CA, Wood FS. Clinical results of a cross-over treatment with pyridoxine and placebo of the carpal tunnel syndrome. Am J Clin Nutr 1979;32:2040–46.

Ellis JM, Kishi T, Azuma J, Folkers K. Vitamin B_6 deficiency in patients with a clinical syndrome including the carpal tunnel defect. Biochemical and clinical response to therapy with pyridoxine. Res Commun Chem Pathol Pharmacol 1976;13:743–57.

Falkenburg SA. Choosing hand splints to aid carpal tunnel syndrome recovery. Occup Health Saf 1987;56:60.

Folkers K, Ellis J, Watanabe T, Saji S, Kaji M. Biochemical evidence for a deficiency of vitamin B_6 in the carpal tunnel syndrome based on a crossover clinical study. Proc Natl Acad Sci USA 1978;75:3410–12.

Folkers K, Wolaniuk A, Vadhanavikit S. Enzymology of the response of the carpal tunnel syndrome to riboflavin and to combined riboflavin and pyridoxine. Proc Natl Acad Sci USA 1984;81:7076–78.

Foster JB. Hydrocortisone and the carpal-tunnel syndrome. Lancet 1960;1:454–56.

Fuhr JE, Farrow A, Nelson HS Jr. Vitamin B_6 levels in patients with carpal tunnel syndrome. Arch Surg 1989;124:1329–30.

Gelberman RH, Aronson D, Weisman MH. Carpal-tunnel syndrome. Results of a prospective trial of steroid injection and splinting. J Bone Joint Surg 1980;62A:1181–84.

Giannini F, Passero S, Cioni R, Paradiso C, Battistini N, Giordano N, Vaccai D, Marcolongo R. Electrophysiologic evaluation of local steroid injection in carpal tunnel syndrome. Arch Phys Med Rehabil 1991;72:738–42.

Goodman HV, Foster JB. Effect of local corticosteroid injection on median nerve conduction in carpal tunnel syndrome. Ann Phys Med 1962;6:287–94.

Goodman HV, Gilliatt RW. The effect of treatment on median nerve conduction in patients with the carpal tunnel syndrome. Ann Phys Med 1961;6:137–55.

Gottlieb NL, Riskin WG. Complications of local corticosteroid injections. JAMA 1980;243:1547–48.

Gray RG, Gottlieb NL. Intra-articular corticosteroids. An updated assessment. Clin Orthop 1983;177:235–63.

Green DP. Diagnostic and therapeutic value of carpal tunnel injection. J Hand Surg 1984;9A:850–54.

Heathfield KWG. Acroparaesthesiae and the carpal-tunnel syndrome. Lancet 1957;2:663–66.

Kasdan ML, Janes C. Carpal tunnel syndrome and vitamin B_6. Plast Reconstr Surg 1987;79:456–62.

Kopell HP. Carpal tunnel compression median neuropathy treated nonsurgically. NY State J Med 1958;58:744–45.

Linskey ME, Segal R. Median nerve injury from local steroid injection in carpal tunnel syndrome. Neurosurgery 1990;26:512–15.

McCallum MJ. Acroparaesthesia in pregnancy. Br Med J 1959;2:1095.

McConnell JR, Bush DC. Intraneural steroid injection as a complication in the management of carpal tunnel syndrome. A report of three cases. Clin Orthop 1990;250:181–84.

Minamikawa Y, Peimer CA, Kambe K, Wheeler DR, Sherwin FS. Tenosynovial injection for carpal tunnel syndrome. J Hand Surg 1992;17A:178–81.

Ozdogan H, Yazici H. The efficacy of local steroid injections in idiopathic carpal tunnel syndrome: a double-blind study. Br J Rheumatol 1984;23:272–75.

Parry GJ, Bredesen DE. Sensory neuropathy with low-dose pyridoxine. Neurology (Minneap) 1985;35:1466–68.

Phalen GS. The carpal-tunnel syndrome. Seventeen years' experience in diagnosis and treatment of six hundred fifty-four hands. J Bone Joint Surg 1966;48A:211–28.

Phalen GS, Kendrick JI. Compression neuropathy of the median nerve in the carpal tunnel. JAMA 1957;164:524–30.

Quin CE. Carpal tunnel syndrome: treatment by splinting. Ann Phys Med 1961;6:72–75.

Roaf R. Compression of the median nerve in the carpal tunnel. Lancet 1947;1:387.

Schaumberg HJ, Kaplan A, Windebank A, Vick N, Rasmus S, Pleasure D, Brown MJ. Sensory neuropathy from pyridoxine abuse: a new megavitamin syndrome. N Engl J Med 1983;309:445–48.

Scheyer RD, Haas DC. Pyridoxine in carpal tunnel syndrome (letter). Lancet 1985;2:42.

Smith GP, Rudge PJ, Peters TJ. Biochemical studies of pyridoxal and pyridoxal phosphate status and therapeutic trial of pyridoxine in patients with carpal tunnel syndrome. Ann Neurol 1984;15:104–7.

Stransky M, Rubin A, Lava NS, Lazaro RP. Treatment of carpal tunnel syndrome with vitamin B_6: a double-blind study. South Med J 1989;82:841–42.

van der Bracht AA. Carpal tunnel syndrome. Br Med J 1958;1:1180–81.

Vasile A, Goldberg R, Kornberg B. Pyridoxine toxicity: report of a case. J Am Osteopath Assoc 1984;83:790–91.

Wolaniuk A, Vadhanavikit S, Folkers K. Electromyographic data differentiate patients with the carpal tunnel syndrome when double blindly treated with pyridoxine and placebo. Res Commun Chem Pathol Pharmacol 1983;41:501–11.

Wood EC. Acroparaesthesia in pregnancy. Br Med J 1959;2:1254.

Wood MR. Hydrocortisone injections for carpal tunnel syndrome. Hand 1980;12:62–64.

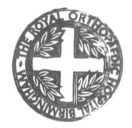

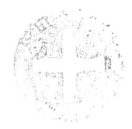

15

Surgical Treatment of Carpal Tunnel Syndrome

Learmonth (1933) first reported the surgical division of the flexor retinaculum to relieve the symptoms of carpal tunnel syndrome. By the late 1940s Cannon and Love (1946), Brain et al. (1947), and Phalen et al. (1950) had reported excellent symptomatic relief of carpal tunnel syndrome symptoms following surgery in small series of patients.

The preceding chapter discusses nonsurgical therapy and indications for electing surgical therapy. This chapter covers surgical technique, postoperative care, results of surgery, and complications of surgery.

TECHNIQUE

The basic concept is simple: complete section of the flexor retinaculum through a palmar incision. A number of variations on the theme are possible regarding details such as anesthesia, location of the incision, care in identifying nerve branches, treatment of the palmaris longus tendon, neurolysis of the median nerve, inspection and debridement of the carpal canal, intraoperative use of steroids, and postoperative care. Dawson et al. (1990), Ariyan and Watson (1977), Heckler and Jabaley (1986), and Conolly (1983) provide descriptions of their personal techniques with photographic illustrations.

Anesthesia

Carpal tunnel surgery may be performed under local or regional anesthesia (Duncan et al. 1987). General anesthesia is used for occasional cases. Most surgeons use a tourniquet to maintain a "bloodless" operative field.

Incision

A curvilinear longitudinal incision in line with the axis of the ring finger is strongly favored (Taleisnik 1973; Ariyan and Watson 1977; Heckler and Jabaley 1986). This minimizes the possibility of injury to the palmar cutaneous branches of the median and ulnar nerves. The operation may be done through a small incision, as outlined in Figure 15.1, but some cases require proximal extension of the incision, and some surgeons routinely use a longer incision (Duncan et al. 1987). The incision is carried down through the palmar aponeurosis to the flexor retinaculum (Denman 1981).

The palmar cutaneous branch leaves the radial side of the median nerve 5 to 8 cm above the distal wrist crease (Carroll and Green 1972; Taleisnik 1973). The nerve typically crosses the distal wrist crease at the tubercle of the navicular bone. The nerve is vulnerable to transection or to encasement in scar if the surgical incision is carried too far laterally. Figure 15.2 shows some of the unusual anomalous paths the nerve may follow; the surgeon must be aware of this even with the recommended longitudinal incision (Das and Brown 1976).

Engber and Gmeiner (1980) reported two cases of painful neuromata in the hypothenar area after carpal tunnel surgery. They demonstrated that the palmar cutaneous branch of the ulnar nerve could follow a variety of courses in the

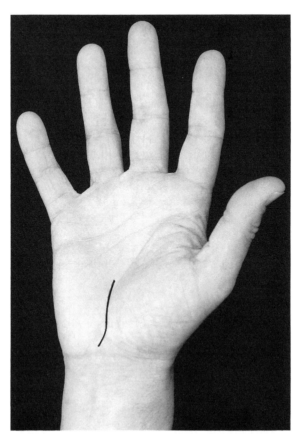

Figure 15.1 Outline of a typical incision for carpal tunnel surgery.

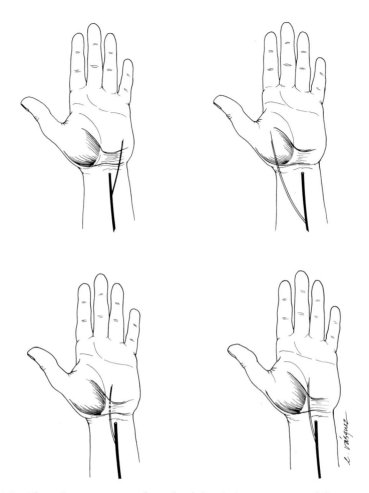

Figure 15.2 The palmar cutaneous branch of the median nerve may follow a variety of courses (see also Figure 1.5). (Reproduced with permission of the publisher from Das SK, Brown HG. In search of complications in carpal tunnel decompression. Hand 1976;8:243–49.)

hypothenar area. This nerve is best avoided if the incision is no more medial than the axis of the ring finger.

The simplest operation is section of the flexor retinaculum without exploration or disturbance of the median nerve or of the contents of the carpal tunnel. Prior to division of the retinaculum, the recurrent thenar motor branch of the median nerve must be identified and protected. The varied possible courses of this branch are illustrated in Chapter 1. The recurrent thenar motor branch is particularly vulnerable to injury when it takes a course through the flexor retinaculum. If the recurrent thenar motor branch is severed at the time of carpal tunnel surgery, the nerve should be primarily repaired; if the nerve laceration is unrecognized, the patient may require reoperation for secondary repair of the severed nerve (Mannerfelt and Hybbinette 1972; Lilly and Magnell 1985; Hybbinette 1986).

The flexor retinaculum must be divided from its most proximal to its most distal extent. Distally, care must be taken not to injure the digital nerves and the superficial palmar arterial arch (Semple and Cargill 1969). Phalen (1966) noted that after complete division the retinaculum will separate by about one-quarter inch.

A number of alternative operative techniques have been suggested but have not gained popularity (Pierce 1976; Fissette et al. 1981; Paine and Polyzoidis 1983; Grundberg 1986; Bergman et al. 1988; Pearl 1989).

Neurolysis

Neurolysis is usually not necessary at the time of carpal tunnel release. Opinion has been divided on its benefits (Phalen 1966; Curtis and Eversmann 1973; Hybbinette and Mannerfelt 1975). The argument for neurolysis is that nerve damage can be assessed and appropriate therapy planned only by inspection of the median nerve through the operating microscope (Palazzi and Palazzi 1980). Neurolysis starts with longitudinal division of the epineurium. Next, the epineurium is dissected away from the nerve fascicles to achieve external neurolysis. The dissection typically spares the dorsal epineurium in an effort to preserve microvascular supply to the nerve. The surgeon may proceed with an internal neurolysis to remove fibrosis between the fascicles. A fascicle that is deformed by scarring or neuroma might be resected and grafted. Some surgeons elect internal neurolysis based on the clinical severity of the median nerve deficit; others make a decision on the extent of neurolysis after inspecting the condition of the nerve at surgery.

Eversmann and Ritsick (1978) recommended internal neurolysis in patients with a preoperative deficit such as thenar atrophy or abnormal sensory examination. In seven patients undergoing carpal tunnel surgery with internal neurolysis, they measured median distal motor latency before release of the flexor retinaculum, after release, and after internal neurolysis. Five of the seven showed a greater improvement in distal motor latency after internal neurolysis than after release of the flexor retinaculum but before neurolysis. Table 15.1 shows the values for the seven patients.

Note that in contrast to the impressive improvement in five of the patients following neurolysis, patients number 5 and 7 showed a deterioration in median distal motor latency following neurolysis. During surgery in eight patients undergoing carpal tunnel release with neurolysis, Yates et al. (1981) measured median distal motor latency and thenar compound muscle action potential amplitude. Three of the patients had a drop in compound muscle potential amplitude after neurolysis, suggesting development of acute partial conduction block.

Even in patients with intraoperative improvement in nerve conduction after internal neurolysis, the electrical improvement does not guarantee that neurolysis leads to a superior clinical outcome. As discussed in Chapter 8, the correlation

Table 15.1 Median distal motor latency intraoperative results (msec)

Patient	Before Surgery	After Ligament Release	After Internal Neurolysis
1	9.7	7.9	6.7
2	8.6	7.1	4.5
3	7.1	6.7	5.1
4	10.1	8.3	5.9
5	4.0	5.1	5.3
6	5.6	5.5	4.6
7	8.3	4.9	5.4
Mean	7.6	6.5	5.4

(Data from Eversmann and Ritsick 1978.)

between nerve conduction results and symptoms is imperfect. Furthermore, internal neurolysis might lead to delayed fibrosis or nerve ischemia that could negate any of the acute benefits proposed by Eversmann and Ritsick.

A number of clinical studies address the effectiveness of neurolysis in carpal tunnel syndrome. Evrard and Tshiakatumba (1977) reported the results of carpal tunnel release accompanied by internal neurolysis in 18 hands. Some 89% of the operations gave excellent or good results; in comparison, they obtained good or excellent results in only 61% of an earlier surgical series of patients not treated with neurolysis. They provided little data on the comparability of the series.

Fissette and Onkelinx (1979) reported a series of 45 carpal tunnel operations in which they inspected the nerve under the microscope and performed an external neurolysis when the nerve was thickened or narrowed. In three cases, they found interstitial fibrosis and proceeded with internal neurolysis. They found no definite advantage with this protocol compared with their own experience with division of the flexor retinaculum without neurolysis.

Lowry and Follender (1988) randomized 50 carpal tunnel operations to flexor retinaculum release alone or to flexor retinaculum release followed by internal neurolysis. All of the patients had severe carpal tunnel syndrome with thenar atrophy or with a fixed median sensory deficit. Three months after surgery, 67% of the patients with neurolysis and 65% of the patients without neurolysis had a good or excellent surgical result. There was no significant difference between the two groups in postoperative median nerve conduction studies or in complication rate.

Holmgren-Larsson et al. randomized 48 patients to ligament division either alone or followed by internal neurolysis (Holmgren-Larsson et al. 1985; Holmgren and Rabow 1987). At immediate postoperative and three-year postoperative follow-up, the two groups had no significant differences in improvement following surgery.

Gelberman et al. initially favored internal neurolysis in patients with carpal tunnel syndrome that was severe enough to result in objective neurologic deficit (Rhoades et al. 1985). They reported excellent clinical results in 36 hands with this technique. They changed their opinion after evaluating 33 additional hands with equally severe neurologic deficit and obtaining equivalent results after section of the retinaculum without neurolysis (Gelberman et al. 1987).

In 63 carpal tunnel decompressions, Mackinnon et al. (1991) randomly assigned which patients would undergo internal neurolysis. In this prospective study, neurolysis added no demonstrable benefit to the surgical outcome.

In summary, division of the flexor retinaculum is extremely effective treatment for most cases of carpal tunnel syndrome. No consistent benefit from neurolysis has been demonstrated.

Flexor Tenosynovectomy

Phalen (1966) advised against routine flexor tenosynovectomy or neurolysis. He performed tenosynovectomy in 4% of his patients, only when the median nerve appeared persistently stretched after section of the ligament. The typical patient who requires tenosynovectomy has carpal tunnel syndrome accompanying rheumatoid arthritis (Straub and Ranawat 1969; Marmor 1971; Nalebuff 1983). Corradi et al. (1989) advocate flexor tenosynovectomy in chronic hemodialysis patients who require surgery for carpal tunnel syndrome. In a small, controlled series, Freshwater and Arons (1978) compared 12 patients treated with release of the flexor retinaculum alone to 14 patients who were treated with flexor retinaculum release, flexor tenosynovectomy, external neurolysis of the median nerve, and intraoperative instillation of steroids. At follow-up two years postoperatively, all 26 patients were asymptomatic. The group with the more extensive surgery had a longer average delay before return to work after surgery.

Palmaris Longus Tendon

Most surgeons do not resect the palmaris longus tendon routinely at the time of carpal tunnel surgery but will optionally resect the tendon on those rare occasions when it appears to compress the median nerve (Phalen 1966; Duncan et al. 1987).

Some surgeons advocate palmaris longus tendon transfer to the thenar muscles to improve opposition in selected patients with severe thenar atrophy (Littler and Li 1967; Braun 1978; Foucher et al. 1991). Other surgeons use various other forearm and hand muscles on those rare occasions when opponensplasty is needed (Inglis et al. 1972; Cooney 1988).

Carpal Tunnel Endoscopy

There is growing experience with endoscopic section of the flexor retinaculum with minimal disturbance of the skin or the palmar aponeurosis (Okutsu et al. 1987, 1989; Chow 1989). Endoscopy facilitates early hand mobilization, but there is little evidence that this improves or detracts from the final operative outcome. Chow (1990) reported the results of endoscopic carpal tunnel surgery in 149 hands. Some 86% of patients returned to work within four weeks of the procedure. In 45 patients tested for grip strength, grip had returned to pre-operative levels within four weeks after surgery. Injury to the digital nerves or to the median nerve proper has been noted as a complication of endoscopic carpal tunnel surgery (Palensky 1991).

Postoperative Care

Various postoperative regimens are used after carpal tunnel surgery, and little data favors one approach over another. Four fifths of hand surgeons apply a compressive dressing after surgery; one fifth do not (Duncan et al. 1987). Some leave the dressing on only 1 day; others for more than 10 days. Four fifths of hand surgeons apply a wrist splint. Surgical opinion is divided on whether the splint should be in extension or neutral position and on duration of splinting. Among those who prescribe a splint, most favor one to three weeks of splinting.

Chaise (1990) randomized 50 patients undergoing carpal tunnel surgery to immediate postoperative active mobilization without splinting or to splinting for 15 to 18 days in 20° of extension. He followed both grip strength and carpal tunnel computed tomography (CT) scanning at 2, 6, and 12 months postoperatively. The patients with active mobilization had a greater deficit in grip strength at follow-up; the grip strength in these patients was most impaired with the wrist flexed. The CT results suggested that healing without the splint allowed greater anterior bowing of the flexor retinaculum with a resulting adverse effect on the stability and strength of the thenar muscles and on the effective grip of the finger flexors.

In a group of patients after carpal tunnel surgery, Groves and Rider (1989) tried supervised hand therapy with resistive exercises and a work simulator between the third and sixth weeks after surgery. The supervised therapy offered little advantage over unsupervised hand activities such as gentle bending, warm soaks, and pursuit of simple daily tasks.

SURGICAL RESULTS

Patients commonly report dramatic improvement in symptoms after carpal tunnel surgery. Relief of intermittent paresthesia and pain and of nocturnal symptoms is often immediate or evident as soon as incisional pain resolves.

Cseuz et al. (1966) provided follow-up data on surgical results in 254 hands. The patients were surveyed by questionnaire, months to years after surgery; their assessments of postoperative results are shown in Table 15.2. Probability of improvement was independent of duration of symptoms or presence or absence of preoperative nerve conduction slowing. Older patients were less likely to obtain good symptomatic relief. Numerous surgical series have confirmed the generally excellent results of this operation (Table 15.3).

Table 15.2 Patient's estimate of postoperative improvement

Number of Patients	Amount of Improvement (%)
144	100
110	75
23	50
8	25
17	0
11	Worse

(Data from Cseuz et al. 1966.)

Prognosis for Recovery of Neurologic Deficit

After surgery, neurologic dysfunction usually improves, but the improvement may take weeks or months. Phalen (1966) reported results in 112 hands with preoperative thenar atrophy that were examined five months or more after surgery (Table 15.4).

The rapidity of recovery correlated with the duration of symptoms, but patients could show excellent motor recovery even if atrophy had been present for three years or more. Of the hands that failed to improve, seven had atrophy for more than 20 years, but six had atrophy for 1 year or less. The single patient with progressive atrophy was reexplored and found to have had incomplete section of the distal flexor retinaculum at the initial operation. Rietz and Onne (1967) also

Table 15.3 Results of carpal tunnel surgery

Series	Number of Hands	Results
Semple and Cargill 1969	150	75% of hands asymptomatic at follow-up two to seven years after surgery
Doyle and Carroll 1968	100	97% of hands relieved of symptoms or significantly better
Farhat et al. 1974	109	65% of hands excellent relief; 30% fair relief
Ariyan and Watson 1977	429	99% of hands improved
Hybbinette and Mannerfelt 1975	465	98% of hands relieved of carpal tunnel syndrome pain
Kulick et al. 1986	130	81% of hands free of symptoms at follow-up two to six years after surgery
Gainer and Nugent 1977	306	51% of hands cured; 31% greatly improved

Table 15.4 Thenar motor status after surgery in 112 patients with thenar atrophy

Normal or Nearly Normal	Partial Improvement	No Improvement	Progressive Atrophy
76 (68%)	16 (14%)	19 (17%)	1 (1%)

(Data from Phalen 1966.)

found that thenar atrophy often improved postoperatively even if present for over two years.

Phalen (1966) followed 200 patients who had impaired median cutaneous sensation prior to surgery. Some 77% had return of normal sensation postoperatively. Prognosis was slightly better in patients without thenar atrophy.

Other Prognostic Factors

Cseuz et al. (1966) found that duration of symptoms, presence of associated diseases, and extent of abnormality of median nerve conduction studies were not good predictors of outcome of carpal tunnel surgery.

Harris et al. (1979) found that patients who had prolonged median distal motor latency were more likely to have a good surgical response than were patients who had a normal median distal motor latency but prolonged median distal sensory latency. Mendelson and Balla (1973) made a similar observation and suggested that this seemingly paradoxical finding might indicate misdiagnoses in some patients with milder nerve conduction abnormalities.

Patients who obtain transient relief of symptoms from steroid injection of the carpal tunnel are more likely to benefit from carpal tunnel surgery than are patients who do not obtain relief from steroid injection (Green 1984; Kulick et al. 1986). Coexistent diffuse peripheral neuropathy does not preclude excellent response of carpal tunnel syndrome to surgery (Clayburgh et al. 1987).

In the series of Tountas et al. (1983), cases of carpal tunnel syndrome that had been labeled as workers' compensation cases were less likely to have good operative results (Table 15.5).

Table 15.5 Carpal tunnel surgery and workers' compensation

Surgical Result	Workers' Compensation	
	Yes (%)	No (%)
Good	66	85
Fair	23	11
Poor	11	4

(Data from Tountas et al. 1983.)

ANALYSIS OF UNSATISFACTORY SURGICAL RESULTS

In every series of carpal tunnel operations, a minority of patients have unsatisfactory results. The operation is now done so frequently that treatment and diagnosis of these patients who have not been cured by initial surgery are becoming common clinical challenges. Patients may be divided into those who have persistent symptoms after surgery, those who have recurrent symptoms of carpal tunnel syndrome after initially successful surgery, and those who have new symptom patterns after surgery. Table 15.6 outlines a differential diagnosis for these patients.

Incomplete Relief of Symptoms with Surgery

In the past the most common cause of incomplete relief of symptoms after surgery has been incomplete division of the flexor retinaculum (Stark 1968; Conolly 1978; MacDonald et al. 1978). Langloh and Linscheid (1972) found that of patients who had a second operation for incomplete section of the flexor retinaculum, 80% had had incomplete relief of symptoms following the first operation or had had recurrent symptoms within three months of the first

Table 15.6 Unsatisfactory results of carpal tunnel surgery

Incomplete Relief of Symptoms with Surgery

Delayed neurologic recovery

Incomplete section of the flexor retinaculum

Multicausal hand symptoms

Recurrent Carpal Tunnel Syndrome After Initial Success

Perineural fibrosis

Progressive tenosynovitis

Unusual canal contents

New Symptom Patterns After Surgery

Postoperative wrist pain

"Reflex sympathetic dystrophy"

Joint stiffness

Loss of hand strength

Bowstringing of flexor tendons

Alterations in carpal arch configuration

Postoperative wound infection

Iatrogenic nerve branch injury

Postoperative tourniquet palsy

operation. Use of a transverse, rather than longitudinal, incision increases the risk of incomplete visualization of the distal extent of the ligament (Phalen 1966; Stark 1968). Now that the importance of complete section to the distal edge of the flexor retinaculum is widely known, this complication should be increasingly uncommon.

Patients who have a preoperative neurologic dysfunction, despite slow or incomplete recovery of nerve function, usually have excellent postoperative relief of pain and paresthesias if the flexor retinaculum is adequately sectioned (Phalen 1966). Worsening of neurologic dysfunction following surgery, however, suggests inadequate decompression of the median nerve or an alternative neurologic diagnosis.

In some patients, pain persists after carpal tunnel surgery because the initial diagnosis was incorrect or incomplete. Either the diagnosis of carpal tunnel syndrome may have been incorrect or the patient may have another condition in addition to carpal tunnel syndrome. Crymble (1968) found this pattern in 20% of 140 patients who underwent carpal tunnel surgery. New diagnoses were made postoperatively after the patients had only partial relief of symptoms; diagnoses included De Quervain's tenosynovitis, ulnar nerve compression at the elbow, tenosynovitis of flexor pollicis longus, and lateral epicondylitis. Conolly (1978) reported patients in whom diagnoses of diffuse peripheral neuropathy or cervical spondylosis became evident after carpal tunnel surgery failed. Eason et al. (1985) found that 81% of their patients with suboptimal surgical results had had coexistent neck pain or X-ray evidence of cervical spondylosis, but the authors do not include control data on the incidence of these common findings in a matched population.

Patients with multicausal hand symptoms such as carpal tunnel syndrome accompanied by Dupuytren's contracture, flexor tenosynovitis, or arthritis of the basal thumb joint are likely to have hand symptoms after carpal tunnel surgery (Bloem et al. 1986). Nissenbaum and Kleinert (1980) found that their patients who had treatment of carpal tunnel syndrome and Dupuytren's contracture in a single operation often had postoperative hand symptoms, but Gonzalez and Watson (1991) reported good results when correcting both conditions at the same operation.

Recurrent Carpal Tunnel Syndrome After Initial Surgical Success

An occasional patient will report that symptoms abated shortly after carpal surgery but that typical symptoms of carpal tunnel syndrome recurred months to years later. Langloh and Linscheid (1972) found that patients with this history often had scar formation in the carpal tunnel or tenosynovial hypertrophy leading to recurrent nerve compression. In 40 wrists reexplored because of recurrent symptoms of carpal tunnel syndrome, Wadstroem and Nigst (1986) found perineural fibrosis in 36 and flexor tenosynovitis in 19.

Six patients in a surgical series of 140 experienced excellent initial relief of symptoms postoperatively but reported recurrent symptoms several months later. At reoperation their retinacula were thickened and had rejoined. The retinacula were resectioned and partially removed, with lasting relief of symptoms (Crymble 1968).

The median nerve can be trapped in the fibrotic retinaculum (Inglis 1980). Sennwald and Hagen (1990) repeated surgery in 12 patients with recurrent pain after initial carpal tunnel release. At reexploration, the median nerves of these patients had migrated anteriorly and were fixed in the scar of the flexor retinaculum. In some cases, they also noted anterior subluxation of the flexor tendons. They suggested that simple section of the flexor retinaculum should be replaced with reconstruction of the ligament using tendon from the palmaris brevis or flexor carpi radialis to allow increase in canal volume without the danger of anterior subluxation of the canal contents.

On rare occasion reexploration will reveal abnormal canal contents that were not recognized at the first operation; reported examples include a ganglion in the canal or chronic granulomatous infection (Kelly et al. 1967; Conolly 1978; Langa et al. 1986).

New Symptom Patterns After Surgery
Postoperative Wrist Pain
Following carpal tunnel surgery the operative scar is often reported as feeling painfully sensitive and uncomfortable. (Farhat et al. 1974). Usually, wrist pain resolves within six months of surgery (Das and Brown 1976). Cseuz et al. (1966) found that 36% of their patients reported unpleasant scar sensitivity when queried months or years postoperatively. Most patients with scar symptoms reported "minor discomfort which did not interfere with their daily activities." Some patients reported scar discomfort for over three years after surgery.

An occasional patient develops a hypertrophic wrist scar (MacDonald et al. 1978; Louis et al. 1985). This is more likely to occur if the initial incision crosses the distal wrist crease at right angles.

Seradge and Seradge (1989) identified five instances among 500 carpal tunnel operations of patients who had persistent hypothenar pain six months after surgery. In these patients, the pain could be induced by ulnar displacement of the pisiform bone. The patients had temporary relief of pain and improvement of grip strength after local anesthetic injection of the piso-triquetrum joint. In all five patients, excision of the pisiform bone relieved the pain.

"Reflex Sympathetic Dystrophy"
On rare occasion, a patient develops chronic pain and autonomic and vasomotor dysfunction in the operated hand after carpal tunnel surgery (Mac-Donald et al. 1978). The hand may be swollen, warm, usually dry. Later, the skin may become cool, pale, or shiny with trophic changes. The patient may describe hyperalgesia and hyperesthesia. If treated early with physical therapy and re-portedly, with sympathetic blockade, symptoms may resolve. Case 3, Chapter 16,

illustrates how histrionic features may complicate evaluation of patients with purported "reflex sympathetic dystrophy."

Three-fourths of MacDonald's patients with this complication had undergone neurolysis. Might neurolysis increase the risk of this complication? We do not have sufficient data to draw conclusions.

As discussed in Chapter 16, the definition and diagnosis of reflex sympathetic dystrophy are fraught with difficulty. Milward et al. (1977) describe a patient who developed hand swelling and "scalding" pain after carpal tunnel surgery. Pain did not improve with stellate ganglion block. When the wrist was reexplored, extensive scar formation was found involving both the median and ulnar nerves, and symptoms improved following neurolysis of both nerves.

Joint Stiffness

Rarely, patients describe increased stiffness in finger joints after carpal tunnel surgery (MacDonald et al. 1978). At the extreme, they may permanently develop contractures of interphalangeal joints (Louis et al. 1985). Active finger use early after surgery should minimize the risk of this complication, and hand physical therapy is the treatment of choice if postoperative joint stiffness develops.

Loss of Hand Strength

There is conflicting opinion on the effect of carpal tunnel surgery on hand strength. Most reviews of surgical results fail to assess postoperative grip strength. A retrospective survey of employees at a meat processing plant who had undergone carpal tunnel surgery found that 78% of the patients complained that grip strength was persistently decreased following surgery; grip strength was not actually measured in this series (Masear et al. 1986). Gartsman et al. (1986) retrospectively measured grip strength in 46 patients examined eight months or more after unilateral carpal tunnel surgery. After correcting for hand dominance, they found that the operated hand was a mean of 12% weaker than the nonoperated hand. Gellman et al. (1989) measured grip and pinch strength before and after carpal tunnel surgery in 24 hands. Six months after surgery, pinch strength was 126%, and grip strength was 116% of preoperative levels. Chaise (1990) found that grip strength, particularly when the wrist was flexed, was more likely to be impaired one year after surgery if the wrist was not splinted for two to three weeks postoperatively.

Fissette et al. (1981) reconstructed the flexor retinaculum at the time of the initial carpal tunnel surgery using a Dacron and silicone sheet. They compared grip strength after surgery in 26 patients who had the surgery with reconstruction and in 27 patients who had division of the flexor retinaculum without reconstruction. The group with reconstruction had consistently stronger grips at 3, 6, 9, and 12 months after surgery. Unfortunately, there is no preoperative data on group comparability; however, the groups did not have consistent postoperative differences in strength of pronation or supination. Fissette et al. argue that reconstruction of the flexor retinaculum was particularly important for maintaining grip strength.

Bowstringing of Flexor Tendons

In rare patients, after division of the flexor retinaculum, the flexor tendons move anteriorly with wrist flexion (MacDonald et al. 1978). When these patients flex their wrists, they may experience pain, a snapping sensation, and paresthesias in a median distribution. The subluxed tendons may be visible on examination of the flexed wrist.

Alterations in Carpal Arch Configuration

There is increasing interest in the effect of carpal tunnel surgery on the configuration of the carpal bones. Gartsman et al. (1986) estimated the transverse carpal diameter by measuring the distance between the palmar tips of the ridge of the trapezium and the hook of the hamate on standardized carpal radiographs. They compared the wrist that had surgery to the contralateral unoperated wrist; 47 of 50 patients had a postoperative increase in the transverse diameter of the canal. The amount of increase correlated with amount of decrease in the patient's grip strength but not with the presence or absence of postoperative wrist pain. The operated wrists did not lose range of flexion or extension.

Richman et al. (1989) used magnetic resonance imaging (MRI) to compare wrist configuration before and after carpal tunnel surgery. They found that after surgery carpal canal volume increased an average of 24%, and the median nerve was displaced an average of 3.5 mm anteriorly. They found that the transverse diameter of the carpal canal was increased six weeks after surgery, but the increase disappeared at later follow-up.

These few studies on grip strength and on carpal configuration after surgery are tantalizing. If grip strength is consistently decreased after surgery, treatment options, particularly for patients who wish to resume vigorous hand use after surgery, need to be reconsidered. More data is needed on the role of flexor retinaculum reconstruction or of postoperative mobilization or splinting on hand function after surgery.

Postoperative Wound Infection

The risk of deep postoperative wound infection after carpal tunnel surgery is small. At the Mayo Clinic the incidence of infection was 0.5% in 3,600 operations (Hanssen et al. 1989). *Staphylococcus aureus* was the most commonly identified organism, but a variety of other bacteria have been found in individual cases. In one case, the offending organism was *Prototheca wickerhamii,* an algaelike organism (Moyer et al. 1990). Risk factors for infection include tenosynovectomy, intraoperative steroid installation, use of a surgical drain, and longer operating time. Sequelae of infection may include scar pain, loss of range of motion, tendon rupture, and swan neck deformity.

Iatrogenic Nerve Branch Injury

The median nerve proper, the recurrent thenar motor branch, the median palmar cutaneous nerve branch, the ulnar palmar cutaneous nerve branch, the superficial radial nerve, and digital nerve branches are all vulnerable to injury at the time of carpal tunnel surgery. When the recurrent thenar motor branch is injured, clinical examination will show thenar weakness with preserved lumbrical and median sensory function. Electromyography (EMG) can confirm the diagnosis and often characterize the nature of the nerve injury. When a sensory branch is injured, local sensory impairment is often accompanied by a painful neuroma and a positive Tinel's sign at the site of nerve injury. Table 15.7 provides references to examples of iatrogenic nerve injuries from carpal tunnel surgery.

Postoperative neuroma of a cutaneous nerve such as the median or ulnar palmar cutaneous branches can improve with surgery.

Postoperative Tourniquet Palsy

Usually, carpal tunnel surgery is completed in less than one hour; therefore, clinical postoperative tourniquet palsies should not occur (Flatt 1972). However, the tourniquet can cause subclinical nerve injury. Nitz and Dobner (1989) performed EMGs in 60 patients three weeks before and three weeks after carpal

Table 15.7 Iatrogenic nerve injury after carpal tunnel surgery

Nerve	Reference
Digital	Das and Brown 1976 Semple and Cargill 1969
Median palmar cutaneous	Louis et al. 1985 MacDonald et al. 1978 Das and Brown 1976 Hybbinette and Mannerfelt 1975 Taleisnik 1973 Carroll and Green 1972
Recurrent thenar motor	Hybbinette 1986 Lilly and Magnell 1985 Das and Brown 1976 Hybbinette and Mannerfelt 1975 Mannerfelt and Hybbinette 1972
Superficial radial	Louis et al. 1985
Ulnar	Favero and Gropper 1987
Ulnar-median digital anastomosis	May and Rosen 1981
Ulnar palmar cutaneous	Engber and Gmeinar 1980

tunnel surgery. Patients were randomized in regard to use of a tourniquet during surgery. Tourniquet time was one hour or less. After surgery, reportedly 77% of patients in whom a tourniquet was used, but only 3% of patients who did not have a tourniquet, had developed fibrillations, positive sharp waves, or bizarre high-frequency discharges in nonthenar muscles distal to the tourniquet.

Crandall and Weeks (1988) described a 24-year-old woman who developed radial, anterior interosseous, and ulnar neuropathies in an arm that had had carpal surgery with use of a tourniquet. The delayed onset of these neuropathies excluded a classic tourniquet palsy, which is apparent immediately postoperatively. They speculated whether the tourniquet had caused subclinical nerve injury that predisposed to the development of the subsequent neuropathies.

SURGICAL REEXPLORATION

Persistent or recurrent carpal tunnel syndrome after carpal tunnel surgery should prompt consideration of surgical reexploration of the carpal tunnel. Patients with postoperative wrist pain or alternative hand diagnoses must be

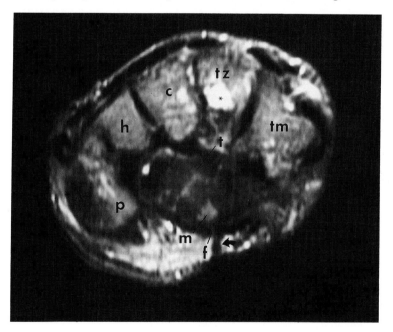

Figure 15.3 Failed carpal tunnel surgery. The axial T2–weighted magnetic resonance (MR) image of the wrist shows abnormalities in a patient who had persistent neuropathic symptoms after carpal tunnel surgery. The *curved arrow* points to postsurgical scarring at the site of the incision. The flexor retinaculum *(f)* appears continuous and shows thickening and volar bowing. The median nerve *(m)* is prominent with high signal intensity, suggesting nerve edema or inflammation. There is an incident intraosseous cyst in the trapezoid. Hamate *(h)*, pisiform *(p)*, capitate *(c)*, trapezoid *(tz)*, trapezium *(tm)*, and flexor tendons *(t)*. (Courtesy of Dr. Stephen F. Quinn.)

separated carefully from those with unrelieved or recurrent carpal tunnel syndrome, since the former are unlikely to benefit from repeated carpal tunnel surgery. Surgery is definitely indicated in patients with progressive median nerve dysfunction.

The timing of improvement in median nerve conduction that follows successful carpal tunnel surgery is reviewed in Chapter 8. Failure of nerve conduction to evolve toward normal as expected after surgery is another indicator of incomplete nerve decompression.

MRI scanning can be particularly helpful to evaluate postoperative symptoms, both to exclude unexpected masses in the carpal canal and to assess the continuity of the flexor retinaculum (Mesgarzadeh et al. 1989; Reicher and Kellerhouse 1990). Figure 15.3 shows an MRI scan of the wrist of a patient who had recurrent symptoms of median nerve compression after carpal tunnel surgery. The MRI finding of an intact or refibrosed flexor retinaculum was matched by the surgical finding of fibrotic scarring at the site of previous section of the ligament. Following the reexploration, the patient had relief of the symptoms of median nerve compression.

When patients for reexploration are chosen with care, the majority improve after the second surgery (Langloh and Linscheid 1972; Wadstroem and Nigst 1986). A decision to repeat carpal tunnel surgery requires careful consideration of the differential diagnosis, and most patients with hand symptoms after carpal tunnel surgery do not need reexploration.

REFERENCES

Ariyan S, Watson HK. The palmar approach for the visualization and release of the carpal tunnel. An analysis of 429 cases. Plast Reconstr Surg 1977;60:539–47.

Bergman RS, Murphy BJ, Foglietti MA. Clinical experience with the CO_2 laser during carpal tunnel decompression. Plast Reconstr Surg 1988;81:933–38.

Bloem JJ, Pradjarahardja MC, Vuursteen PJ. The post-carpal tunnel syndrome. Causes and prevention. Neth J Surg 1986;38:52–55.

Brain WR, Wright AD, Wilkinson M. Spontaneous compression of both median nerves in the carpal tunnel. Lancet 1947;1:277–82.

Braun RM. Palmaris longus tendon transfer for augmentation of the thenar musculature in low median palsy. J Hand Surg 1978;3:488–91.

Cannon BW, Love JG. Tardy median palsy; median neuritis; median thenar neuritis amenable to surgery. Surgery 1946;20:210–16.

Carroll RE, Green DP. The significance of the palmar cutaneous nerve at the wrist. Clin Orthop 1972;83:24–28.

Chaise F. Immediate active mobilization or rigid postoperative immobilization of the wrist in carpal tunnel syndrome. Comparative analysis of a series of 50 patients (in French). Rev Rhum Mal Osteoartic 1990;57:435–39.

Chow JCY. Endoscopic release of the carpal ligament: a new technique for carpal tunnel syndrome. Arthroscopy 1989;5:19–24.

Chow JCY. Endoscopic release of the carpal ligament for carpal tunnel syndrome: 22 month clinical result. Arthroscopy 1990;6:288–96.

Clayburgh RH, Beckenbaugh RD, Dobyns JH. Carpal tunnel release in patients with diffuse peripheral neuropathy. J Hand Surg 1987;12A:380–83.

Conolly WB. Pitfalls in carpal tunnel decompression. Aust NZ J Surg 1978;48:421–25.

Conolly WB. Color atlas of treatment of carpal tunnel syndrome. Oradell, NJ: Medical Economics Books, 1983.

Cooney WP. Tendon transfer for median nerve palsy. Hand Clin 1988;4:155–65.

Corradi M, Paganelli E, Pavesi G. Internal neurolysis and flexor tenosynovectomy: adjuncts in the treatment of chronic median nerve compression at the wrist in hemodialysis patients. Microsurgery 1989;10:248–50.

Crandall RE, Weeks PM. Multiple nerve dysfunction after carpal tunnel release. J Hand Surg 1988;13A:584–89.

Crymble B. Brachial neuralgia and the carpal tunnel syndrome. Br Med J 1968;3:470–71.

Cseuz KA, Thomas JE, Lambert EH, Love JG, Lipscomb PR. Long-term results of operation for carpal tunnel syndrome. Mayo Clin Proc 1966;41:232–41.

Curtis RM, Eversmann WW Jr. Internal neurolysis as an adjunct to the treatment of the carpal-tunnel syndrome. J Bone Joint Surg 1973;55A:733–40.

Das SK, Brown HG. In search of complications in carpal tunnel decompression. Hand 1976;8:243–49.

Dawson DM, Hallett M, Millender LH. Carpal tunnel syndrome. In: Entrapment neuropathies. 2nd ed. Boston: Little, Brown, 1990; 25–92.

Denman EE. The anatomy of the incision for carpal tunnel decompression. Hand 1981;13:17–28.

Doyle JR, Carroll RE. The carpal tunnel syndrome. A review of 100 patients treated surgically. Calif Med 1968;108:263–67.

Duncan KH, Lewis RC Jr, Foreman KA, Nordyke MD. Treatment of carpal tunnel syndrome by members of the American Society for Surgery of the Hand: results of a questionnaire. J Hand Surg 1987;12A:384–91.

Eason SY, Belsole RJ, Greene TL. Carpal tunnel release: analysis of suboptimal results. J Hand Surg 1985;10B:365–69.

Engber WD, Gmeiner JG. Palmar cutaneous branch of the ulnar nerve. J Hand Surg 1980;5:26–29.

Eversmann WW Jr, Ritsick JA. Intraoperative changes in motor nerve conduction latency in carpal tunnel syndrome. J Hand Surg 1978;3:77–81.

Evrard H, Tshiakatumba MB. Intraneural neurolysis (in French.) Acta Orthop Belg 1977;43:186–90.

Farhat SM, Kahn EA, Child MA. The carpal tunnel syndrome. Surg Neurol 1974;2:285–88.

Favero KJ, Gropper PT. Ulnar nerve laceration—a complication of carpal tunnel decompression: case report and review of the literature. J Hand Surg 1987;12B:239–41.

Fissette J, Boucq D, Lahaye T, Onkelinx A. Effects of reconstruction of the anterior annular carpal ligament using a silicone sheet in surgery of the carpal tunnel syndrome (in French). Acta Orthop Belg 1981;47:375–81.

Fissette J, Onkelinx A. Treatment of carpal tunnel syndrome. Comparative study with and without epineurolysis. Hand 1979;11:206–10.

Flatt AE. Tourniquet time in hand surgery. Arch Surg 1972;104:190–92.

Foucher G, Malizos C, Sammut D, Marin Braun F, Michon J. Primary palmaris longus transfer as an opponensplasty in carpal tunnel syndrome. J Hand Surg 1991;16B:56–60.

Freshwater MF, Arons MS. The effect of various adjuncts on the surgical treatment of carpal tunnel syndrome secondary to chronic tenosynovitis. Plast Reconstr Surg 1978;61:93–96.

Gainer JV Jr, Nugent GR. Carpal tunnel syndrome: report of 430 operations. South Med J 1977;70:325–28.

Gartsman GM, Kovach JC, Crouch CC, Noble PC, Bennett JB. Carpal arch alteration after carpal tunnel release. J Hand Surg 1986;11A:372–74.

Gelberman RH, Pfeffer GB, Galbraith RT, Szabo RM, Rydevik B, Dimick, M. Results of treatment of severe carpal-tunnel syndrome without internal neurolysis of the median nerve. J Bone Joint Surg 1987;69A:896–903.

Gellman H, Kan D, Gee V, Kuschner SH, Botte MJ. Analysis of pinch and grip strength after carpal tunnel release. J Hand Surg 1989;14A:863–64.

Gonzalez F, Watson HK. Simultaneous carpal tunnel release and Dupuytren's fasciectomy. J Hand Surg 1991;16B:175–78.

Green DP. Diagnostic and therapeutic value of carpal tunnel injection. J Hand Surg 1984;9A:850–54.

Groves EJ, Rider BA. A comparison of treatment approaches used after carpal tunnel release surgery. Am J Occup Ther 1989;43:398–402.

Grundberg AB. Guyon's canal decompression (letter). J Hand Surg 1986;11A:454.

Hanssen AD, Amadio PC, DeSilva SP, Ilstrup DM. Deep postoperative wound infection after carpal tunnel release. J Hand Surg 1989;14A:869–73.

Harris CM, Tanner E, Goldstein MN, Pettee DS. The surgical treatment of the carpal-tunnel syndrome correlated with preoperative nerve-conduction studies. J Bone Joint Surg 1979;61A:93–98.

Heckler FR, Jabaley ME. Evolving concepts of median nerve decompression in the carpal tunnel. Hand Clin 1986;2:723–36.

Holmgren H, Rabow L. Internal neurolysis or ligament division only in carpal tunnel syndrome. II. A 3 year follow-up with an evaluation of various neurophysiological parameters for diagnosis. Acta Neurochir (Wien) 1987;87:44–47.

Holmgren-Larsson H, Leszniewski W, Linden U, Rabow L, Thorling J. Internal neurolysis or ligament division only in carpal tunnel syndrome—results of a randomized study. Acta Neurochir (Wien) 1985;74:118–21.

Hybbinette CH. Severance of thenar branch (letter). J Hand Surg 1986;11A:613.

Hybbinette CH, Mannerfelt L. The carpal tunnel syndrome. A retrospective study of 400 operated patients. Acta Orthop Scand 1975;46:610–20.

Inglis AE. Two unusual operative complications in the carpal-tunnel syndrome. A report of two cases. J Bone Joint Surg 1980;62A:1208–9.

Inglis AE, Straub LR, Williams CS. Median nerve neuropathy at the wrist. Clin Orthop 1972;83:48–54.

Kelly PJ, Karlson AG, Weed LA, Lipscomb PR. Infection of synovial tissues by mycobacteria other than *Mycobacterium tuberculosis*. J Bone Joint Surg 1967;49A:1521–30.

Kulick MI, Gordillo G, Javidi T, Kilgore ES Jr, Newmayer III WL. Long-term analysis of patients having surgical treatment for carpal tunnel syndrome. J Hand Surg 1986;11A:59–66.

Langa V, Posner MA, Hoffman S, Steiner GC. Carpal tunnel syndrome secondary to tuberculous tenosynovitis. Bull Hosp Joint Dis 1986;46:137–42.

Langloh ND, Linscheid RL. Recurrent and unrelieved carpal-tunnel syndrome. Clin Orthop 1972;83:41–47.

Learmonth JR. Treatment of diseases of peripheral nerves. Surg Clin North Am 1933;13:905–13.

Lilly CJ, Magnell TD. Severance of the thenar branch of the median nerve as a complication of carpal tunnel release. J Hand Surg 1985;10A:399–402.

Littler JW, Li CS. Primary restoration of thumb opposition with median nerve decompression. Plast Reconstr Surg 1967;39:74–75.

Louis DS, Greene TL, Noellert RC. Complications of carpal tunnel surgery. J Neurosurg 1985;62:352–56.

Lowry WE Jr, Follender AB. Interfascicular neurolysis in the severe carpal tunnel syndrome. A prospective, randomized, double-blind, controlled study. Clin Orthop 1988;227:251–54.

MacDonald RI, Lichtman DM, Hanlon JJ, Wilson JN. Complications of surgical release for carpal tunnel syndrome. J Hand Surg 1978;3:70–76.

Mackinnon SE, McCabe S, Murray JF, Szalai JP, Kelly L, Novak C, Kin B, Burke GM. Internal neurolysis fails to improve the results of primary carpal tunnel decompression. J Hand Surg 1991;16A:211–18.

Mannerfelt L, Hybbinette CH. Important anomaly of the thenar motor branch of the median nerve. A clinical and anatomical report. Bull Hosp Joint Dis 1972;33:15–21.

Marmor L. Surgery of rheumatoid hand and wrist. Semin Arthritis Rheum 1971;1:7–24.

Masear VR, Hayes JM, Hyde AG. An industrial cause of carpal tunnel syndrome. J Hand Surg 1986;11A:222–27.

May JW Jr, Rosen H. Division of the sensory ramus communicans between the ulnar and median nerves: a complication following carpal tunnel release. A case report. J Bone Joint Surg 1981;63A:836–38.

Mendelson B, Balla J. Results of surgical treatment of the carpal tunnel syndrome. Proc Aust Assoc Neurol 1973;9:129–32.

Mesgarzadeh M, Schneck CD, Bonakdarpour A, Mitra A, Conaway D. Carpal tunnel: MR imaging. Part II. Carpal tunnel syndrome. Radiology 1989;171:749–54.

Milward TM, Stott WG, Kleinert HE. The abductor digiti minimi muscle flap. Hand 1977;9:82–85.

Moyer RA, Bush DC, Dennehy JJ. *Prototheca wickerhamii* tenosynovitis. J. Rheumatol. 1990;17:701–4.

Nalebuff EA. Rheumatoid hand surgery—update. J Hand Surg 1983;8A:678–82.

Nissenbaum M, Kleinert HE. Treatment considerations in carpal tunnel syndrome with coexistent Dupuytren's disease. J Hand Surg 1980;5:544–47.

Nitz AJ, Dobner JJ. Upper extremity tourniquet effects in carpal tunnel release. J Hand Surg 1989;14A:499–504.

Okutsu I, Ninomiya S, Natsuyama M, Takatori Y, Inanami H, Kuroshima N, Hiraki S. Subcutaneous operation and examination under universal endoscope. Nippon Seikeige-ka Gakkai Zasshi 1987;61:491–98.

Okutsu I, Ninomiya S, Takatori Y, Ugawa Y. Endoscopic management of carpal tunnel syndrome. Arthroscopy 1989;5:11–18.

Paine KW, Polyzoidis KS. Carpal tunnel syndrome. Decompression using the Paine retina-culotome. J Neurosurg 1983;59:1031–36.

Palazzi S, Palazzi JL. Neurolysis in compressive neuropathies. Int Surg 1980;65:509–14.

Palensky FJ. Dear Doctor letter of 28 Feb 1991, from 3M Orthopedic Products.

Pearl RM. Use of the laser in treatment of carpal tunnel syndrome (letter). Plast Reconstr Surg 1989;83:577.

Phalen GS. The carpal-tunnel syndrome. Seventeen years' experience in diagnosis and treatment of six hundred fifty-four hands. J Bone Joint Surg 1966;48A:211–28.

Phalen GS, Gardner WJ, La Londe AA. Neuropathy of the median nerve due to compression beneath the transverse carpal ligament. J Bone Joint Surg 1950;32A:109–12.

Pierce RO. A different surgical approach for carpal tunnel syndrome. J Natl Med Assoc 1976;68:252.

Reicher MA, Kellerhouse LE. Carpal tunnel disease, flexor and extensor tendon disorders. In: Reicher MA, Kellerhouse LE, eds. MRI of the wrist and hand. New York: Raven Press, 1990; 49–68.

Rhoades CE, Mowery CA, Gelberman RH. Results of internal neurolysis of the median nerve for severe carpal-tunnel syndrome. J Bone Joint Surg 1985;67A:253–56.

Richman JA, Gelberman RH, Rydevik BL, Hajek PC, Braun RM, Gylys-Morin VM, Berthoty D. Carpal tunnel syndrome: morphologic changes after release of the transverse carpal ligament. J Hand Surg 1989;14A:852–57.

Rietz KA, Onne L. Analysis of sixty-five operated cases of carpal tunnel syndrome. Acta Chir Scand 1967;133:443–47.

Semple JC, Cargill AO. Carpal-tunnel syndrome. Results of surgical decompression. Lancet 1969;1:918–19.

Sennwald G, Hagen K. Decompression of the carpal tunnel. Apropos of 16 reoperated cases. Schweiz Med Wochenschr 1990;120:931–35.

Seradge H, Seradge E. Piso-triquetral pain syndrome after carpal tunnel release. J Hand Surg 1989;14A:858–62.

Stark WA. Carpal tunnel syndrome, failure of surgery. J Indiana State Med Assoc 1968;61:1547–50.

Straub LR, Ranawat CS. The wrist in rheumatoid arthritis. Surgical treatment and results. J Bone Joint Surg 1969;51A:1–20.

Taleisnik J. The palmar cutaneous branch of the median nerve and the approach to the carpal tunnel. An anatomical study. J Bone Joint Surg 1973;55A:1212–17.

Tountas CP, MacDonald CJ, Meyerhoff JD, Bihrle DM. Carpal tunnel syndrome. A review of 507 patients. Minn Med 1983;66:479–82.

Wadstroem J, Nigst H. Reoperation for carpal tunnel syndrome. A retrospective analysis of forty cases. Ann Chir Main 1986;5:54–58.

Yates SK, Hurst LN, Brown WF. Physiological observations in the median nerve during carpal tunnel surgery. Ann Neurol 1981;10:227–29.

16

Median Nerve "Causalgia"

The term *causalgia* (from the Greek *kausos*—"burning"—and *algos*—"pain") was used by Weir Mitchell (1872) in his descriptions of painful limbs that he investigated in Civil War veterans. He described a number of cases of causalgia following median nerve injury.

Causalgia is defined in different ways by different authors (International Association for the Study of Pain [IASP] 1986; Abram et al. 1989; Bonica 1990; see Ochoa and Verdugo 1993). Common features of several definitions of causalgia include chronic pains and hyperalgesias, often associated with sensory, motor, and autonomic signs, resulting from nerve trauma (or disease). After Weir Mitchell, the term was also used by Leriche (1916), Doupe et al. (1944), Livingston (1947), Nathan (1947), Loh and Nathan (1978), and then many others to describe patients with chronic pains and sensorimotor manifestations, usually associated with vasomotor changes. Some of the patients seemed responsive to sympathetic blocks or sympathectomy.

Clinicians assessing the hand and its innervation are routinely confronted by cases of chronic burning hand pain, commonly associated with positive and/or negative motor, sensory, or autonomic manifestations, strongly suggesting "neuropathic" dysfunction. In these patients, the clinical challenge is to determine:

1. the presence or absence of detectable peripheral nerve dysfunction
2. the relationship of the positive and negative clinical phenomena to nerve dysfunction, when present
3. the legitimate role of the sympathetic system as a possible cause of pain

This diagnostic exercise calls for special zeal because

1. most nerve injuries do not lead to causalgia
2. refined electrophysiologic methods can detect subtle subclinical local nerve dysfunction, which may be misconstrued as the authentic basis for the clinical symptoms (see Gilliatt 1978)
3. in many patients with a picture of "causalgia" and presumed nerve injury, the absence of nerve injury can be convincingly demonstrated

SENSORY PATHOPHYSIOLOGY IN NERVE DYSFUNCTION

Most patients with nerve injury develop sensory dysfunction. A minority of patients develop chronic spontaneous pains after nerve injury. Gentle stimulation of the symptomatic area may also induce pain with abnormal ease (hyperalgesia; allodynia). Both in the peripheral and the central nervous system, a number of hypothetical or proven pathophysiologic phenomena may be responsible for these positive sensory findings.

1. *Sensitization of nerve endings* of high threshold sensory units that normally respond only to potentially damaging stimuli (nociceptors) may lead to the experience of pain, spontaneously or in response to normally nonpainful stimulus energy. This mechanism was envisioned half a century ago by Sir Thomas Lewis to explain certain clinical observations. He proposed that the vasomotor phenomena and "tenderness of the skin in causalgia are all due to the release of substances peripherally; the release is supposed to bring the corresponding skin into a condition similar to what has been called erythralgic skin" (Lewis 1942, 92). He further hypothesized that, the mechanism of the pain is release into the skin of a substance which lowers the threshold of the pain nerve endings to various forms of stimulation (Lewis 1936). Others subsequently supported Lewis's hypothesis on the grounds of experience with their own patients (Jung 1941). Note that the term *causalgia* was being applied loosely by Lewis to signify the presence of a burning pain associated with vasodilatation; associated hyperalgesia improved if the temperature of the skin was lowered. Lewis (1936) stated that the condition does not have to do with abnormality of the vasomotor system. The neurosecretory process that lowered the threshold of the pain nerve endings and changed the vasomotor tone would be an affair of sensory nerves, which he termed "nocifensor." Basic research on antidromic vasodilation and neurogenic inflammation now endorses many of Lewis's ideas (Chahl et al. 1984). Furthermore, rigorous research methods have demonstrated that in a subset of causalgic patients there is indeed sensitization of nociceptors and antidromic nociceptor-dependent vasodilatation as the basis for the painful and vasomotor phenomena (Ochoa 1986a, 1986b; Cline et al. 1989) (Figure 16.1).

However, this specific pathophysiologic basis for causalgia applies only to a subset of chronic pain patients who have the variant termed "erythralgia" (Lewis 1936) or "ABC syndrome" (Ochoa 1986a). While animal or human models of erythralgia or ABC syndrome are readily reproduced in the laboratory by application to tissues of substances that "irritate" nociceptor nerve fibers (Culp et al. 1989), and while repetitive experimental excitation of nociceptor peripheral nerve fibers in humans does cause antidromic vasodilation and pain (see Colorplate 10.1C and D), there is not yet a self-perpetuating animal model of erythralgia or ABC syndrome that can be generated by experimentally disturbing peripheral nerve trunks rather than nerve terminals. Certain features of Bennett's model of painful nerve injury, however, suggest elements of ABC syndrome (Bennett and Ochoa 1991).

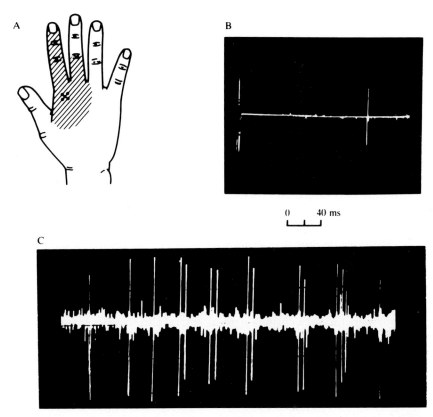

Figure 16.1 **A,** Within the *hatched area* of hyperalgesia, the receptive field of an identified C-nociceptor is marked *(cross)*. **B,** Intradermal electrical stimulation in the receptive field evoked a slowly conducted unitary response recorded with a microelectrode in the superficial radial nerve (conduction velocity of 1.25 m/sec). **C,** Intraneural recording of C-unit response to nine consecutive gentle mechanical stimuli applied to the receptive field. Such low-threshold response of a human polymodal nociceptor to innocuous energy implies sensitization. (Reproduced with permission of Oxford University Press from Cline M, Ochoa JL, Torebjörk HE. Chronic hyperalgesia and skin warming caused by sensitized C-nociceptors. Brain 1989;112:621–47.)

2. *Ectopic impulse generation* from pathologic axons within locally injured nerve trunks definitely contributes to the generation of pain induced by mechanical challenge of the abnormal nerve (sign of Tinel, etc.) and may even contribute to spontaneous pain in patients (Ochoa et al. 1982; Nordin et al. 1984). Whether abnormal foci of increased axonal excitability within locally injured nerve trunks contribute spontaneous pains through electrical or chemical ephaptic cross exaltation from sympathetic efferents is an unresolved matter. After initial popularity (Doupe et al. 1944; Nathan 1947; Devor and Jänig 1981), this theory has received decreasing support (see Ochoa and Verdugo 1993). If causalgic patients

were truly improved by ablation of sympathetic innervation, this idea would have clinical backing. However, these concepts deserve reconsideration because the sympathetic pathophysiology is purely hypothetical, and the sympathetic blocks may relieve pain through placebo effect, whether or not the pain is associated with nerve injury. In our experience, placebo-controlled sympathetic block does not relieve pain through suppression of sympathetic function in patients with chronic pain associated with bona fide nerve injury (Verdugo et al. 1991).

3. There has been rigorous experimental research in the last decade on *secondary central nervous system derangements following nerve injury.* Morphologic, histochemical, neurophysiologic, cellular, and molecular biologic studies have shown that a host of changes may occur in dorsal horns, and more rostrally, that may contribute to the pathogenesis of some components of the painful syndrome (Devor and Wall 1981; Simone et al. 1989; and many others now). However, while such experimental changes are found consistently, patients with nerve injury infrequently develop chronic painful syndromes.

ROLE OF THE SYMPATHETIC NERVOUS SYSTEM

Many patients with chronic painful limb syndromes have changes in limb temperature, skin color, and texture, and, to a lesser extent, sweat pattern of the symptomatic area. These vasomotor and sudomotor abnormalities have focused attention on the sympathetic nervous system in patients with causalgia.

The autonomic phenomena, particularly the vasomotor deviations, may indeed be a consequence of changes in sympathetic nervous system activity. However,

1. the sympathetic activity may be a physiologic reflex response to pain rather than a pathologic state
2. excessive activity of sympathetic end organs may be the consequence of sympathetic denervation supersensitivity rather than of hyperactivity of sympathetic nerves
3. the vasomotor phenomena may be entirely unrelated to the sympathetic system; they may reflect antidromic vasodilatation mediated by sensory nociceptive fibers (see Colorplate 10.1C and D.)
4. regardless of the physiology of the vasomotor phenomena, the assumption that sympathetic actions determine the pain is not rigorously founded (Ochoa 1986a, 1990, 1991a, 1991b; Ochoa and Verdugo, 1993).

In sum, vasomotor changes are not always of sympathetic origin, and sympathetic function need not be the cause of pain.

Observations of vasomotor and sudomotor abnormalities in chronic pain patients led to trials of sympatholytic therapies. Reports that sympathetic blocks or sympathectomy may transiently improve pain in causalgic patients were followed by almost a century of treatment of patients by sympatholysis. Neither the pathophysiology of the transient responses to blocks nor the long-term value of this therapy has been rigorously assessed (Ochoa 1991a, 1992, 1991c, 1991d; Ochoa and Verdugo 1993).

Another important source of mystification of the idea of sympathetic participation in chronic painful syndromes has been the progressive mis-understanding of the writings by classic authors. For example, Weir Mitchell (1872) actually wrote that causalgia was an affair of somatic nerves, foreign to the sympathetic system. Livingston (1947, 215) explicitly stated, "In seeking for a clue as to what this unknown alternative might be, one might start by abandon-ing, for the time being, the assumption that the activities of the sympathetic nerves represent the essential factor in either the cause or the cure of the causalgic syndrome." Leriche's (1916) Corporal G., who had a severe neurovascular lesion at left retroclavicular level, did not have "reflex sympathetic dystrophy" by current IASP criteria: What Leriche severed for therapy was his patient's humeral perivascular sympathetic innervation, and what he cured were probably ischemic ulcers, not neuropathic pain (Ochoa and Verdugo 1993).

"REFLEX SYMPATHETIC DYSTROPHY"

Convictions on the supposed role of the sympathetic nervous system in some patients with chronic limb pain led to introduction of the diagnostic term *reflex sympathetic dystrophy* (RSD) (see Bonica 1990). Attempts to define RSD have taken varied approaches:

1. Emphasize chronic pain in the absence of nerve injury. A multiauthor attempt published by the IASP (1986, S–29; emphasis added) defines RSD as "continuous pain in a portion of an extremity after trauma which may include fracture but *does not involve a major nerve,* associated with *sympathetic hyperactivity.* . . . The pain is described as burning, continuous, exacerbated by movement, cutaneous stimulation, or stress." This definition does not mention a motor component (other than disuse atrophy) or significant sensory components (other than pain exacerbated by "cutaneous stimulation").

2. Include overt motor and sensory nerve dysfunction among the diagnostic criteria (Abram et al. 1990; Jänig et al. 1991). If motor and sensory neurologic dysfunction are necessary components of RSD, the definition of RSD is so similar to classic definitions of causalgia that the terminology becomes redundant (Ochoa and Verdugo 1993).

3. Offer a compromise definition that tries to include patients with and without nerve injury and to avoid the debate on the importance of the sympa-thetic nervous system in the pathogenesis of the clinical phenomena. The Con-sensus Statement on RSD Definition by Jänig et al. (1991, 373; emphasis added) states that "RSD is a descriptive term meaning a *complex disorder or a group of disorders* that may develop *as a consequence of trauma* affecting the limbs, *with or without an obvious nerve lesion* . . . it consists of *pain and related sensory abnormalities, abnormal blood flow* and sweating, *abnormalities in the motor*

system and changes in structure of both superficial and deep tissues . . . it is agreed that the name reflex sympathetic dystrophy is used in a descriptive sense and *does not imply specific underlying mechanisms.*" This definition logically abandons the therapeutic connotations in *RSD* and specific pathophysiologic assumptions regarding the role of the sympathetic system in pain. However, by retaining the term *sympathetic,* it invites indiscriminate assault to that system in seeking pain relief for any of a broad variety of conditions. We prefer to abandon the term *RSD* because the meanings and roles of *reflex, sympathetic,* and *dystrophy* in the clinical syndrome are all unestablished.

ANIMAL MODELS

The science behind the concepts of causalgia, RSD, and sympathetically maintained pain (SMP) is surprisingly biased. There are excellent animal models of nerve injury (Bennett and Xie 1988; Seltzer et al. 1990). However, there is insufficient evidence that they provide legitimate models of human RSD or SMP. In man, chronic pain following nerve injury is rare, so the multiple primary peripheral and secondary central nervous system abnormalities consistently demonstrated following experimental nerve injury in animals must include idiosyncrasies inadequate to explain the uncommon and multifaceted human pain syndromes. The specific pathology and pathophysiology of the animal nerve injury models (Jänig 1991) are unlikely to represent the universal pathology and pathophysiology of human RSD and related syndromes. Currently, there are no authentic animal models for RSD. Given the all-embracing consensus definition of RSD by Jänig et al. (1991), it would be surprising if a unitary animal model could be found for that diffuse complex. Moreover, to the extent that psychologic mechanisms are so intrinsic to some of the human conditions, it is hard to conceive an appropriate animal model for them. Observations on normal animal physiology have shown activation of tactile sensory receptors by sympathetic efferent discharge (Roberts 1986). However, in humans the sympathetic system does not activate low-threshold mechanoreceptors (Dotson et al. 1990), so this animal model does not establish the validity of the concept of SMP for humans.

PSYCHOLOGIC FACTORS

It is well known that the psyche always participates in the human experience of pain. Older methods of investigation of neurologic function frequently did not allow determination of the relative roles of nerve injury and psychologic mechanisms in chronic posttraumatic syndromes that were associated with pains and motor and/or sensory phenomena. The French master neuropsychiatrists attributed the clinical presentation of a subset of such patients to hysteria (Charcot 1877, 1889; Déjérine 1901). In 1944, Doupe et al. reemphasized that chronic posttraumatic causalgic syndromes might be caused by either organic or psychogenic dysfunction. By present standards, an unmeasurable percentage of previously described "causalgic" patients must have had no nerve injury at all.

However, debate on proportions of organic versus psychogenic causalgia remains current (Merskey 1988; Weintraub 1988; Ochoa 1991c).

PLACEBO-CONTROLLED EVALUATION OF SYMPATHETIC BLOCK

The incidence of placebo response in patients with chronic causalgiform syndromes is twice as high (Verdugo and Ochoa 1991) as the placebo response in the general population (Evans 1974). Sympathetic blocks are typically not controlled for placebo pain response (see Ochoa 1991a, 1991b, Ochoa and Verdugo 1993). When controlled, efficacy of the active drug is found to be no better than placebo (Glynn and Jones 1990; Glynn 1991; Verdugo et al. 1991). These observations reemphasize the importance of psychologic mechanisms in patients with causalgiform pain syndromes. They also call for reevaluation of theories on the pathogenesis of the syndrome that assume that these pain patients are specifically responsive to sympathetic blockade.

For example, Roberts (1986, 298) introduced the term "sympathetically maintained pain" to describe patients with "a) a history of physical trauma on the painful areas; b) the presence of a continuous burning pain together with mechanical hyperalgesia-allodynia (painful sensation to touch); and c) relief from the pain during sympathetic block." In his original paper, Roberts summarized SMP as "pain relieved during sympathetic block." Subsequently, others have defined SMP as "that aspect of pain that is dependent on sympathetic efferent activity in the painful part" (Raja et al. 1991, 691) or as "all pain syndromes that can be relieved by sympathetic blockade" (Treede et al. 1991, 377).

The proposed pathophysiologic basis for SMP assumes that sympathetic efferent activity supplying a symptomatic limb naturally activates receptors of low-threshold (tactile) mechanoreceptors (Roberts 1986; Roberts and Kramis 1991). Such afferent input would impinge on previously sensitized *wide dynamic range* neurons in the spinal dorsal horn assumed to be capable of evoking pain. Spontaneous pain would be a consequence of natural, tonic sympathetic efferent activity that through low-threshold mechanoreceptors would excite the secondarily abnormal, pain-evoking, wide dynamic range neurons. Mechanical hyperalgesia-allodynia would be the consequence of natural activation by external stimuli of normally responsive low-threshold mechanoreceptor tactile units, again impinging on the same hypothetically sensitized central neurons.

The concept of SMP can be fairly criticized on two fronts: First, it heavily relies on the volunteered testimony of an individual concerning a subjective experience in response to a medical intervention that combines pharmacologic and placebo effects. These two effects are traditionally not separated by those who perform sympathetic blocks. This flaw is magnified by the inordinately high incidence of placebo responders among these patients (Verdugo and Ochoa 1991). In other words, the strongest clinical support for the idea of SMP, the patients' subjective report of pain improvement following a ritualistic intervention that may remove pain by nonspecific mechanisms, has little current scientific weight. Clinical evidence against the existence of SMP is that sympathectomy and sympathetic blocks do not cure patients with causalgia, RSD, or SMP (Ochoa 1991a, 1991b; Ochoa and Verdugo 1993).

Second, there is no demonstrable activation of low-threshold mechano-receptor units in symptomatic parts of patients when the sympathetic system has been effectively recruited by reflex maneuvers (Dotson et al. 1990). Moreover, while one subtype of mechanical hyperalgesia in patients is undoubtedly mediated by large-caliber afferents, there are several alternative hypotheses to explain this observation, and in some patients, the hyperalgesia is definitely mediated by sensitized peripheral nociceptors, rather than by normal low-threshold tactile units (Ochoa et al. 1989).

In summary, for causalgia as defined by the IASP (1986)—that is, for the painful syndrome following organic nerve injury—multiple different pathophys-iologic processes may be operant throughout the length of sick primary sensory units and also in second- or higher-order neurons in the sensory pathway. Clearly, more than one mechanism can contribute to the complex painful syndrome in any one case. The idea of a critical role of the sympathetic system in maintaining the pains following nerve injury in humans is not supported by rigorous evidence. Presence of organic nerve injury does not prove organic origin for the sensory syndrome.

We emphasize that causalgia, RSD, and SMP are purely descriptive terms. To the extent that they are given different meanings by different authors and practitioners, they cause confusion. Moreover, they perpetuate the illusion of understanding causes, mechanisms, and cures for these chronic painful syn-dromes (Ochoa 1990, 1991a, 1991b; Ochoa and Verdugo 1993). These terms should be updated. At this point, keeping in mind the urgent need to formulate solid concepts to effectively assess and treat patients with causalgia-RSD-SMP, one of Dr. Samuel Johnson's (1773, 354) lighthearted quotes may be applicable to our currently biased notions:

> A cucumber should be well sliced, and dressed with pepper and vinegar, and then thrown out, as good for nothing.

PATIENT EVALUATION

With or without nerve injury, patients may develop a chronic posttraumatic syndrome of pains and neuromuscular and autonomic dysfunctions. The neurologic assessment should document the level of function of each category of nerve fiber systems. This must rely not just on conventional nerve conduction studies, which only detect normality versus deficit and only for large-caliber fibers. Documentation of the physiologic status of nerve fibers must include quantitative somatosensory thermotest (see Chapter 9) and quantitative auto-nomic testing (see Chapter 10) to evaluate small-caliber nerve fiber function and to differentiate normal from deficient or excessive function. Where available, microneurographic recording may prove the critical test (Cline et al. 1989) (see Figure 16.1).

Differentiating between an organic basis and a psychologic basis for the patient's symptoms and signs starts with routine physical and neurologic history and examination. At times further studies are needed to explicitly demonstrate that muscle weakness, spasms, sensory loss, hyperalgesia, and pains are of cerebral, rather than of neuromuscular origin. Strategies for this involve refined subspecialty testing. Criteria do not just rely on absence of organic neuromuscular dysfunction or on presence of psychologic dysfunction. Nor do they rely on a menu of traditional but controverted clinical phenomena (Gould et al. 1986). In "weak" muscles, electromyographic evidence of *un*impaired volitional drive of upper motor neurons, with recruitment of full interference pattern interrupted by pauses of decruitment, in absence of pain, is strongly suggestive of psychogenic origin. So is the disappearance of neuromuscular motor or sensory *deficit* following diagnostic block (Verdugo and Ochoa, 1992) (Colorplate 16.2).

A traditional handicap in our ability to assess the real nature of many patients with the picture of RSD, whether in absence or in presence of nerve injury, is that these patients are usually not evaluated by neurologists for what is essentially a neurologic picture of pain, motor phenomena, sensory phenomena, and apparent neurovascular phenomena involving the peripheral nervous system. General practitioners, orthopedists, and anesthesiologists usually care for these patient, bypassing the necessary and complex specialized neurologic evaluation. When patients with RSD but without specific nerve trauma are evaluated thoroughly to assess function in subpopulations of nerve fibers, they often have no *pertinent* peripheral nerve dysfunction; express subjective responses to medical interventions that are, in some two thirds, voided by placebo effect (Verdugo and Ochoa 1991); and display psychologically mediated numbness and/or hyperalgesia and psychologically mediated weakness and/or "dystonic" muscle spasms.*

THREE CLINICAL CASES OF "CAUSALGIA-REFLEX SYMPATHETIC DYSTROPHY"
Case 1. Rapid Development of ABC Syndrome After Nerve Trauma

The young man in Figure 16.3 was seen in the summer of 1989. Symptoms started five months earlier, immediately after a gunshot wound to the right upper arm, with the bullet exiting in the medial upper arm. "I heard the shot coming from within the car that fled. I felt burning and pins and needles in the hand and some of my fingers. When I rubbed the skin, I felt pain and tingling in the area which was numb and burning. My hand was weak. I thought the shot hit me in the hand, but there was nothing there; there was blood pouring down my elbow." In the emergency room, two hours after injury, "the right hand became swollen and hot; it was just those parts [of the skin] which were tingling and burning that became hot and red." The initial pain was severe enough for him to require narcotics. The hand remained "definitely tender to touch and, at the same time,

---

*Ochoa, Verdugo, Campero, and Comstock, unpublished.

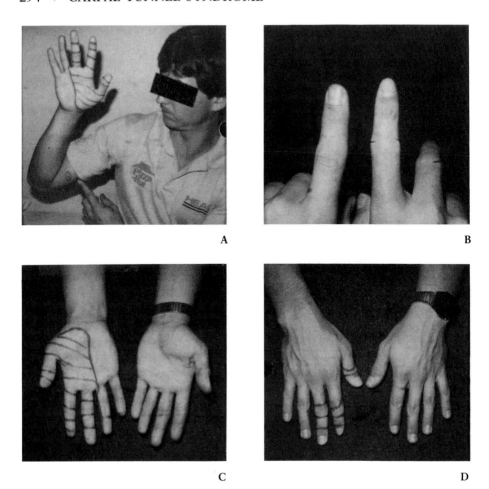

Figure 16.3 **A,** Patient points to bullet exit site in medial upper arm. The *circle* enclosing the scar defines the point of Tinel's sign. **B,** Dystrophic features of right index finger. **C-D,** The *hatched areas* of skin on volar and dorsal aspects of hands and digits delineate well defined sensory dysfunction combining hyperalgesia and hypoesthesia to all modalities. The area corresponds to usual median nerve territory.

numb." He described the sensory symptoms as confined to the median nerve territory of palm and fingers, splitting the ring finger. A few days after the injury, he started noticing a Tinel's sign at the site of bullet exit.

A few weeks after the injury, he first noticed thinning of the muscles in the forearm. Early after injury, he had become aware of thermal dependence of his painful syndrome when he discovered that while in bed his pain would lessen if the arm was kept outside of the covers. Subsequently, he realized that in a sauna his pains would be much worse, but in a cold pool, they would significantly improve. The spontaneous burning pain was the most temperature-dependent symptom; the touch-induced tingling and pain seemed to be less influenced by cold immersion. The sign of Tinel was not influenced by temperature.

From clinical, electrodiagnostic, and thermographic assessment, the referring doctor from Florida established the diagnosis of local nerve injury to median nerve, with axonal involvement and hypothesized development of an ABC syndrome. As shown in Figure 16.3B, with time the affected fingers, particularly the index, became tapered and moderately "dystrophic."

When seen in Portland, months after the injury, the sign of Tinel remained close to the scar of bullet exit (Figure 16.3A). The area of abnormal cutaneous sensation was strictly confined to textbook median nerve territory and included hypoesthesia to all submodalities and mechanical hyperalgesia of both dynamic and static subtypes (Ochoa et al. 1989) (see Figure 16.3A, C, and D). The symptomatic burning hand was hypothermic to touch and to thermography, particularly the skin of the most symptomatic index and middle fingers. Residual ability to vasodilate in response to reflex sympathetic maneuvers revealed a degree of autonomic control on the cold skin. Therefore, the switch from a "hot" to a "cold" symptomatic state meant interjection of vasoconstriction, either as a consequence of partial sympathetic denervation supersensitivity or engagement of exaggerated sympathetic vasoconstrictor neural outflow, or a combination of both.

Perhaps the most remarkable feature in this patient, who might have been one of Weir Mitchell's soldiers with "causalgia," and who by modern criteria has RSD with clear dystrophic features in the symptomatic parts, is the development almost immediately after injury of an erythralgic or ABC syndrome, characterized by vasodilatation, heat and mechanical hyperalgesia, and significant improvement by passive cooling. The locally irritated polymodal nociceptors-in-continuity probably discharged ectopically—orthodromically evoking spontaneous burning pain, while antidromically evoking vasodilatation and perhaps sensitization of peripheral receptors.

Another striking feature is the similarity between this case and many features of Bennett's animal model of nerve injury (Bennett and Xie 1988). Indeed, vasodilatation leading eventually to vasoconstriction, spontaneous pain behavior, mechanical hyperalgesia, thermal hyperalgesia, and even dystrophic features are shared by the experimental animal state. The mechanical hyperalgesia in the particular animal model of Bennett (and in the ABC syndrome) is probably explained on the grounds of nociceptor sensitization, since myelinated fibers are practically devastated and therefore A-fiber–mediated hyperalgesia could not apply (Ochoa 1990). In this patient, however, the mechanical hyperalgesia was dichotomized into two phenomenological types, one (dynamic) mediated by myelinated fibers, the other (static) by unmyelinated. The striking dynamic mechanical hyperalgesia was rapidly abolished by A-fiber blocks. In retrospect, it was abolished too rapidly. The effect may well have been a placebo response. Since this dynamic mechanical hyperalgesia developed immediately following injury, we suspect that rather than reflecting instantaneous development of secondary dorsal horn pathophysiologic changes, the hyperalgesia simply reflects echo and amplification and reverberations at the site of injury as a result of ephapses (Rasminsky 1982).

Unfortunately, the patient could not tolerate microneurography intended to explore a) the basis for the Tinel sign, b) the kind of afferent activity recorded during elicitation of mechanical hyperalgesia, c) whether any of such activity was reflected antidromically after elicitation, and d) possible presence of ectopic discharge in C nociceptors.

Case 2. Painful Digital Nerve Injury with Distal Neuropathic Pain Mechanism

This worker suffered a deep cut by broken glass on the radial border of the right palm in May 1991 (Colorplate 16.4A). He immediately felt painful tingling in the index finger, associated with a combination of diminution of sensory acuity and painful hypersensitivity to gentle mechanical skin stimulation. Shortly after the injury, a plastic surgeon microscopically repaired a digital nerve in the palm.

When seen six months after the injury, he continued to complain of constant local pain in the region of the scar, associated with a local sign of Tinel. Lightly touching the lateral aspect of the right index finger continued to induce a weird, unpleasant sensation, and pressure in the same area induced a sharp pain, "like someone is sticking a needle." Colorplate 16.4A shows the patient puzzled by concurrence of painful exaggeration (red) next to diminution (black) of sensitivity to touching the symptomatic skin. Cold temperature would increase the painful symptoms, and the hand always felt cold to the patient and was diffusely cold thermographically (see Colorplate 16.4B).

A sham "block" of the right median nerve at wrist level revealed no placebo response. In contrast, lidocaine block caused multimodality sensory loss in "classic" median nerve territory, while abolishing Tinel's sign, hyperalgesia, and spontaneous pain (see Colorplate 16.4C). The corresponding territory of skin warmed up considerably, as shown in the thermogram (see Colorplate 16.4D). Note remarkable matching between anesthetic and vasodilated areas.

In this case, the positive and negative sensory phenomena, including multimodality hypoesthesia, mechanical hyperalgesia, Tinel's sign, and spontaneous pain, were all in complete harmony with the anatomically proven local nerve injury. The positive sensory phenomena were erased by anesthetic nerve block proximal to the injury but not by placebo block. The locally abnormal nerve physiology therefore must explain the whole of the sensory syndrome. Indeed, the spontaneous and the stimulus induced pains must be sustained by activity coming from below the site of nerve block. The diffuse hypothermia affecting the whole of the symptomatic hand, rather than just the territory of the affected nerve, is consistent with recruitment of somatosympathetic vasoconstrictor reflex; the vasodilatation in response to blockade of sympathetic vasoconstrictor efferent outflow at wrist level indicates its abolition.

This case is to be contrasted with the next.

Case 3. Histrionic Pain Syndrome Following Carpal Tunnel Surgery

The unfortunate patient shown in Colorplate 16.2 developed classical carpal tunnel syndrome on the left side. Clinical and electrodiagnostic testing were clearly abnormal. She underwent surgical decompression of the median nerve at carpal tunnel level in spring 1989. The surgeon was sufficiently impressed with the gigantic median nerve to biopsy a nerve fascicle. As shown in Figure 16.5, the nerve specimen was profoundly abnormal, with marked depopulation of myelinated fibers.

Following surgery, she complained of a new, extremely severe pain (grade 10 in the 10-point scale) in the whole hand. There was also mechanical hyperalgesia, both of the static and dynamic subtypes. She reported that cooling might abolish the pain but not the mechanical hyperalgesia, and that the hand tended to become "red or pink." In addition, she claimed profound sensory loss all the way up to elbow level (see Colorplate 16.2A, hatched area). A hypothetical organic explanation for the new pain syndrome was that it might be caused by surgical trauma to an anomalous nerve that supplied the whole hand or, alternatively, that it might be a nerve injury that became complicated by "centralization," as has been proposed for RSD-SMP.

Local anesthetic diagnostic block of the median nerve, supplemented by thermography, clarified the issue. As compared with a normal symmetric baseline thermogram (see Colorplate 16.2B), the post-lidocaine-block thermogram (see Colorplate 16.2D) showed objective warming (paralytic vasodilatation) confined to the typical normal left median nerve territory. This correlated with deep, legitimate anesthesia in the same territory (see Colorplate 16.2C). But the blocked

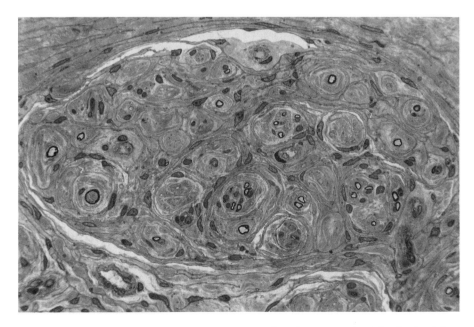

Figure 16.5 Light micrograph of cross section of median nerve fascicle obtained from patient shown in Colorplate 16.2 during carpal tunnel surgery on the affected left hand. Severe dropout of myelinated fibers is obvious.

nerve did not supply sympathetic fibers to the nonmedian areas of the hand that she had described as extremely painful and hyperalgesic. At the same time, the hypothesis of centralization was not supported, but rather dismissed, because the diagnostic block intriguingly abolished the long glove of deep anesthesia. In other words, this medical intervention took away the deficit. This miraculous recovery is not explicable in terms of organic dysfunction (Verdugo and Ochoa 1992). Furthermore, the anesthesia was of psychological nature: on multiple occasions, while blindfolded, the patient punctually announced with a "no" every stimulus to an anesthetic part.

In summary, this RSD case is complex. Of course, the patient did have histologically proven nerve pathology, but beyond doubt, she also had a psychogenic sensory syndrome. Without thorough investigation, the bizarre sensory profile might have erroneously been attributed to hypothetical secondary spinal cord changes.

REFERENCES

Abram SE, Blumberg H, Boas RA, Haddox JD, Jänig W, Kruescher H, Racz GB, Raj PP, Roberts WJ, Stanton-Hicks M, et al. Proposed definition of reflex sympathetic dystrophy. In: Stanton-Hicks M, Wilfrid J, Boas RA, eds. Reflex sympathetic dystrophy. Boston: Kluwer Academic Publishers, 1990;207–10.

Bennett GJ, Ochoa JL. Thermographic observations on rats with experimental neuropathic pain. Pain 1991;45:61–67.

Bennett GJ, Xie Y-K. A peripheral mononeuropathy in rat that produces disorders of pain sensation like those seen in man. Pain 1988;33:87–107.

Bonica JJ. The management of pain. Vol 1. Philadelphia: Lea & Febiger, 1990.

Chahl LA, Szolcsányi J, Lembeck F, eds. Antidromic vasodilatation and neurogenic inflammation. Budapest: Akademiai Kiado, 1984.

Charcot JM. (Clinical) lectures on the diseases of the nervous system. Vols 1, 3. New Sydenham Society, London, Special Edition (1985), Critchley M, ed. The Classics of Neurology and Neurosurgery Library. Birmingham, AL: Gryphon Editions, 1877, 1889.

Cline M, Ochoa JL, Torebjörk HE. Chronic hyperalgesia and skin warming caused by sensitized C nociceptors. Brain 1989;112:621–47.

Culp WJ, Ochoa JL, Cline M, Dotson R. Heat and mechanical hyperalgesia induced by capsaicin: cross modality threshold modulation in human C-nociceptors. Brain 1989;112:1317–31.

Déjérine PJ. Sémiologie du système nerveux. In: Traité de pathologie générale. Paris: Masson et Cie, 1901;559–1168.

Devor M, Jänig W. Activation of myelinated afferents ending in a neuroma by stimulation of the sympathetic supply in the rat. Neurosci Lett 1981;24:43–47.

Devor M, Wall PD. Plasticity in the spinal cord sensory map following peripheral nerve injury in rats. J Neurosci 1981;148:679–84.

Dotson R, Ochoa JL, Cline M, Roberts W, Yarnitsky D, Simone D, Marchettini P. Sympathetic effects on human low threshold mechanoreceptors (abstract). Soc Neurosci 1990;16:1280.

Doupe J, Cullen CH, Chance GQ. Post-traumatic pain and the causalgic syndrome. J Neurol Neurosurg Psychiatry 1944;7:33–48.

Evans FJ. The placebo response in pain reduction. Adv Neurol 1974;4:289–96.

Gilliatt RW. Sensory conduction studies in the early recognition of nerve disorders. Muscle Nerve 1978;1:352–59.

Glynn CJ, (1991) in Ochoa JL. Controversies on chronic somatic pain and the sympathetic system. A five year chronicle. In: Hamann W, Wedley JR, eds. Physiological mechanisms of pain and pharmacology of analgesia, London: Gordon and Breach, 1992.

Glynn CJ, Jones PC. An investigation of the role of clonidine in the treatment of reflex sympathetic dystrophy. In: Stanton-Hicks M, Wilfrid J, Boas RA, eds. Reflex sympathetic dystrophy. Boston: Kluwer Academic Publishers, 1990;187–96.

Gould R, Miller BL, Goldberg MA, Benson DF. The validity of hysterical signs and symptoms. J Nerv Ment Dis 1986;174:593–97.

International Association for the Study of Pain (IASP). Classification of chronic pain. Descriptions of chronic pain syndromes and definitions of pain terms. Prepared by the Subcommittee on Taxonomy. Pain Suppl (3) 1986.

Jänig W. Experimental approach to reflex sympathetic dystrophy and related syndromes. Pain 1991;46:241–45.

Jänig W, Blumberg H, Boas RA, Campbell JN. The reflex sympathetic dystrophy syndrome: consensus statement and general recommendations for diagnosis and clinical research. In: Bond MR, Charlton JE, Woolf CJ, eds. Proceedings of the VIth world congress on pain. Amsterdam: Elsevier, 1991;373–76.

Johnson SJ. Quoted by James Boswell in Life of Johnson. (L.F. Powell's revision of G.B. Hill's edition.) p. 354, 1773, Oxford Dictionary of Quotations. Oxford University Press, 1979: 280.

Jung R. Die allgemeine Symptomatologie der Nervenverletzungen und ihre Physiologischen grundlagen. Nervenarzt 1941;14:493–516.

Leriche R. De la causalgie, envisagée comme une névrite du sympathique et de son traitement par la dénudation et l'excision des plexus nerveux péri-arteriels. Presse Méd 1916;24:178–80.

Lewis T. Vascular disorders of the limbs, described for practitioners and students. London: Macmillan, 1936;93.

Lewis T. Pain. London: Macmillan, 1942.

Livingston WK. Pain mechanisms. New York: Macmillan, 1947;209–23.

Loh L, Nathan PW. Painful peripheral states and sympathetic blocks. J Neurol Neurosurg Psychiatry 1978;41:664–71.

Merskey H. Regional pain is rarely hysterical. Arch Neurol 1988;45:915–18.

Mitchell SW. Injuries of nerves and their consequences. 1872; Reprinted, New York: Dover Publications, 1965.

Nathan PW. On the pathogenesis of causalgia in peripheral nerve injuries. Brain 1947;70:145–70.

Nordin M, Nyström B, Wallin U, Hagbarth K-E. Ectopic sensory discharges and paresthesiae in patients with disorders of peripheral nerves, dorsal roots and dorsal columns. Pain 1984;20:231–45.

Ochoa JL. The newly recognized painful ABC syndrome: thermographic aspects. Thermology 1986a;2:65–107.

Ochoa JL. Unmyelinated fibers, microneurography, thermography and pain. (abstract). Ninth annual continuing education course B, American Association of Electromyography and Electrodiagnosis, Rochester, 1986b;29–34.

Ochoa JL. Neuropathic pains, from within: personal experiences, experiments, and reflections on mythology. In: Dimitrijevic MR, ed. Recent achievements in restorative neurology. Altered sensation and pain. Basel, Switzerland: Karger, 1990;100–111.

Ochoa JL. Afferent and sympathetic roles in chronic "neuropathic" pains: confessions on misconceptions. In: Besson JM, Guilbaud G, eds. Lesions of primary afferent fibers as a tool for the study of clinical pain. Amsterdam: Elsevier, 1991a.

Ochoa JL. Controversies on chronic somatic pain and the sympathetic system. A five year chronicle. In: Hamann W, Wedley JR, eds. Physiological mechanisms of pain and pharmacology of analgesia, April, 1991. London: Gordon and Breach, 1991b.

Ochoa JL. A dangerous diagnosis to be given (editorial). Eur J Pain 1991c;12(3):63–64.

Ochoa JL, Roberts WJ, Cline MA, Dotson R, Yarnitsky D. Two mechanical hyperalgesias in human neuropathy (abstract). 1989;15:472.

Ochoa JL, Torebjörk HE, Culp WJ, Schady W. Abnormal spontaneous activity in single sensory nerve fibers in humans. Muscle Nerve 1982;5:S74–S77.

Ochoa JL, Verdugo R. Reflex sympathetic dystrophy. Definitions and history of the ideas. A critical review of human studies. In: Low PA, ed. The evaluation and management of clinical autonomic disorders. Boston: Little, Brown, 1993.

Raja SN, Treede R-D, Davis K, Campbell J. Systemic alpha-adrenergic blockade with phentolamine: a diagnostic test for sympathetically maintained pain. Anesthesiology 1991;74:691–98.

Rasminsky M. Ectopic excitation, ephatic excitation and autoexcitation in peripheral nerve fibers of mutant mice. In: Culp WJ, Ochoa J, eds. Abnormal nerves and Muscles as Impulse Generators. New York: Oxford University Press, 1982.

Roberts WJ. A hypothesis on the physiological basis for causalgia and related pains. Pain 1986;24:297–311.

Roberts WJ, Kramis RC. Sympathetically dependent pain: physiology and clinical expression. In: Wynn-Parry CB, ed. Management of pain in the hand and wrist. London: Churchill Livingstone, 1991;14–27.

Seltzer Z, Dubner R, Shir Y. A novel behavioral model of neuropathic pain disorders produced by partial sciatic nerve injury in rats. Pain 1990;43:205–18.

Simone DA, Baumann TK, Collins JG, LaMotte RH. Sensitization of cat dorsal horn neurons to innocuous mechanical stimulation after intradermal injection of capsaicin. Brain 1989;486:185–89.

Treede RD, Raja SN, Davis KD, Meyer RA, Campbell JN. Evidence that peripheral α-adrenergic receptors mediate sympathetically maintained pain. In: Bond MR, Charlton JE, Woolf CJ, eds. Proceedings of the VIth world congress on pain. Amsterdam: Elsevier, 1991;377–82.

Verdugo R, Ochoa JL. High incidence of placebo responders among chronic neuropathic pain patients (abstract). Ann Neurol 1991;30:294.

Verdugo R, Rosenblum S, Ochoa J. Phentolamine sympathetic blocks mislead diagnosis (abstract) Soc Neurosci 1991;17:107.

Verdugo RJ, Ochoa J. Hypoesthesia erased by somatic nerve block, or placebo: a pseudoneuropathic, psychogenic sign, in causalgia/RSD. (abstract) Soc Neurosci 1992; 18:287.

Weintraub MI. Regional pain is usually hysterical. Arch Neurol 1988;45:914–15.

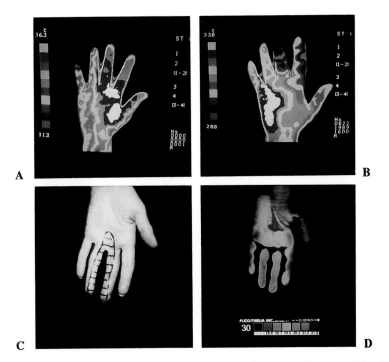

Colorplate 10.1 Thermograms displaying three typical patterns determined by different kinds of abnormal nerve function (see text pp. 185–186).

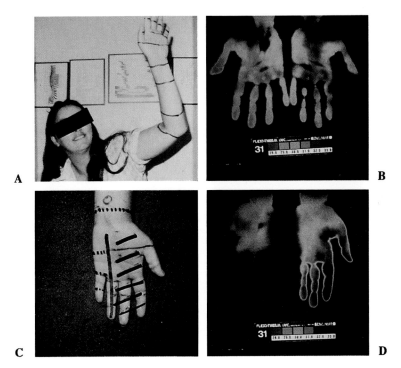

Colorplate 16.2 Usefulness of combined local anesthetic block/thermography in assessing abnormal neurophysiology of cold painful limb (see text p. 296).

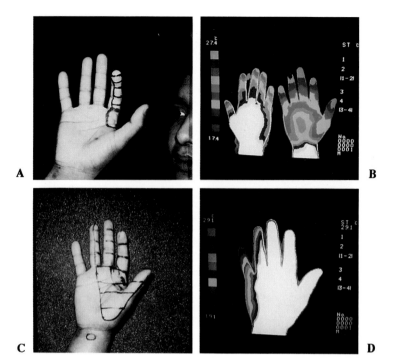

Colorplate 16.4 Usefulness of combined local anesthetic block-thermography in differentiating organic versus psychogenic sensory profiles (see text p. 296).

17

Median Neuropathy Proximal to the Carpal Tunnel

From its formation by the medial and lateral cords of the brachial plexus to its entrance into the carpal tunnel, the median nerve runs a gauntlet of potential injuries and compressions. Nonetheless, the total prevalence of proximal median neuropathies is only a small fraction of the prevalence of carpal tunnel syndrome. Figure 17.1 shows the sites and Table 17.1 shows the relative prevalences of median nerve compression at these sites reported in one series; most clinicians will find that this overestimates the incidence of median neuropathies proximal to the carpal tunnel (Gessini et al. 1983a).

Laceration and repair of the median nerve are amply covered in textbooks of peripheral nerve surgery (Seddon 1972; Omer and Spinner 1980; Mackinnon and Dellon 1988). We shall discuss other proximal median neuropathies, starting in the distal forearm and tracing the nerve to the brachial plexus.

MEDIAN NEUROPATHY IN THE DISTAL FOREARM

Median nerve compression in the distal forearm has been called "pseudo-carpal-tunnel syndrome." It is usually discovered on those rare occasions when a patient presents with features indicative of carpal tunnel syndrome, but the contents of the carpal tunnel are found to be normal at the time of flexor retinaculum release. In these patients the surgeon should trace the course of the median nerve over its first few centimeters into the distal forearm in search of an unusual site of nerve compression. For example, median nerve compression has been reported to occur from a bifid palmaris longus tendon, some 5 cm proximal to the tunnel, or by a muscle body of flexor digitorum sublimis in the middle of an anomalously bifid median nerve (Baruch and Hass 1977; Dorin and Mann 1984). A lipoma on the anterior wrist, proximal to the carpal tunnel and superficial to the median nerve, may cause symptoms of median nerve compression (Phalen et al. 1971).

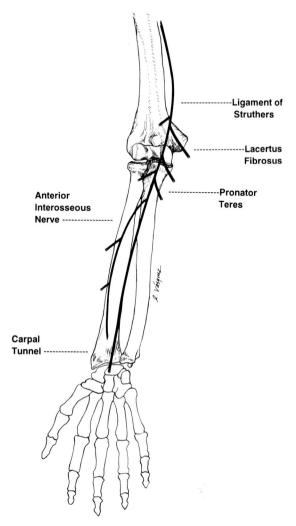

Ligament of
Struthers

Lacertus
Fibrosus

Pronator
Teres

Anterior
Interosseous
Nerve

Carpal
Tunnel

Figure 17.1 Potential sites of compression of the median nerve. The relative incidence of compression at these sites is shown in Table 17.1.

Pseudocarpal-tunnel syndrome may develop acutely following trauma. For example, marked median neuropathy developed over 36 hours after a tire fell on the dorsum of a patient's hand and forearm. At surgery the median nerve was compressed against the forearm fascia by flexor digitorum superficialis muscle (Gardner 1970).

The median nerve can be injured with distal radial or ulnar fractures. For example, Sumner and Khuri (1984) reported a case of median nerve entrapment in an epiphyseal fracture-dislocation of the distal radioulnar joint. In this case the entrapment was corrected acutely, and clinical nerve injury was prevented. In

Table 17.1 Sites of median nerve compression in 238 cases of median neuropathy

Site of Compression	Number of Cases
Carpal tunnel	201
Pronator teres	21
Anterior interosseous nerve	3
Lacertus fibrosus	2
Ligament of Struthers	1

(Data From Gessini et al. 1983a.)

some patients who acutely develop symptoms of median nerve compression following Colles' fracture, the median nerve may be compressed by a hematoma beneath the fascia of the distal forearm (Lewis 1978).

MEDIAN PALMAR CUTANEOUS NEUROPATHY

The anatomy of the palmar cutaneous branch of the median nerve is discussed in Chapter 1. Isolated compression or injury of this nerve branch is very unusual. There are case reports of its compression by ganglion, atypical palmaris longus muscle, or fascia of flexor digitorum superficialis (Stellbrink 1972; Gessini et al. 1983b; Buckmiller and Rickard 1987; Shimizu et al. 1988). It may be injured with surgery of the volar wrist, particularly with surgery for carpal tunnel release (Carroll and Green 1972).

There is no well-established method to study nerve conduction in the median palmar cutaneous nerve. Lum and Kanakamedala (1986) proposed studying nerve conduction of the median palmar cutaneous nerve using a pair of surface recording electrodes over the thenar eminence while stimulating the nerve antidromically. With stimulation 10 cm proximal to the recording electrode, mean latency to the negative peak of the nerve action potential was 2.6 msec. Mean amplitude of the evoked response was 12 μV. However, Dumitru et al. (1989) showed that the nerve action potential recorded by this method did not reliably originate from the palmar cutaneous nerve. They found that this nerve action potential persisted after the median palmar cutaneous nerve was blocked by local anesthetic but disappeared after the median nerve was blocked by local anesthetic injection in the palm.

ANTERIOR INTEROSSEOUS NEUROPATHY

Anterior interosseous nerve palsy is of interest for its distinctive clinical presentation and varied etiologies. The anatomy of the anterior interosseous nerve is discussed in Chapter 1. Palsy limited to the distribution of this nerve was described by Kiloh and Nevin (1952)—hence the eponym "Kiloh-Nevin syndrome." They reported two cases of sudden onset of focal weakness without preceding trauma. A 52-year-old man presented with painless weakness of flexor pollicis longus and of flexor digitorum profundus to index and middle fingers. A

28-year-old man awoke with pain along the lateral forearm and weakness of flexor pollicis longus. Within months, both patients recovered spontaneously. Kiloh and Nevin postulated that these patients had a variant of acute brachial plexitis.

Anterior interosseous nerve palsy represents much less than 1% of median neuropathies. Two cases were seen at the Mayo Clinic in seven years compared with 39 cases of pronator syndrome (Hartz et al. 1981).

Clinical Presentation

The hallmark of anterior interosseous nerve palsy is weakness limited to flexor pollicis longus, flexor digitorum profundus to the index finger, and pronator quadratus. Occasionally, flexor digitorum profundus to the middle finger may be weakened. In the classic posture, the patient extends the distal phalangeal joints of the thumb and index finger when trying to pinch these two fingers together (Figure 17.2). The normal hand can form a circle with this pinch. The palsy may be partial with clinical weakness limited to flexor pollicis longus or to flexor digitorum profundus to the index finger (Hill et al. 1985; Conway and Thomas 1990). To test pronator quadratus while minimizing the action of pronator teres, pronation is tested with the elbow flexed.

In the presence of Martin-Gruber anastomosis, motor axons may travel with the median nerve into the forearm, accompany the anterior interosseous

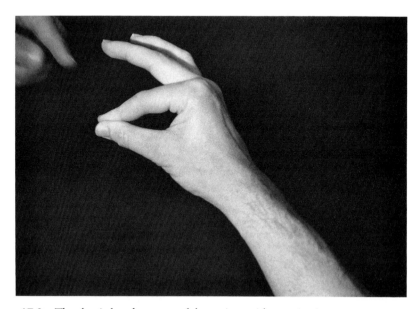

Figure 17.2 The classic hand posture of the patient with anterior interosseous nerve palsy results from paresis of flexor pollicis longus and flexor digitorum profundus to the index finger.

nerve, cross to join the ulnar nerve proximal to the wrist, and innervate ulnar intrinsic hand muscles, particularly adductor pollicis and first dorsal interosseous (Mannerfelt 1966). The diagnostically puzzling combination of weakness of ulnar-innervated hand muscles and muscles classically innervated by the anterior interosseous nerve may be found if anterior interosseous nerve palsy occurs in a patient with Martin-Gruber anastomosis.

Patients with isolated anterior interosseous nerve palsy have no associated sensory loss. Pain in the wrist or forearm is a variable symptom.

Causes

Anterior Interosseous Nerve Compression

Anterior interosseous nerve palsy may be caused by chronic isolated compression of the anterior interosseous nerve (Fearn and Goodfellow 1965). Symptoms of compression may develop gradually or, in relation to a forearm strain or injury, more abruptly. The patients typically have elbow and forearm pain associated with forearm tenderness to deep pressure. Paresthesias, such as "pins and needles," should be absent. Weakness confined to muscles supplied by the anterior interosseous nerve develops gradually and may lag behind the painful symptoms in appearance.

Clinical clues to anterior interosseous nerve compression, in addition to the characteristic pattern of weakness, may be a positive Tinel's sign over the nerve in the forearm and an increase in elbow pain elicited by pronating the forearm against resistance, then extending the elbow while keeping the fingers and wrist hyperflexed ("modified Mills test") (Rask 1979). A rare patient may note weakness in muscles innervated by the anterior interosseous nerve that develops with excessive forearm use and resolves within days of stopping the excessive activity (Hill et al. 1985).

The site of nerve compression can be confirmed only with surgery. Possible compressing structures include a fibrous band (the arcuate ligament of Fearn and Goodfellow [1965]), the heads of pronator teres, or an accessory head of flexor pollicis longus ("Gantzer's muscle") (Figure 17.3) (Spinner 1970; Megele 1988). However, in many patients these structures are present as asymptomatic anatomic variants. Dellon (1986) reported that 16 of 31 cadaver arms had a fibrous arch crossing the anterior interosseous nerve. The arch may originate from the flexor digitorum superficialis or from either head of pronator teres. In 10% of cadavers, the anterior interosseous nerve branches from the median nerve proximal to the distal edge of the pronator teres (Johnson et al. 1979). An accessory head of flexor pollicis longus originates from the medial humeral epicondyle and crosses to the lateral forearm between the median nerve and the anterior interosseous nerve in most individuals (Mangini 1960). The mere presence of one of these structures crossing the anterior interosseous nerve does not prove pathologic compression.

Peters and Todd (1983) described a very unusual occurrence: compression of the anterior interosseous nerve by a metastasis from bronchogenic carcinoma.

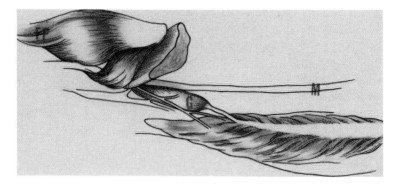

Figure 17.3 Gantzer's muscle *(G)*, an accessory head of flexor pollicis longus, may compress the anterior interosseous nerve (unlabeled). *M*, median nerve; *FP*, flexor and pronator muscles. Forearm; distal is toward the right. (Reproduced with permission of the publisher from Dellon AL, Mackinnon SE. Musculoaponeurotic variations along the course of the median nerve in the proximal forearm. J Hand Surg 1987;12B:359–63.)

Anterior Interosseous Nerve Trauma

Trauma may lead to isolated anterior interosseous nerve injury. Spinner and Schreiber (1969) described six cases of anterior interosseous nerve palsy occurring after *supracondylar humeral fractures* in children. In each case the evidence of neuropathy was limited to weakness of flexor pollicis longus and flexor digitorum profundus, and recovery occurred within eight weeks. They noted that at the level of the fracture median nerve fascicles destined for the anterior interosseous nerve are situated posteriorly and in close proximity to motor fascicles for pronator teres and flexor digitorum superficialis and to sensory fascicles. Therefore, partial direct contusion of the median nerve would be unlikely to selectively paralyze flexor pollicis longus and flexor digitorum profundus. In cadavers, they found that supracondylar fracture with posterior displacement placed tension on the anterior interosseous nerve at the level of the proximal third of the forearm and suggested that nerve stretching at this point in the forearm was the probable mechanism of nerve injury. A case of documented anterior interosseous nerve avulsion at its origin from the median nerve in association with an open humeral fracture gives credence to this hypothesized mechanism (Collins and Weber 1983). Anterior interosseous nerve injuries are not always this severe. Injury may be neurapraxic, allowing motor recovery a few weeks following open reduction of the supracondylar fracture (Moehring 1986).

Anterior interosseous nerve palsy has been noted as a delayed effect following *posterior dislocation of the elbow* (Beverly and Fearn 1984). The anterior interosseous nerve may also be injured in association with *forearm fractures*. It may occur following ulnar fracture with ipsilateral dislocation of the radial head ("Monteggia fracture") and, more rarely, with less severe fractures of the proximal ulna (Warren 1963; Engber and Keene 1983; Mirovsky et al. 1988; Geissler et al. 1990). The Monteggia fracture is more commonly accompanied by posterior interosseous nerve injury. Hope (1988) reported an anterior interosseous nerve palsy appearing within the first three weeks after open reduction and internal fixation of a radial fracture. A bone holding forceps was used at surgery, and cadaver studies suggested that the forceps might have temporarily compressed the anterior interosseous nerve during surgery.

Penetrating *injuries of the forearm* may lacerate the anterior interosseous nerve directly. Closed forearm injury can lead to anterior interosseous neuropathy as a delayed effect of the injury due to secondary scarring and nerve compression (Spinner 1970).

Anterior interosseous nerve palsy has also been reported secondary to *thrombosis of the anterior interosseous artery* or as a sequel of *Volkmann's contracture* of the forearm. External pressure on the forearm can cause anterior interosseous nerve palsy; examples include pressure on the forearm during surgery with the patient prone, compression by an arm sling applied for treatment of acromioclavicular joint dislocation, compression by the strap of a heavy purse carried across the forearm, and constriction by a tight band wrapped around the forearm to treat "tennis elbow" (Spinner 1970; Albanese et al. 1986; O'Neill et al. 1990; Enzenauer and Nordstrom 1991).

Neuralgic Amyotrophy

In the syndrome of neuralgic amyotrophy, patients present with acute arm pain and focal weakness. In some patients, weakness may be limited to the distribution of the anterior interosseous nerve. In their series of 136 patients with neuralgic amyotrophy or acute brachial plexitis, Parsonage and Turner (1948) noted that flexor pollicis longus and flexor digitorum profundus were at times preferentially weakened in patients with the syndrome. They noted a single case in which the motor abnormality was limited to flexor pollicis longus and flexor digitorum profundus to the index finger and assumed that this presentation was part of the spectrum of neuralgic amyotrophy. Kiloh and Nevin (1952) considered their two cases of isolated anterior interosseous nerve palsy as a "neuritis" analogous to the cases of Parsonage and Turner. Features linking Kiloh and Nevin's cases to neuralgic amyotrophy were sudden, often painful, onset and spontaneous but delayed motor recovery beginning more than one year after onset of symptoms. Other patients may have sudden onset of pain and focal anterior interosseous nerve weakness and recover more rapidly (Smith and Herbst 1974). The following cases that bridge the gap between neuralgic amyotrophy and isolated anterior interosseous nerve neuritis are instructive:

Case 1
A 31-year-old man developed right antecubital pain and weakness of flexor digitorum profundus to the right index finger 11 days after an illness characterized by headache, fever, and malaise (Dunne et al. 1987). Five days later he developed similar pain on the left, with weakness in left flexor digitorum profundus and flexor pollicis longus. Tenderness adjacent to the biceps tendon interfered with elbow extension. Clues to disease beyond the territory of the anterior interosseous nerves were slight tingling of the thumbs, decreased sensation

reported at the tip of the left thumb, and decreased appreciation of pinprick over the upper lateral right arm. Using a needle recording electrode in the pronator quadratus and stimulating in the antecubital fossa, the distal motor latency of the anterior interosseous nerve was prolonged at 6.8 msec over 24 cm on the left and was unobtainable on the right.

Electromyographic examination with a needle electrode showed increased insertional activity, fibrillations, and reduced interference pattern bilaterally in pronator quadratus, flexor pollicis longus, and flexor digitorum profundus. The left pronator teres and flexor carpi radialis showed similar abnormalities.

Cytomegalovirus (CMV) infection was diagnosed based on CMV-specific serology and CMV isolation from the urine. After five months, he had partially recovered strength.

Case 2

A 20-year-old man presented with a left anterior interosseous nerve palsy coincident with a myalgic flu-like illness (Rennels and Ochoa 1980). Motor abnormalities were initially limited to the anterior interosseous nerve distribution, but hyperesthesia in both arms and asymmetrically depressed deep tendon reflexes hinted at more diffuse neurologic involvement. Light taping in the antecubital fossa elicited intense forearm pain. Sixteen days later he developed weakness in the right serratus anterior. Recovery of left-hand strength was first noted 19 months following onset of symptoms and was nearly complete by 23 months following onset.

These cases match the cases of isolated anterior interosseous neuritis in sudden onset and prominent pain and indicate that in some instances while the anterior interosseous nerve may be preferentially involved, the neuropathy is actually more widespread. In these two cases, there was electromyographic evidence of axonal degeneration, and the delayed recovery is consistent with axonal regeneration over a distance similar to the distance from brachial plexus to forearm using the approximation of 1 mm of axonal regrowth daily. However, the hypothesis that the pathology is a patchy process in the brachial plexus rather than in the anterior interosseous nerve itself is unproven.

In fact, other cases compatible with neuralgic amyotrophy show axonopathy of multiple arm nerves, suggesting a mononeuritis multiplex rather than a brachial plexitis (England and Sumner 1987). Cases may show isolated denervation in pronator teres, sensory change in a palmar cutaneous pattern, or more complete median neuropathy proximal to the branch to pronator teres. In some cases, time to reinnervation favors lesions in the arm or forearm rather than the brachial plexus. The anatomically noncommittal label "neuralgic amyotrophy," rather than "brachial plexitis," is appropriate to this condition because of the varied sites of nerve pathology.

The differentiation between anterior interosseous nerve compression and anterior interosseous neuralgic amyotrophy is challenging at times. Sudden onset of proximal pain, rapid evolution of weakness, subtle neuropathy beyond the innervation of the anterior interosseous nerve, and electromyographic evidence of axonal interruption favor the diagnosis of neuralgic amyotrophy. Note that in the above cases nerve sensitivity to percussion in the forearm can be prominent in neuralgic amyotrophy and is not a reliable indicator of focal nerve compression. In problematic cases a meticulous search, both by neurologic examination and electromyography (EMG), for evidence of neuropathy beyond the distribution of the anterior interosseous nerve may resolve the issue. When neuropathy is clearly restricted to the anterior interosseous nerve, clinical judgment becomes especially important. Retrospective reading of case reports of anterior interosseous nerve compression suggests that some patients are unnecessarily explored for compressive lesions. For example, Miller-Breslow et al. (1990) describe two cases of anterior interosseous nerve palsy in which they found no pathology at surgery; they warn other surgeons of the danger of overhasty surgical exploration when neuralgic amyotrophy is a likely diagnosis.

Differential Diagnosis

The importance of a careful clinical and electromyographic evaluation is highlighted by the "pseudo–anterior interosseous nerve syndrome." At times a partial median neuropathy with injury in the vicinity of the antecubital space, proximal to the takeoff of the anterior interosseous nerve, may masquerade as an anterior interosseous nerve syndrome. Phlebotomy and cutdown for catheterization are typical causes of this type of injury (Schneck 1960; Finelli 1977; Saeed and Gatens 1983). Only subtle findings may document more widespread median nerve involvement. For example, a 55-year-old man presented two days following right antecubital cardiac catheterization with forearm and hand discomfort and weakness restricted to the right flexor pollicis longus and flexor digitorum profundus (Wertsch et al. 1985). The clues to more widespread median nerve involvement were a 4-mm diameter area of sensory loss at the tips of the right index finger and thumb and mild asymmetries of nerve conduction comparing right and left median nerves. Electromyographic needle exam of median-innervated muscles showed sharp waves and fibrillations in flexor pollicis longus and pronator quadratus but was otherwise normal. At exploration dense fibrosis was noted around the median nerve in the antecubital space at the site of previous cutdown for catheterization, whereas the anterior interosseous nerve itself was normal.

Katirji (1986) reported a similar case in a 30-year-old man who sustained a posterior elbow dislocation that was reduced without surgery. Weakness limited to flexor pollicis longus and flexor digitorum profundus developed a few weeks later, and sensory exam was normal. Median motor and sensory conduction studies to the hand were normal and symmetric except that the thenar compound muscle action potential was 6.6 mV on the symptomatic side compared with 16.0 mV contralaterally. The most convincing evidence of more extensive median nerve injury were neuropathic abnormalities on needle EMG involving not only flexor pollicis longus, pronator quadratus, and flexor digitorum profundus but also, to a lesser extent, abductor pollicis brevis, pronator teres, and flexor digitorum superficialis. At antecubital exploration, scarring was found around the median nerve.

These cases of pseudo–anterior interosseous nerve syndrome are consistent with the fascicular organization of the median nerve (Figure 17.4); the fibers destined for the anterior interosseous nerve are grouped discretely in the posterior portion of the median nerve (Jabaley et al. 1980). For more than 93 mm above the medial epicondyle, the anterior interosseous nerve can be microdissected free from the main median nerve since the epineurium divides the two nerve bundles.

Rupture of flexor pollicis longus or flexor digitorum profundus tendons or rare congenital absence of one of these muscles may easily be confused with anterior interosseous nerve palsy. Tendon rupture may occur spontaneously, particularly in patients with rheumatoid arthritis. Confusion is heightened because a partial anterior interosseous nerve palsy may present with weakness clinically evident in only a single muscle. Electrodiagnosis should be helpful in making the distinction.

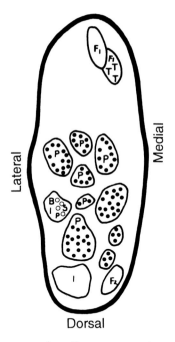

Figure 17.4 Fascicular anatomy of median nerve at the antecubital level. The fibers destined for the anterior interosseous nerve *(I)* are predominantly dorsal so that partial nerve injury favoring the posterior aspect of the nerve may cause a "pseudo–interosseous nerve syndrome." Other fibers: *P*, palmar cutaneous; *T*, pronator teres; F_1, proximal common flexors; F_2, distal common flexors; *round dots*, mixed fibers; *S*, flexor digitorum superficialis; *B*, cutaneous fibers from the second interspace. (Reproduced with permission of the publishers from Sunderland S. The intraneural topography of the radial, median and ulnar nerves. Brain 1945;68:243–98; and Sunderland S. The median nerve. Anatomical and physiological considerations. In: Nerves and nerve injuries. 2nd ed. Edinburgh: Churchill Livingstone, 1978;674.)

Electrodiagnosis

Nerve conduction studies of the anterior interosseous nerve are limited to assessment of motor conduction. A number of different techniques have been proposed.

The compound muscle action potential of pronator quadratus can be recorded with surface electrodes while the median nerve is stimulated at the antecubital space with the forearm pronated and the elbow flexed 90° (Mysiw and Colachis 1988). The active recording electrode is placed on the dorsum of the forearm 3 cm proximal to the ulnar styloid with the reference electrode at the ulnar styloid. The distance from stimulus site in the antecubital space to the recording electrode may vary from 17 to 28 cm. Table 17.2 shows the normal values for this technique based on Mysiw and Colachis's study of 26 normal individuals.

Nakano et al. (1977) reported normative data on latency obtained by recording in the pronator quadratus with a needle electrode. With stimulation in the ventromedial arm adjacent to the biceps tendon, mean latency was 5.1 msec, with a 95% confidence limit of 6.0 msec. With stimulation in the forearm 10 cm distal to the lateral epicondyle, mean latency was 3.6 msec with a 95% confidence limit of 4.4 msec. Nakano et al. studied seven patients with anterior interosseous nerve palsy; all had prolonged duration of muscle action potential, and five had prolonged motor latency.

Rosenberg (1990) proposed recording the muscle action potential from pronator quadratus with a monopolar active intramuscular electrode using a surface reference electrode. With stimulation of the median nerve proximal to the antecubital fossa, the latencies to the pronator quadratus and abductor pollicis brevis are measured, and the ratio of these latencies is used to compare anterior interosseous nerve and median nerve conductions.

The compound muscle action potential of the flexor pollicis longus may be recorded using an active surface electrode over the lateral distal third of the anterior forearm (Craft et al. 1977). The active electrode should be placed three eighths of the distance between the distal wrist crease and the antecubital crease

Table 17.2 Normal values for anterior interosseous nerve conduction

	Mean	Range	Standard Deviation	Maximum Side-to-Side Variation
Distal normal motor latency	3.6 msec	2.8–4.4 msec	0.4 msec	0.4 msec
CMAP amplitude	3.1 mV	2.0–5.5 mV	0.8 mV	25%
CMAP duration	7.8 msec	5.6–10.5 msec	1.3 msec	

CMAP = Compound muscle action potential. (Data from Mysiw and Colachis 1988.)

with the reference electrode placed distally over the flexor pollicis longus tendon. Ideally, the body of flexor pollicis longus should be palpated to confirm electrode placement, but this is not always possible if the flexor pollicis longus is severely paretic. With stimulation of the median nerve just proximal to the elbow, the amplitude of the compound muscle action potential ranged from 3.8 to 7.5 mV, and the latency ranged from 1.8 to 3.6 msec in 25 normal women.

Electrodiagnostic study of patients with suspected anterior interosseous nerve palsy should include motor and sensory studies of the main trunk of the median nerve, which should be normal (O'Brien and Upton 1972). Electromyographic needle electrode examination should be performed to confirm localization of the abnormality to the muscles supplied by the anterior interosseous nerve. If neuropathic abnormalities are noted in ulnar-innervated hand intrinsic muscles, nerve stimulation may be needed to check for a Martin-Gruber anastomosis. Electromyographic needle electrode examination is also helpful in characterizing the degree of axonal interruption contributing to the anterior interosseous nerve dysfunction.

Treatment

Appropriate treatment will, of course, vary with cause. Some patients with compressive neuropathy will improve with decreased forearm use. In some cases, this may be imposed by casting the arm in supination (Rask 1979). If no improvement occurs in four to eight weeks, many surgeons favor forearm exploration for correction of entrapment (Mills et al. 1969; Spinner 1970; Stern 1984). If the clinical presentation suggests gradual development of compressive symptoms and if the EMG shows evidence of axonal interruption, surgical exploration should not be delayed. If the clinical presentation favors neuralgic amyotrophy, decompressive surgery is obviously without value, and improvement may take up to two years.

In patients with persistent weakness in flexor pollicis longus or flexor digitorum profundus, tendon transfer surgery may be of value. Spinner (1970) suggests releasing the flexor digitorum superficialis tendon of the ring finger and attaching it to the flexor pollicis longus tendon. The tendon of the brachioradialis or the flexor digitorum profundus of ring or middle finger can be transferred to the flexor digitorum profundus tendon of the index finger.

Terminal Branch of Anterior Interosseous Nerve

Dellon et al. (1984) reported a series of 12 patients with the diagnosis of focal injury to the terminal branch of the anterior interosseous nerve. This branch of the nerve provides sensory innervation of the anterior radiocarpal and intercarpal joints. The patients complained of dull, aching volar wrist pain, exacerbated by some wrist movements, particularly hyperextension. The symptoms developed and became chronic following hyperextension wrist injuries. Unfortunately, no neurologic or electrophysiologic testing can confirm the diagnosis.

Dellon et al. suggest a diagnostic test of terminal anterior interosseous nerve block with injection of local anesthetic at the interosseous membrane after piercing the pronator quadratus. A positive test includes pain relief and normal grip testing after the block. Treatment is resection of the terminal anterior interosseous nerve.

The patients reportedly had long-standing good to excellent response to surgery. Evaluation of the diagnosis and of results of treatment is complicated because many of the patients had concomitant treatment of other problems including carpal tunnel surgery and ganglionectomy and because many of the patients had unresolved litigation or workers' compensation claims.

MEDIAN NEUROPATHY IN THE ANTECUBITAL SPACE AND PROXIMAL FOREARM
Compression by Normal or Anomalous Anatomic Structures

The pronator syndrome, specifically defined as resulting from median nerve compression by the pronator teres muscle, was described by Seyffarth (1951). We now recognize that the median nerve may be compressed at a variety of sites as it enters the forearm. The pronator teres is the most common of these sites. Other possible points of nerve compression include a tendinous origin of flexor digitorum superficialis, the lacertus fibrosus, or the ligament of Struthers (Figures 17.5–17.7). The anatomy of the course of the median nerve through the antecubital space and into the forearm is reviewed in Chapter 1.

Clinical Presentation
Pronator syndrome presents with aching forearm distress and muscle fatigability, often related to repetitive forearm pronation. Intermittent, but vaguely localized, numbness in the hand, especially in the thumb and index finger, may be present at the time of use-induced distress. Nocturnal awakening with pain or paresthesia is not characteristic of pronator syndrome. Symptoms typically develop insidiously and are often present for months prior to diagnosis. Occasionally, symptoms appear more abruptly following a specific sprain or episode of heavy forearm use or focal trauma (Hartz et al. 1981). Pronator syndrome is much rarer than carpal tunnel syndrome. Reported clinical series are relatively small (Morris and Peters 1976; Johnson et al. 1979; Hartz et al. 1981). Males are more commonly affected in some series, whereas females predominate in others. Typically, the dominant arm is symptomatic.

Physical Examination Findings
The key abnormality on physical examination is found on palpation of the ventral forearm over the pronator teres. This muscle originates at or proximal to the medial epicondyle and crosses to the proximal forearm at about a 45° angle to insert on the radius 7 to 10 cm distal to the lateral epicondyle. The muscle may

Figure 17.5 In this patient the median nerve *(M)* is crossed by two arches, one formed by the flexor digitorum superficialis *(FDS)* and the other formed by the superficial head of pronator teres *(PT)*. Left arm; distal is toward the right. Other patients may have no crossing arch or a single arch. (Reproduced with permission of the publisher from Dellon AL, Mackinnon SE. Musculoaponeurotic variations along the course of the median nerve in the proximal forearm. J Hand Surg 1987;12B:359–63.)

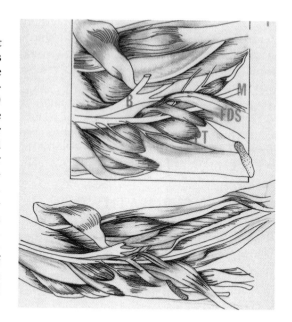

feel firm, tender, or enlarged. Hartz et al. (1981) found tenderness at this point in 37 of 39 patients. Patients may also note tenderness over the thenar eminence (Seyffarth 1951). A Tinel's sign may be elicited over the median nerve in the proximal forearm in about one half the cases (Hartz et al. 1981; Werner et al. 1985). A misleading finding may be a positive Phalen's wrist flexion test (Hartz et al. 1981).

The proximal forearm at the level of the pronator teres may be visibly

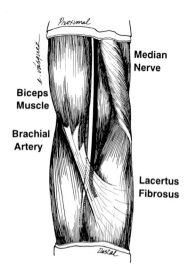

Figure 17.6 The lacertus fibrosus, a fascial band that stretches between the biceps tendon and the proximal ulna, may potentially compress the median nerve.

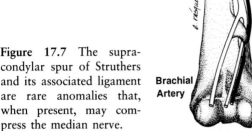

Figure 17.7 The supra-condylar spur of Struthers and its associated ligament are rare anomalies that, when present, may compress the median nerve.

Median Nerve

Ligament of Struthers

Brachial Artery

enlarged. If the lacertus fibrosus is responsible for the compression, it may create a depressed contour in the antecubital space.

Median nerve entrapment by the ligament of Struthers or by the supra-condylar process of the humerus is much rarer than entrapment by the pronator muscle (Barnard and McCoy 1946; Kessel and Rang 1966; Rofes-Capo et al. 1981; Gessini et al. 1983a; Suranyi 1983; Al-Qattan and Husband 1991). These entrapments along the distal humerus may be clinically suspected and distinguished from entrapments in the antecubital space or proximal forearm if there is concomitant arterial compression, if symptoms are increased with elbow extension with the arm supinated, or if a supracondylar process is visible on humeral radiographs (Symeonides 1972). However, occasionally symptoms increase with elbow flexion (Bilge et al. 1990). Very rarely, the ulnar nerve may also be compressed by the supracondylar process (Thomsen 1977; Mittal and Gupta 1978). In many cases a clinical distinction of site of median nerve compression is impossible until the course of the nerve is surgically explored.

In the larger series of pronator syndrome collected by orthopedists and hand surgeons, objective sensory loss is usually absent and motor impairment in the median distribution is subtle or absent (Johnson et al. 1979; Hartz et al. 1981). A smaller series from a neurology group found muscle weakness and sensory loss in most patients with the diagnosis (Morris and Peters 1976). Did the neurologists do a more thorough neuromuscular exam? Did the orthopedists overdiagnose the syndrome? Did the neurologists not make the diagnosis until the syndrome was more advanced? The third hypothesis may explain at least part of the discrepancy: In chronic compressive neuropathies, the expected pattern is for intermittent pain and paresthesias to precede objective neurologic deficit. The second hypothesis also merits consideration; there is no standard test to prove the diagnosis, and distinguishing mild cases of pronator syndrome from other causes of forearm pain is challenging.

On rare occasions, *focal "dystonia,"* manifested as involuntary hand posturing, induced or increased by action, has been reported in patients with purported proximal median neuropathy (Scherokman et al. 1986).

Provocative Tests

A number of provocative tests have been recommended in an attempt to localize median compression in the forearm (Figure 17.8) (Spinner 1980):

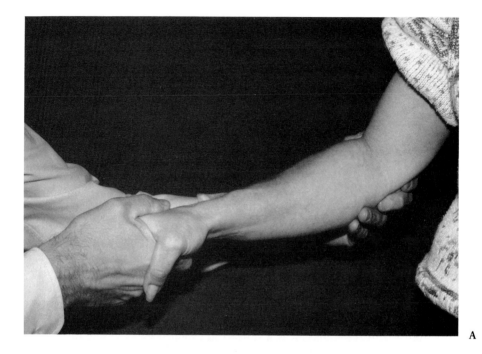

A

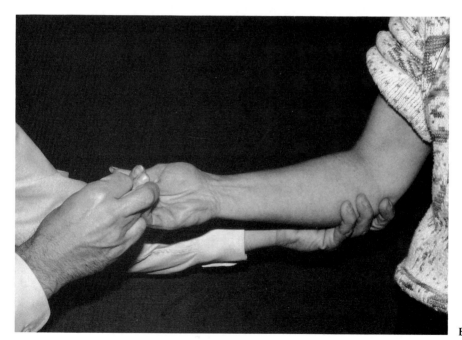

B

Figure 17.8 Spinner (1980) recommends three provocative tests for median nerve entrapment in the forearm: resisted pronation **A,** resisted flexion of the proximal interphalangeal joint of the middle finger **B,** and sustained elbow flexion with the forearm supinated **C.**

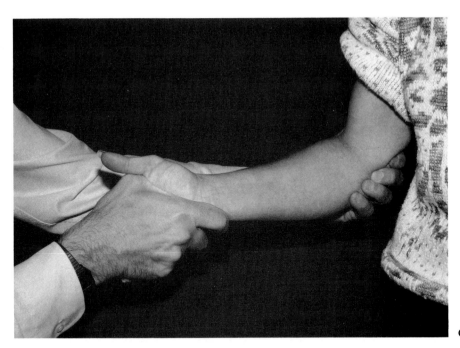

C

1. When forearm pain and hand paresthesias are increased with resisted pronation or with elbow extension with the forearm pronated, the entrapment is probably at the level of the pronator teres.
2. When forearm pain and hand paresthesias are increased by resisted flexion of the proximal interphalangeal joint of the middle finger, entrapment at the arch formed by the flexor digitorum superficialis is the favored diagnosis.
3. When forearm pain and hand paresthesias are increased by maintaining elbow flexion (with the forearm supinated) against resistance, the expected level of entrapment is at the lacertus fibrosus.

The specificity of each test is improved if elicitation of paresthesias in the median cutaneous distribution, rather than pain alone, is used as the criterion for a positive test. In 39 patients reported by Hartz et al. (1981), 30 had paresthesias provoked by test 1, and 14 had paresthesias provoked by test 2. The correlation between which test was positive and the surgically identified site of entrapment was imperfect. There is little data available on the false-positive rates for these provocative tests. Extrapolating from the false-positive incidence of Phalen's wrist flexion test in carpal tunnel syndrome, from the high incidence of potential sites of median nerve compression in the asymptomatic forearm, and from the possibility that musculoskeletal pains may confuse the results, abundant false-positive results on these forearm provocative tests should be anticipated (Dellon 1986; Gellman et al. 1986).

Electrodiagnosis

Median nerve conduction studies may show abnormalities in patients with median nerve entrapment in the forearm. Median motor conduction velocity to the abductor pollicis brevis may be slowed in the forearm with a normal distal motor latency (Morris and Peters 1976). Median motor latency between the antecubital space and flexor digitorum profundus or flexor digitorum superficialis may be prolonged, or median sensory conduction may be slowed across the site of entrapment (Buchthal et al. 1974). All 18 patients reported by Buchthal et al. and Morris and Peters had deteriorated to the stage of clinical weakness in median-innervated muscles; two thirds of the patients showed an abnormality in motor or sensory median nerve conduction, but each test was not done in every patient. In comparison, the incidence of median nerve conduction abnormalities in the larger clinical series was quite low, and abnormalities, when present, were usually not of value in localizing the site of compression; even intraoperative median nerve conduction studies usually failed to demonstrate localized slowing of nerve conduction (Johnson et al. 1979; Hartz et al. 1981).

The sensitivity of nerve conduction tests may possibly be improved by combining them with provocative maneuvers (Werner et al. 1985). In nine patients with a clinical diagnosis of pronator syndrome, routine median motor nerve conduction to the thenar eminence was normal, but three of the patients showed abnormalities when nerve conduction was repeated during isometric forearm pronation. In one patient the abnormality was a 40% drop in the compound muscle action potential amplitude (CMAP) and a 0.5-msec increase in the motor latency with antecubital median nerve stimulation. In two patients the change was a 20% drop in the CMAP amplitude. In these three patients the abnormalities were reversed following surgical decompression.

In a minority of patients, electromyographic needle examination may show neuropathic changes in median-innervated hand or forearm muscles (Buchthal et al. 1974; Hartz et al. 1981; Werner et al. 1985). Although the median nerve branches to the pronator teres usually leave the nerve before its site of entrapment by the pronator, some branching to the pronator teres may occur distal to the entrapment, and neuropathic changes on electromyography of pronator teres are seen on rare occasion in pronator syndrome (Aiken and Moritz 1987). On occasion, nerve branches to flexor carpi radialis and flexor digitorum superficialis leave the median nerve proximal to the site of entrapment, and these muscles may be normal on EMG even though other median-innervated muscles are abnormal (Gessini et al. 1987).

Treatment

Initial nonsurgical therapy should include avoiding those arm activities that induce symptoms, antiinflammatory medication, physical therapy, or forearm immobilization. Local steroid infiltration of the pronator teres may be symptomatically successful therapy even if objective neurologic abnormalities are present (Morris and Peters 1976).

If surgery is undertaken, the course of the median nerve through the antecubital space from the ligament of Struthers to the flexor digitorum superficialis must be explored. Clinical findings do not reliably localize the exact site of entrapment, and multiple sites of entrapment may be present. The most optimistic view of surgery is provided by Johnson et al. (1979), who claim only 4 failures in 51 operations. They, however, do not precisely describe their follow-up criteria.

In the Mayo Clinic series of 36 operations, 8 patients had complete relief of symptoms; 20 patients had good relief of symptoms to the extent that they could return to previous activities; 5 patients had some relief of symptoms but persistence of some residual disability; and 3 patients did not improve (Hartz et al. 1981). Postoperative immobilization for two to three weeks, followed by gradual mobilization and strengthening exercises with six weeks of avoidance of strenuous arm use, undoubtedly contributed to the improvement. The Mayo Clinic surgical series is uncontrolled; the therapeutic value of the postoperative protocol, without surgery, is unknown.

The course of recovery following nerve decompression will depend on the severity of median nerve injury. If there has been no axonal interruption, both positive and negative sensorimotor symptoms should resolve quickly, and neurologic function should recover within a few weeks (Eversmann 1986). Persistent forearm pain should prompt reconsideration of the differential diagnosis. Incomplete exploration and decompression of the nerve should be considered; for example, if the surgical scar does not extend above the elbow flexion crease, inadequate evaluation for ligament of Struthers would be suspected. An alternative or additional site of nerve entrapment must be considered; for example, carpal tunnel syndrome may coexist with pronator syndrome. Persistent forearm pain associated with forearm paresthesias or sensory loss raises the possibility of injury to the lateral antebrachial cutaneous nerve at the time of surgery.

A word of caution: persistent pain in a limb, as opposed to recurrent use-induced mechanosensitive pain, is much less commonly due to organic nerve damage than assumed by surgical specialists (see Chapter 16).

Differential Diagnosis

Differential diagnostic categories of compressive median neuropathies in the antecubital space and forearm can be categorized as follows.

Rarer Median Neuropathies of the Forearm

Case reports document a variety of unusual causes of median nerve compression in the antecubital space. A persistent median artery may compress the median nerve in the forearm (Gainor and Jeffries 1987; Jones and Ming 1988). A child born with "congenital ring constrictions" may develop forearm nerve entrapments from the remnants of the constricting rings (Marlow et al. 1981).

Patients may develop median neuropathy after placement of forearm vascular shunts for hemodialysis; in some patients the neuropathy appears ischemic as demonstrated by resolution of symptoms when the shunt remains in place but is closed (Matolo et al. 1971). Other patients develop scarring around the shunt that compresses the median nerve (Zamora et al. 1986). A brachial pseudo-aneurysm may develop at the antecubital end of the shunt and cause nerve compression (Ergungor et al. 1989).

In anticoagulated patients, acute median neuropathy may develop from antecubital hematomas following brachial arterial puncture for blood gas testing or even following repeated venipunctures (Macon and Futrell 1973; Luce et al. 1976; Blankenship 1991). These patients may require urgent surgical decompression. Another potential mechanism for median nerve compression in anticoagulated patients is an acute syndrome of the biceps brachii compartment following rupture of the biceps tendon (McHale et al. 1991).

An acute median injury in the antecubital area has also been reported in children following reduction of elbow dislocations (Matev 1976; Hallett 1981; Strange 1982; Floyd et al. 1987). The nerve may be entrapped in the elbow joint, and acute surgical nerve release is indicated. If diagnosis is delayed, chronic median nerve dysfunction may result (Boe and Holst-Nielsen 1987).

Following forearm injury of various types, patients may develop a compartment syndrome characterized by increased pressure in the fascial compartment of the volar forearm (Mubarak and Hargens 1981). If left untreated, Volkmann's contracture may develop with dysfunction arising both from direct muscle necrosis and from nerve damage. The median, ulnar, and radial nerves may be injured in forearm compartment syndromes, but the median nerve is the most vulnerable. The nerve may be injured through direct nerve trauma, from focal compression or epineurial scarring, or from nerve ischemia secondary to the high compartment pressure (Holmes et al. 1944; Moberg 1960).

The median nerve is the nerve most commonly injured by electrical burns of the arm (DiVincenti et al. 1969; Solem et al. 1977).

The median basilic vein in the antecubital space crosses just anterior to the median nerve (Pask and Robson 1954). Thrombophlebitis in this vein can cause a secondary median neuropathy (Oh and Kim 1967). The median nerve can be damaged if medication intended for intravenous administration through this vein is inadvertently injected into the nerve (Seddon 1972; Hudson et al. 1980).

Following greenstick fracture of the proximal ulna, the median nerve can be progressively entrapped at the fracture site as callus develops (Nunley and Urbaniak 1980).

Median nerve compression neuropathy may result from improper positioning during anesthesia or from prolonged arm constriction by a tourniquet (Parks 1973; Bolton and McFarlane 1978). The pathology of tourniquet paralysis is discussed in Chapter 12.

Median Neuropathy with Multiple Mononeuropathies

Vasculitis and other focal nerve ischemia can cause median mononeuropathy, either in isolation or as part of mononeuritis multiplex (Figure 17.9). These ischemic neuropathies should be particularly suspected when focal lesions develop suddenly at sites other than common areas of nerve compression. In mononeuritis multiplex the first nerve affected is somewhat more likely to be in the legs than in the arms; nonetheless, eventual median nerve involvement is common. For example, among 12 patients with nonsystemic vasculitic mononeuritis multiplex, 6 had median neuropathies (Dyck et al. 1987). In another series, 26% of patients with mononeuritis multiplex had sensory or motor deficits in the median nerve distribution (Hellmann et al. 1988).

Proximal median mononeuropathy may occur acutely in sickle cell pain crisis (Shields et al. 1991). Bilateral median neuropathy has been reported complicating sarcoidosis (Kömpf et al. 1976). Hemophiliacs may develop focal nerve compression by hemorrhages, often without obvious trauma (Ehrmann et al. 1981). A patient with idiopathic thrombocytopenic purpura developed mononeuropathies of multiple nerves, including the median; at autopsy, multiple intraneural hemorrhages were found (Greenberg and Sonoda 1991).

Some other causes of multiple mononeuropathies such as diabetes, leprosy, and hereditary liability to pressure palsies are discussed in Chapters 5 and 6.

Median Neuropathies at Other Sites

Carpal tunnel syndrome is a much commoner cause of forearm pain than is pronator syndrome. Criteria favoring pronator syndrome are focal tenderness over the pronator muscle, weakness of forearm muscles, and diurnal persistence of pain. In theory, proximal median neuropathies should have sensory changes not only in the fingers but also over the thenar eminence, since the recurrent palmar sensory branch leaves the median nerve proximal to the carpal tunnel; in practice this sensory distinction is rarely reliable. Criteria favoring carpal tunnel syndrome are a typical nocturnal or rest-induced pattern of sensory symptoms; motor findings, when present, limited to thenar muscles and lumbricals; and sensory changes, when present, limited to digital nerves. In patients with pronator syndrome, an initial erroneous diagnosis of carpal tunnel syndrome is common; at times both conditions coexist.

The rare median neuropathies originating in the axilla or upper arm must be distinguished from pronator syndrome. These are discussed later in this chapter.

Other Neuropathic Syndromes of the Forearm

Compression of the lateral antebrachial cutaneous nerve in the antecubital space is rare and may present with forearm pain and antecubital tenderness (Nunley and Howson 1989). The tenderness in a typical case will be located lateral to the biceps tendon in the antecubital space rather than over the pronator muscle. Paresthesias and sensory signs on examination will be localized to the lateral forearm, rather than to the hand, but the sensory territory of the anterior branch of the nerve may overlap the territory of the median palmar cutaneous nerve. Motor deficit will be absent. Elbow extension may be limited by pain when the forearm is pronated—a finding that may be confused with a positive provocative test for pronator syndrome.

Other neuropathic processes that need consideration include ulnar neuropathy, radial or posterior interosseous neuropathy, brachial plexopathies, and cervical radiculopathy. Ulnar or radial neuropathies should be distinguishable by

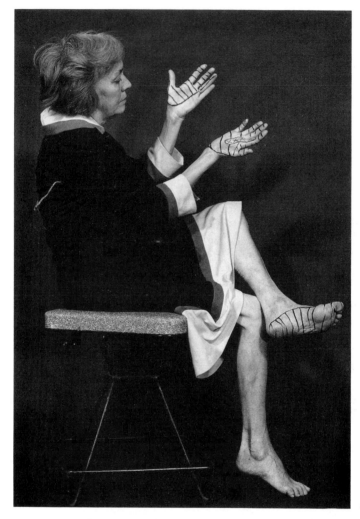

A

Figure 17.9 **A,** Areas of sensory deficit in one patient with mononeuritis multiplex including the median, ulnar, and posterior tibial nerves. **B,** Electron micrograph of this patient's biopsied nerve. Note the cellular exudate adjacent to epineural blood vessel, and eosinophil at the corner. The clinical diagnosis was asthma and allergic granulomatosis and angiitis (Churg-Strauss syndrome).

their specific patterns of motor and sensory impairment. Tinel's sign may be localized over the course of the appropriate nerve. Brachial plexopathies, when predominantly affecting the lateral cord of the brachial plexus, may cause diagnostic difficulty. Fortunately, isolated disease of this part of the plexus is rare.

The problem of distinguishing neuralgic amyotrophy from median neuropathy is discussed earlier in regard to the anterior interosseous nerve. A 36-year-old woman described by Swiggett and Ruby (1986) exemplifies the difficulty of

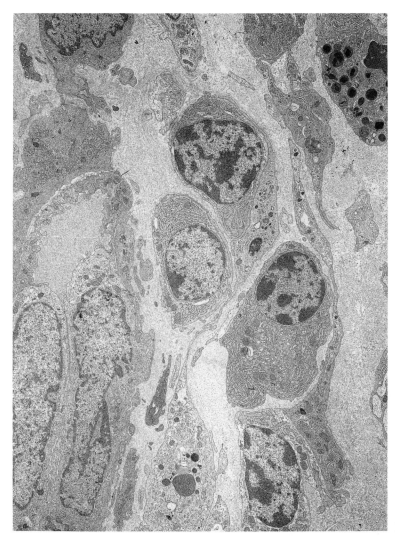

B

making this distinction. She had sudden onset of pain followed over 10 days by weakness in both median and ulnar muscles and no sensory changes. The authors present this patient as an example of median nerve compression by the lacertus fibrosus, but neuralgic amyotrophy might be considered in the differential diagnosis based on the timing of symptoms and the involvement of more than one nerve.

Cervical radiculopathy may present with forearm pain, particularly when the sixth or seventh cervical roots are implicated. Clues favoring cervical radiculopathy include neck pain, reproduction of forearm pain with neck movements ("Spurling's sign"), sensory signs on the dorsum of the hand beyond the distribution of the median nerve, and appropriate changes in tendon reflexes. When muscle weakness is present, the distinction should be relatively easy: Radiculopathic weakness of median-innervated forearm muscles is almost invariably accompanied by triceps weakness since these muscles receive innervation from both the sixth and seventh cervical roots.

Nonneuropathic Syndromes of the Forearm

Focal tenderness in the forearm without focal neurologic dysfunction introduces a differential diagnosis of a variety of localized soft tissue problems. The localization of tenderness should allow separation of lateral epicondylitis from focal sprain or strain of the pronator teres or forearm flexor muscles. A greater diagnostic challenge is separating pronator syndrome from ventral forearm musculoligamentous pains. If pronator syndrome is defined as median neuropathy caused by compression of the nerve at the level of the pronator teres, the clinical diagnosis must require some evidence of median nerve dysfunction such as weakness, sensory change, or reproduction of cutaneous paresthetic symptoms by provocative tests.

MEDIAN NEUROPATHY IN THE UPPER ARM

Supracondylar fractures of the humerus, especially in children, may injure the median nerve (Lipscomb and Burleson 1955; Culp et al. 1990). The nerve injury may be limited to the median nerve or may involve the ulnar or radial nerves as well. If the brachial artery is also compromised by the injury, emergency surgical exploration of the neurovascular bundle is often necessary (Karlsson et al. 1986). If circulation is intact, but the median nerve is injured, some patients show gradual recovery from components of neurapraxic injury, and others require delayed nerve exploration for neurolysis or secondary nerve repair.

A rarer site of traumatic median neuropathy is at the level of midhumerus associated with greenstick humeral fracture. The median neuropathy may worsen as the fracture heals, reflecting nerve entrapment in fracture callus (Macnicol 1978).

Acute median nerve traumatic transection may occur anywhere along the course of the nerve. In the upper arm, trauma that transects the median nerve usually injures the ulnar nerve as well. In the distal few centimeters of the upper arm, the median and ulnar nerves are separated as the ulnar nerve courses posteriorly and medially to run behind the medial epicondyle, whereas the median nerve pursues its antecubital course. Isolated median nerve laceration has been reported 6 cm or less above the medial epicondyle (Boswick and Stromberg 1967). The brachial artery is often transected with the same injury. Primary nerve repair is advisable where possible (Birch and Raji 1991). Recovery of protective hand sensation may take 18 to 26 months. Motor recovery in median forearm muscles may begin within 6 to 12 months. Thenar motor recovery is less likely to occur and may require tendon transfer surgery to reconstitute thumb opposition.

MEDIAN NEUROPATHY IN THE AXILLA

Infraclavicular nerve compression isolated to the median nerve is extremely rare. Reported causes include nerve compression by aberrant axillary arch muscles, vascular anomalies, thickening of the deltopectoral fascia, or a single case of a large infraclavicular lipoma (Mayfield 1970; Spinner 1976, 1980; Weinzweig and Browne 1988). The clinical picture includes weakness or sensory changes in the median distribution and exacerbation of neurologic findings by shoulder abduction or external rotation. Spinner (1980) has emphasized that sensation may be spared and paralysis may be partial, involving particularly forearm muscles. This pattern reflects preferential damage of nerve fibers from the lateral cord of the brachial plexus.

Cases of median nerve compression in the axilla are so unusual that reported cases deserve critical reading. For example, Spinner (1976) describes a case in which paralysis was confined to the right flexor pollicis longus. The patient was a 25-year-old woman who presented with acute onset of severe right shoulder pain 10 days preceding the weakness. She had tenderness and a Tinel's sign over the neurovascular bundle at the level of the coracoid process, distinguishing the case from an anterior interosseous nerve palsy. When her axilla was surgically explored, the median nerve was penetrated by an anomalous posterior circumflex artery and vein. These vessels were ligated. Postoperatively pain was quickly relieved, but weakness took four months to resolve. The case was interpreted as an unusual entrapment of the median nerve in the axilla caused by the vascular anomaly. We present an alternative hypothesis: The sudden onset, prominence of pain, and rapid development of severe weakness are strongly suggestive of neuralgic amyotrophy. The course of clinical recovery, with pain clearing relatively quickly but motor recovery taking many months, is also a feature of neuralgic amyotrophy. Neurovascular anomalies of the median nerve in relation to brachial vessels occur asymptomatically in 8% of the population (Miller 1939).

Acute median neuropathy may evolve over hours or a few days following axillary arteriography or axillary block anesthesia (Stall et al. 1966; Carroll and Wilkins 1970; Molnar and Paul 1972; Westcott and Taylor 1972; Lyon et al. 1975; O'Keefe 1980; Groh et al. 1990). The mechanism may be hematoma or pseudoaneurysm formation in the neurovascular bundle that includes the axillary artery and median nerve. While the neuropathy may be limited to the median nerve, the radial, ulnar, and musculocutaneous nerves are in close proximity to the median nerve at this level and may also be injured.

An acute compressive neuropathy, isolated to the proximal median nerve, may occur as a "sleep" palsy, but it is much rarer than the well-known radial nerve "Saturday night" palsy. In Marinacci's (1967) report of 67 patients with "pressure neuropathy from 'hanging arm,'" only 9 patients had neuropathy limited to the median nerve. The typical patients awaken from sleep with paralysis including all median-innervated muscles and with sensory changes in the median distribution (Roth et al. 1982). There is often a history of preceding stupor, usually from heavy alcohol use the previous night. Recovery may occur quickly or over the course of many months. Nerve conduction studies may show conduction block in the median nerve just distal to the anterior border of the axilla formed by the pectoralis muscle. The ulnar nerve may be clinically spared, and ulnar motor nerve conduction may confirm absence of conduction block with stimulation at Erb's point. The median nerve compression occurs in the proximal arm, after the median and ulnar nerves separate, while the median nerve is in the brachial canal of the arm.

On rare occasion the median nerve may be injured by dislocations of the shoulder or fractures of the proximal humerus (Blom and Dahlback 1970). Joint and bone injuries at this level are much more likely to affect the axillary rather than the median nerve.

The median nerve may be injured by inadvertent injection of local anesthetic into the nerve during attempted nerve block in the axilla (Hudson 1987).

SUMMARY

Familiarity with the proximal median neuropathies, uncommon though they are, is important. They are included in the differential diagnosis of cases presenting with arm pain, weakness, or sensory change. Their diagnosis and management require knowledge of median nerve anatomy and careful attention to details of clinical presentation.

REFERENCES

Aiken BM, Moritz MJ. Atypical electromyographic findings in pronator teres syndrome. Arch Phys Med Rehabil 1987;68:173–75.

Albanese S, Buterbaugh G, Palmer AK, Lubicky JP, Yuan HA. Incomplete anterior interosseous nerve palsy following spinal surgery. A report of two cases. Spine 1986;11: 1037–38.

Al-Qattan MM, Husband JB. Median nerve compression by the supracondylar process: a case report. J Hand Surg 1991;16B:101–3.

Barnard LB, McCoy SM. The supracondyloid process of the humerus. J Bone Joint Surg 1946;28:845–50.

Baruch A, Hass A. Anomaly of the median nerve (letter). J Hand Surg 1977;2:331–32.

Beverly MC, Fearn CB. Anterior interosseous nerve palsy and dislocation of the elbow. Injury 1984;16:126–28.

Bilge T, Yalaman O, Bilge S, Çokneseli B, Barut Ş. Entrapment neuropathy of the median nerve at the level of the ligament of Struthers. Neurosurgery 1990;27:787–89.

Birch R, Raji ARM. Repair of median and ulnar nerves. J Bone Joint Surg 1991;73B:154–57.

Blankenship JC. Median and ulnar neuropathy after streptokinase infusion. Heart Lung 1991;20:221–23.

Blom S, Dahlback LO. Nerve injuries in dislocations of the shoulder joint and fractures of the neck of the humerus: a clinical and electromyographic study. Acta Chir Scand 1970;136:461.

Boe S, Holst-Nielsen F. Intra-articular entrapment of the median nerve after dislocation of the elbow. J Hand Surg 1987;12B:356–58.

Bolton FB, McFarlane RM. Human pneumatic tourniquet paralysis. Neurology 1978;28:787–93.

Boswick JA, Stromberg WB Jr. Isolated injury of the median nerve above the elbow. J Bone Joint Surg 1967;49A:653–58.

Buchthal F, Rosenfalck A, Trojaborg W. Electrophysiological findings in entrapment of the median nerve at wrist and elbow. J Neurol Neurosurg Psychiatry 1974;37:340–60.

Buckmiller JF, Rickard TA. Isolated compression neuropathy of the palmar cutaneous branch of the median nerve. J Hand Surg 1987;12A:97–99.

Carroll RE, Green DP. The significance of the palmar cutaneous nerve at the wrist. Clin Orthop 1972;83:24–28.

Carroll SE, Wilkins WW. Two cases of brachial plexus injury following percutaneous arteriograms. Can Med Assoc J 1970;102:861–62.

Collins DN, Weber ER. Anterior interosseous nerve avulsion. Clin Orthop 1983;181:175–78.

Conway RR, Thomas R. Isolated complete denervation of the flexor pollicis longus. Arch Phys Med Rehabil 1990;71:406–7.

Craft S, Currier DP, Nelson RM. Motor conduction of the anterior interosseous nerve. Phys Ther 1977;57:1143–47.

Culp RW, Osterman AL, Davidson RS, Skirven T, Bora FW Jr. Neural injuries associated with supracondylar fractures of the humerus in children. J Bone Joint Surg 1990;72A:1211–14.

Dellon AL. Musculotendinous variations about the medial humeral epicondyle. J Hand Surg 1986;11B:175–81.

Dellon AL, Mackinnon SE. Musculoaponeurotic variations along the course of the median nerve in the proximal forearm. J Hand Surg 1987;12B:359–63.

Dellon AL, Mackinnon SE, Daneshvar A. Terminal branch of anterior interosseous nerve as source of wrist pain. J Hand Surg 1984;9B:316–22.

DiVincenti FC, Moncrief JA, Pruitt BA Jr. Electrical injuries: a review of 65 cases. J Trauma 1969;9:497–507.

Dorin D, Mann RJ. Carpal tunnel syndrome associated with abnormal palmaris longus muscle. South Med J 1984;77:1210–11.

Dumitru D, Walsh NE, Ramamurthy S. The premotor potential. Arch Phys Med Rehabil 1989;70:537–40.

Dunne JW, Prentice DA, Stewart-Wynne EG. Bilateral anterior interosseous nerve syndromes associated with cytomegalovirus infection. Muscle Nerve 1987;10:446–48.

Dyck PJ, Benstead TJ, Conn DL, Stevens JC, Windebank AJ, Low PA. Nonsystemic vasculitic neuropathy. Brain 1987;110:843–54.

Ehrmann L, Lechner K, Mamoli B, Novotny C, Kow K. Peripheral nerve lesions in hemophilia. J Neurol 1981;225:175–82.

Engber WD, Keene JS. Anterior interosseous nerve palsy associated with a Monteggia fracture. A case report. Clin Orthop 1983;174:133–37.

England JD, Sumner AJ. Neuralgic amyotrophy: an increasingly diverse entity. Muscle Nerve 1987;10:60–68.

Enzenauer RJ, Nordstrom DM. Anterior interosseous nerve syndrome associated with forearm band treatment of lateral epicondylitis. Orthopedics 1991;14:788–90.

Ergungor MF, Kars HZ, Yalin R. Median neuralgia caused by brachial pseudoaneurysm. Neurosurgery 1989;24:924–25.

Eversmann WW Jr. Complications of compression or entrapment neuropathies. In: Boswick JA Jr, ed. Complications in hand surgery. Philadelphia: WB Saunders, 1986; 99–115.

Fearn CBd'A, Goodfellow JW. Anterior interosseous nerve palsy. J Bone Joint Surg 1965;47B:91–93.

Finelli PF. Anterior interosseous nerve syndrome following cutdown catheterization. Ann Neurol 1977;1:205–6.

Floyd WE, Gebhardt MC, Emans JB. Intra-articular entrapment of the median nerve after elbow dislocation in children. J Hand Surg 1987;12A:704–7.

Gainor BJ, Jeffries JT. Pronator syndrome associated with a persistent median artery. A case report. J Bone Joint Surg 1987;69:303–4.

Gardner RC. Confirmed case and diagnosis of pseudocarpal-tunnel (sublimis) syndrome. N Engl J Med 1970;282:858.

Geissler WB, Fernandez DL, Graca R. Anterior interosseous nerve palsy complicating a forearm fracture in a child. J Hand Surg 1990;15A:44–47.

Gellman H, Gelberman RH, Tan AM, Botte MJ. Carpal tunnel syndrome. An evaluation of the provocative diagnostic tests. J Bone Joint Surg 1986;68A:735–37.

Gessini L, Jandolo B, Pietrangeli A. Entrapment neuropathies of the median nerve at and above the elbow. Surg Neurol 1983a;19:112–16.

Gessini L, Jandolo B, Pietrangeli A. The pronator teres syndrome. Clinical and electrophysiological features in six surgically verified cases. J Neurosurg Sci 1987;31:1–5.

Gessini L, Jandolo B, Pietrangeli A, Senese A. Compression of the palmar cutaneous nerve by ganglions of the wrist. J Neurosurg Sci 1983b;27:241–43.

Greenberg MK, Sonoda T. Mononeuropathy multiplex complicating idiopathic thrombocytopenic purpura. Neurology 1991;41:1517–18.

Groh GI, Gainor BJ, Jeffries JT, Brown M, Eggers GWN Jr. Pseudoaneurysm of the axillary artery with median-nerve deficit after axillary block anesthesia. J Bone Joint Surg 1990;72A:1407–8.

Hallett J. Entrapment of the median nerve after dislocation of the elbow. J Bone Joint Surg 1981;63B:408–12.

Hartz CR, Linscheid RL, Gramse RR, Daube JR. The pronator teres syndrome: compressive neuropathy of the median nerve. J Bone Joint Surg 1981;63A:885–90.

Hellmann DB, Laing TJ, Petri M, Whiting-O'Keefe Q, Parry GJ. Mononeuritis multiplex: the yield of evaluations for occult rheumatic diseases. Medicine 1988;67:145–53.

Hill NA, Howard FM, Huffer BR. The incomplete anterior interosseous nerve syndrome. J Hand Surg 1985;10A:4–16.

Holmes W, Highet WE, Seddon HJ. Ishaemic nerve lesions occurring in Volkmann's contracture. Br J Surg 1944;32:259–75.

Hope PG. Anterior interosseous nerve palsy following internal fixation of the proximal radius. J Bone Joint Surg 1988;70B:280–82.

Hudson AR. Nerve injection injuries. In: Terzis JK, ed. Microreconstruction of nerve injuries. Philadelphia: WB Saunders, 1987;173–79.

Hudson A, Kline D, Gentili F. Peripheral nerve injection injury. In: Omer GE Jr, Spinner M, eds. Management of peripheral nerve problems. Philadelphia: WB Saunders, 1980; 639–53.

Jabaley ME, Wallace WH, Heckler FR. Internal topography of major nerves of the forearm and hand: a current view. J Hand Surg 1980;5:1–18.

Johnson RK, Spinner M, Shrewsbury MM. Median nerve entrapment syndrome in the proximal forearm. J Hand Surg 1979;4:48–51.

Jones NF, Ming NL. Persistent median artery as a cause of pronator syndrome. J Hand Surg 1988;13A:728–32.

Karlsson J, Thorsteinsson T, Thorleifsson R, Arnason H. Entrapment of the median nerve and brachial artery after supracondylar fractures of the humerus in children. Arch Orthop Trauma Surg 1986;104:389–91.

Katirji MB. Pseudo-anterior interosseous nerve syndrome (letter). Muscle Nerve 1986;9:266–67.

Kessel L, Rang M. Supracondylar spur of the humerus. J Bone Joint Surg 1966;48:765–69.

Kiloh LG, Nevin S. Isolated neuritis of the anterior interosseous nerve. BMJ 1952;1:850–851.

Kömpf D, Neundörfer B, Kayser-Gatchalian C, Meyer-Wahl L, Raust K. Mononeuritis multiplex bei Boeckscher Sarkoidose. Nervenarzt 1976;47:687.

Lewis MH. Median nerve decompression after Colles's fracture. J Bone Joint Surg 1978;60B:195–96.

Lipscomb PR, Burleson RJ. Vascular and neural complications in supracondylar fractures of the humerus in children. J Bone Joint Surg 1955;37A:487–92.

Luce EA, Futrell JW, Wilgis EFS, Hoopes JE. Compression neuropathy following brachial arterial puncture in anticoagulated patients. J Trauma 1976;16:717–21.

Lum PB, Kanakamedala R. Conduction of the palmar cutaneous branch of the median nerve. Arch Phys Med Rehabil 1986;67:805–6.

Lyon BB, Hansen BA, Mygind T. Peripheral nerve injury as a complication of axillary arteriography. Acta Neurol Scand 1975;51:29–36.

Mackinnon SE, Dellon AL. Surgery of the peripheral nerves. New York: Thieme Medical Publishers, 1988.

Macnicol MF. Roentgenographic evidence of median nerve entrapment in a greenstick humeral fracture. A case report. J Bone Joint Surg 1978;60A:998–1000.

Macon WL, Futrell JW. Median-nerve neuropathy after percutaneous puncture of the brachial artery in patients receiving anticoagulants. N Engl J Med 1973;288:1396.

Mangini U. Flexor pollicis longus muscle—its morphology and clinical significance. J Bone Joint Surg 1960;42A:467–70.

Mannerfelt L. Studies on the hand in ulnar nerve paralysis. Acta Orthop Scand [Suppl] 1966;87.

Marinacci AA. The value of electromyogram in the diagnosis of pressure neuropathy from "hanging arm." Electromyogr Clin Neurophysiol 1967;7:5–10.

Marlow N, Jarratt J, Hosking G. Congenital ring constrictions with entrapment neuropathies. J Neurol Neurosurg Psychiatry 1981;44:247–49.

Matev I. A radiological sign of entrapment of the median nerve in the elbow joint after posterior dislocation. J Bone Joint Surg 1976;58B:353–55.

Matolo N, Kastagir B, Stevens LE, Chrysanthakopolulos S, Weaver DH, Klinkman H. Neurovascular complications of brachial arteriovenous fistula. Am J Surg 1971;121:716–19.

Mayfield FH. Compression syndromes of the shoulder girdle and arms. In: Vinken PJ, Bruyn GW, eds. Handbook of clinical neurology. Diseases of the nerves. New York: American Elsevier, 1970;441.

McHale KA, Geissele A, Perlik PD. Compartment syndrome of the biceps brachii compartment following rupture of the long head of the biceps. Orthopedics 1991;14:787–88.

Megele R. Anterior interosseous nerve syndrome with atypical nerve course in relation to the pronator teres. Acta Neurochir (Wien) 1988;91:144–46.

Miller RA. Observations upon the arrangement of the axillary artery and brachial plexus. Am J Anat 1939;64:143–63.

Miller-Breslow A, Terrono A, Millender LH. Nonoperative treatment of anterior interosseous nerve paralysis. J Hand Surg 1990;15A:493–96.

Mills RH, Mukherjee K, Bassett IB. Anterior interosseous nerve palsy. Br Med J 1969;2:555.

Mirovsky Y, Hendel D, Halperin N. Anterior interosseous nerve palsy following closed fracture of the proximal ulna. A case report and review of the literature. Arch Orthop Trauma Surg 1988;107:61–64.

Mittal RL, Gupta BR. Median and ulnar-nerve palsy: an unusual presentation of the supracondylar process. J Bone Joint Surg 1978;60A:557–58.

Moberg E. Examination of sensory loss by the ninhydrin printing test in Volkmann's contracture. Bull Hosp Joint Dis 1960;21:296–303.

Moehring HD. Irreducible supracondylar fracture of the humerus complicated by anterior interosseous nerve palsy. Clin Orthop 1986;228–32.

Molnar W, Paul DJ. Complications of axillary arteriotomies. Radiology 1972;104:269–76.

Morris HH, Peters BH. Pronator syndrome: clinical and electrophysiological features in seven cases. J Neurol Neurosurg Psychiatry 1976;39:461–64.

Mubarak SJ, Hargens AR. Compartment syndromes and Volkmann's contracture. Philadelphia: WB Saunders, 1981.

Mysiw WJ, Colachis III SC. Electrophysiologic study of the anterior interosseous nerve. Am J Phys Med Rehabil 1988;67:50–54.

Nakano KK, Lundergran C, Okihiro MM. Anterior interosseous nerve syndromes. Diagnostic methods and alternative treatments. Arch Neurol 1977;34:477–80.

Nunley II JA, Howson P. Lateral antebrachial nerve compression. In: Szabo RM, ed. Nerve compression syndromes. Thorofare, NJ: Slack, 1989;201–8.

Nunley JA, Urbaniak JR. Partial bony entrapment of the median nerve in a greenstick fracture of the ulna. J Hand Surg 1980;5:557–59.

O'Brien MD, Upton AR. Anterior interosseous nerve syndrome. A case report with neurophysiological investigation. J Neurol Neurosurg Psychiatry 1972;35:531–36.

Oh SJ, Kim KW. Thrombophlebitis-induced median neuropathy. South Med J 1967;67:1041–42.

O'Keefe DM. Brachial plexus injury following axillary arteriography. Case report and review of the literature. J Neurosurg 1980;53:853–57.

Omer GE Jr, Spinner M, eds. Management of peripheral nerve problems. Philadelphia: WB Saunders, 1980.

O'Neill DB, Zarins B, Gelberman RH, Keating TM, Louis D. Compression of the anterior interosseous nerve after use of a sling for dislocation of the acromioclavicular joint. A report of two cases. J Bone Joint Surg 1990;72A:1100–1102.

Parks BJ. Postoperative peripheral neuropathies. Surgery 1973;74:348–57.

Parsonage MJ, Turner JWA. Neuralgic amyotrophy: the shoulder-girdle syndrome. Lancet 1948;1:973–78.

Pask EA, Robson JG. Injury to the median nerve. Anaesthesia 1954;9:94–95.

Peters WJ, Todd TR. Anterior interosseous nerve compression syndrome: from metastatic bronchogenic carcinoma to the forearm. Plast Reconstr Surg 1983;72:706–7.

Phalen GS, Kendrick JI, Rodriguez JM. Lipomas of the upper extremity. Am J Surg 1971;121:298–306.

Rask MR. Anterior interosseous nerve entrapment: (Kiloh-Nevin syndrome) report of seven cases. Clin Orthop 1979;142:176–81.

Rennels GD, Ochoa J. Neuralgic amyotrophy manifesting as anterior interosseous nerve palsy. Muscle Nerve 1980;3:160–64.

Rofes-Capo S, Ramirez-Ruiz G, Bordas-Sales JL, Gomez-Bonfills J, Lopez-de-Vega J. Median nerve compression on the level of the ligament of Struthers. Case report. Acta Orthop Belg 1981;47:884–89.

Rosenberg JN. Anterior interosseous/median nerve latency ratio. Arch Phys Med Rehabil 1990;71:228–30.

Roth G, Ludy J-P, Egloff-Baer S. Isolated proximal median neuropathy. Muscle Nerve 1982;5:247–49.

Saeed MA, Gatens PF. Anterior interosseous nerve syndrome: unusual etiologies. Arch Phys Med Rehabil 1983;64:182.

Scherokman B, Husain F, Cuetter A, Jabbari B, Maniglia E. Peripheral dystonia. Arch Neurol 1986;43:830–32.

Schneck SA. Peripheral and cranial nerve injuries resulting from general surgical procedures. Arch Surg 1960;81:855–59.

Seddon H. Surgical disorders of the peripheral nerves. Baltimore: Williams & Wilkins, 1972.

Seyffarth H. Primary myosis in the m. pronator teres as cause of lesion of the n. medianus (the pronator syndrome). Acta Psychiatr Neurol Scand 1951;251–54.

Shields RW Jr, Harris JW, Clark M. Mononeuropathy in sickle cell anemia: anatomical and pathophysiological basis for its rarity. Muscle Nerve 1991;14:370–74.

Shimizu K, Iwasaki R, Hoshikawa H, Yamamuro T. Entrapment neuropathy of the palmar cutaneous branch of the median nerve by the fascia of flexor digitorum superficialis. J Hand Surg 1988;13A:581–83.

Smith BH, Herbst BA. Anterior interosseous nerve palsy. Arch Neurol 1974;30:330–31.

Solem L, Fischer RP, Strate RG. The natural history of electrical injury. J Trauma 1977;17:487–92.

Spinner M. The anterior interosseous-nerve syndrome, with special attention to its variations. J Bone Joint Surg 1970;52A:84–94.

Spinner M. Cryptogenic infraclavicular brachial plexus neuritis (preliminary report). Bull Hosp Joint Dis 1976;37:98–104.

Spinner M. Management of nerve compression lesions of the upper extremity. In: Omer GE Jr, Spinner M, eds. Management of peripheral nerve problems. Philadelphia: WB Saunders, 1980;569–592.

Spinner M, Schreiber SN. Anterior interosseous-nerve paralysis as a complication of supracondylar fractures of the humerus in children. J Bone Joint Surg 1969;51A:1584–90.

Stall A, van Voorthuisen AE, van Dijk LM. Neurological complications following arterial catheterisation by the axillary approach. Br J Radiol 1966;39:115–16.

Stellbrink G. Compression of the palmar branch of the median nerve by atypical palmaris longus muscle. Handchirurgie 1972;4:155–57.

Stern MB. The anterior interosseous nerve syndrome (the Kiloh-Nevin syndrome). Report and follow-up study of three cases. Clin Orthop 1984;187:223–27.

Strange FGStC. Entrapment of the median nerve after dislocation of the elbow. J Bone Joint Surg 1982;64B:224–25.

Sumner JM, Khuri MD. Entrapment of the median nerve and flexor pollicis longus tendon in an epiphyseal fracture-dislocation of the distal radioulnar joint: a case report. J Hand Surg 1984;9A:711–14.

Sunderland S. The intraneural topography of the radial, median and ulnar nerves. Brain 1945;68:243–98.

Sunderland S. The median nerve. Anatomical and physiological considerations. In: Nerves and nerve injuries. 2nd ed. Edinburgh: Churchill Livingstone, 1978.

Suranyi L. Median nerve compression by Struther's ligament. J Neurol Neurosurg Psychiatry 1983;46:1047–49.

Swiggett R, Ruby LK. Median nerve compression neuropathy by the lacertus fibrosis: report of three cases. J Hand Surg 1986;11A:700–703.

Symeonides PP. The humerus supracondylar process syndrome. Clin Orthop 1972;82:141–43.

Thomas DF. Kiloh-Nevin syndrome. J Bone Joint Surg 1962;44B:962.

Thomsen PB. Processus supracondyloidea humeri with concomitant compression of the median nerve and ulnar nerve. Acta Orthop Scand 1977;48:391–93.

Warren JD. Anterior interosseous nerve palsy as a complication of forearm fractures. J Bone Joint Surg 1963;45B:511–12.

Weinzweig N, Browne EZ Jr. Infraclavicular median nerve compression caused by a lipoma. Orthopedics 1988;11:1077–78.

Werner CO, Rosen I, Thorngren KG. Clinical and neurophysiologic characteristics of the pronator syndrome. Clin Orthop 1985;197:231–36.

Wertsch JJ, Sanger JR, Matloub HS. Pseudo-anterior interosseous nerve syndrome. Muscle Nerve 1985;8:68–70.

Westcott JL, Taylor PT. Transaxillary selective four-vessel arteriography. Radiology 1972;104:277–81.

Zamora JL, Rose JE, Rosario V, Noon GP. Double entrapment of the median nerve in association with PTFE hemodialysis loop grafts. South Med J 1986;79:638–40.

18

Median Neuropathy Distal to the Carpal Tunnel

DIGITAL NERVES

The digital nerves are the most commonly injured peripheral nerves, both because of the vulnerability of the hand to injuries and because of the location of the proper digital nerves about 3 mm below the skin. For example, of 100 orthopedists who were surveyed, 15 had injured their own digital nerves severely enough to cause at least transient focal sensory loss (Roberts and Allan 1988). Extensive discussion of the treatment and prognosis of digital nerve lacerations and treatment of posttraumatic neuromas is available in hand surgery or peripheral nerve surgery texts (Dellon 1981).

Clinical Presentation

Digital nerve injury that is severe enough to interrupt nerve function causes sensory disturbance in the distribution of the injured nerve. For a proper digital nerve, this disturbance is typically along the volar surface of the ipsilateral half of the finger. Sensation at the finger pulp may or may not be affected, depending on the degree of overlap at the pulp of fibers from the contralateral proper digital nerve. Sensation on the dorsal fingertip will be affected unless the injury is distal to the takeoff of the dorsal branch of the proper digital nerve.

Digital nerve injury is often accompanied by disturbance of blood flow to the finger both because the digital nerve supplies sympathetic fibers to the finger and because the digital artery accompanies the digital nerve, so that the nerve and artery may be damaged by the same injury.

Injury to a common digital nerve causes sensory disturbance in two adjoining half-fingers and in the web space between them. A proximal, partial median nerve injury that selectively damages the fascicles that carry fibers to a common digital nerve can cause the same pattern of sensory dysfunction (Figure 18.1).

333

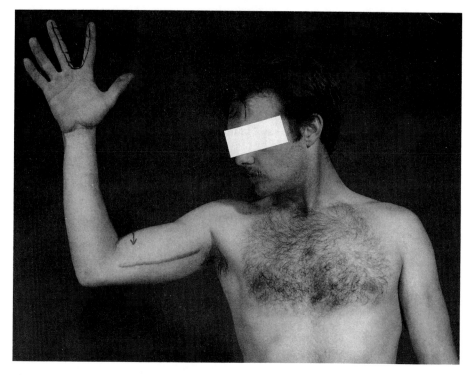

Figure 18.1 Pattern of sensory loss in a patient with a partial median nerve injury in the upper arm. The *arrow* points to the site of penetrating trauma. The sensory loss was confined to the territory of a single common digital nerve, suggesting injury to a single nerve fascicle.

Causes

The proper digital nerves, because of their location between skin and bone, are frequently compressed by objects held in the hand. Repeated compression can lead to development of a "neuroma" in continuity. Pathologically, these are not truly neuromas since there is proliferation of epineurial fibrous tissue rather than of a knot of regenerating nerve fibers (Dobyns et al. 1972). Symptoms include focal thickening of the nerve and surrounding connective tissue. Tinel's sign may be elicitable over the neuroma. The patient may have paresthesia or sensory loss distal to the neuroma.

The ulnar digital nerve of the thumb is the most common site of a compression neuroma. A typical cause is nerve irritation by the thumb hole of a bowling ball—hence, the diagnosis of "bowler's thumb" (Siegel 1965; Marmor 1966; Howell and Leach 1970; Dobyns et al. 1972; Minkow and Bassett 1972). Similar injury may occur from use of a variety of objects including scissors, baseball bats, staple guns, tennis rackets, and axes (Howell and Leach 1970; Rayan and O'Donoghue 1983). The ulnar digital nerve of the thumb may be compressed by a hand splint (Rayan and O'Donoghue 1983).

Cessation of repeated compression is often sufficient treatment of a compression neuroma; occasionally, patients are treated surgically with external neurolysis or by constructing a protective muscle flap over the neuroma (Howell and Leach 1970; Rayan and O'Donoghue 1983).

Digital nerves may also be compressed by abnormal masses in the hand or by external trauma. Kopell and Thompson (1976) describe patients who developed digital neuropathies after forced finger hyperextension, after blunt repeated hand trauma with the palm extended, with arthritis of a metacarpalphalangeal joint, with abnormalities of the tendons near a proximal interphalangeal joint, or even after a particularly crushing handshake. Table 18.1 gives additional examples.

Digital neuropathy is a rare complication in patients with rheumatoid arthritis. The patients usually have a coexistent distal sensory neuropathy in the feet, and at times, more than one digit nerve in the hands is affected (Pallis and Scott 1965).

Nerve tumors of the digital nerves are discussed in Chapter 19.

Both nerves and sensory receptors in the fingers can be injured by prolonged finger exposure to high-frequency vibration (Hjortsberg et al. 1989). The typical patients are dentists and dental technicians who work with tools vibrating at 15,000 to 30,000 Hz. The patients develop numb fingers with increased thresholds to quantitative sensory testing of vibratory function and to heat and cold on quantitative thermotest. Digital nerve conduction studies are normal. The

Table 18.1   Case reports: digital nerve compression

Cause	Reference
Cysts of the flexor tendon sheath	Howell and Leach 1970
Digital osteophytes	Howell and Leach 1970
Dupuytren's contracture	Howell and Leach 1970
Flute playing	Cynamon 1981
Hand clapping	Shields and Jacobs 1986
Osteochondroma, third metacarpal	Richmond 1973
Pacinian corpuscle	Gama and Franca 1980 Cameron 1976 Zweig and Burns 1968
Palmar lipoma	Oster et al. 1989 Paarlberg et al. 1972 Schmitz and Keeley 1957
Posttraumatic palmar aneurysm	Tyler and Stein 1988 O'Connor 1972
Sandblasting injury	Belsole et al. 1982
Sclerodermatous calcinosis	Polio and Stern 1989

thermotest results suggest that the vibration damages small myelinated and unmyelinated fibers. The abnormalities on vibratory testing might be explained by damage to mechanoreceptor end organs or by subtle damage to larger myelinated fibers. This response to high-frequency vibration is distinct from the effect of low-frequency vibration discussed in Chapter 13 under "Vibration Exposure and Carpal Tunnel Syndrome."

Digital Nerve Conduction Studies

Median sensory nerve conduction studies between a finger and the wrist are discussed in Chapter 5. Whether done orthodromically, stimulating the finger, or antidromically, recording from the finger, the studies combine the conduction of both digital nerves of the finger. If conduction is impaired in one proper digital nerve, the sensory nerve action potential may have decreased amplitude (Shields and Jacobs 1986). Slowed conduction in one proper digital nerve can result in a bifid appearance of the sensory nerve action potential (Jablecki and Nazemi 1982).

TERMINAL MOTOR BRANCHES

When the median nerve is injured distal to the departure of the recurrent thenar motor branch, the patient may lose motor function of the median-innervated lumbricals and sensation from the digital branches of the median nerve while retaining function of the thenar muscles (Busis et al. 1986).

The recurrent thenar motor branch can be selectively injured in the palm. Typical case reports are listed in Table 18.2.

Widder and Shons (1988) described a patient with bilateral carpal tunnel syndrome but with thenar atrophy on only one side. At the time of carpal tunnel surgery, the recurrent thenar motor branch on the side with thenar atrophy was compressed between the flexor retinaculum and a prominent superficial palmar branch of the radial artery.

The median nerve fascicles that form the recurrent thenar motor branch are

Table 18.2 Causes of thenar motor branch neuropathy

Cause	Reference
Puncture wound	Yates et al. 1981
Complication of carpal tunnel surgery	Hybbinette 1986 Lilly and Magnell 1985 Dals and Brown 1976 Mannerfelt and Hybbinette 1972
Repeated blunt palmar trauma	Lemmi et al. 1966
Compression by a palmar ganglion	Kato et al. 1991
Compression by a palmar artery	Widder and Shons 1988

usually located on the anterior surface of the median nerve. The differential diagnosis of thenar motor branch injury includes more proximal partial median nerve injury of these anterior fascicles (Perotto and Delagi 1979; Yates et al. 1981).

REFERENCES

Belsole RJ, Nolan M, Eichberg RD. Sandblasting injury of the hand. J Hand Surg 1982;7:523–25.

Busis NA, Logigian EL, Shahani BT. Electrophysiologic assessment of a median nerve injury in the palm. Muscle Nerve 1986;9:208–10.

Cameron S. Two rare cases of nerve entrapment. J Bone Joint Surg 1976;58B:266.

Cynamon KB. Flutist's neuropathy. N Engl J Med 1981;305:961.

Das SK, Brown HG. In search of complications in carpal tunnel decompression. Hand 1976;8:243–49.

Dellon AL. Evaluation of sensibility and re-education of sensation in the hand. Baltimore: Williams & Wilkins, 1981.

Dobyns JH, O'Brien ET, Linscheid RL, Farrow GM. Bowler's thumb: diagnosis and treatment. J Bone Joint Surg 1972;54A:751–55.

Gama C, Franca LCM. Nerve compression by Pacinian corpuscles. J Hand Surg 1980;5:208–10.

Hjortsberg U, Rosén I, Orbaek P, Lundborg G, Balogh I. Finger receptor dysfunction in dental technicians exposed to high-frequency vibration. Scand J Work Environ Health 1989;15:339–44.

Howell AE, Leach RE. Bowler's thumb. J Bone Joint Surg 1970;52A:379–81.

Hybbinette CH. Severance of thenar branch (letter). J Hand Surg 1986;11A:613.

Jablecki C, Nazemi R. Unsuspected digital nerve lesions responsible for abnormal median sensory responses. Arch Phys Med Rehabil 1982;63:135–38.

Kato H, Ogino T, Nanbu T, Nakamura K. Compression neuropathy of the motor branch of the median nerve caused by palmar ganglion. J Hand Surg 1991;16A:751–52.

Kopell HP, Thompson WAL. Peripheral entrapment neuropathies. 2nd ed. Malabar, FL: RE Krieger, 1976.

Lemmi H, Amick LD, Canale DJ. Median acromotor neuropathy (pseudo carpal tunnel syndrome): report of a case. Arch Phys Med Rehabil 1966;47:306–9.

Lilly CJ, Magnell TD. Severance of the thenar branch of the median nerve as a complication of carpal tunnel release. J Hand Surg 1985;10A:399–402.

Mannerfelt L, Hybbinette CH. Important anomaly of the thenar motor branch of the median nerve. A clinical and anatomical report. Bull Hosp Joint Dis 1972;33:15–21.

Marmor L. Bowler's thumb. J Trauma 1966;6:282–84.

Minkow FV, Bassett III FH. Bowler's thumb. Clin Orthop 1972;83:115–17.

O'Connor RL. Digital nerve compression secondary to palmar aneurysm. Clin Orthop 1972;83:149–50.

Oster LH, Blair WF, Steyers CM. Large lipomas in the deep palmar space. J Hand Surg 1989;14A:700–704.

Paarlberg D, Linscheid RL, Soule EH. Lipomas of the hand. Including a case of lipoblastomatosis in a child. Mayo Clin Proc 1972;47:121–24.

Pallis CA, Scott JT. Peripheral neuropathy in rheumatoid arthritis. Br Med J 1965;1:1141–47.

Perotto AO, Delagi EF. Funicular localization in partial median nerve injury at the wrists. Arch Phys Med Rehabil 1979;60:165–69.

Polio JL, Stern PJ. Digital nerve calcification in CREST syndrome. J Hand Surg 1989;14A:201–3.

Rayan GM, O'Donoghue DH. Ulnar digital compression neuropathy of the thumb caused by splinting. Clin Orthop 1983;175:170–72.

Richmond DA. Uncommon causes of nerve compression with hand symptoms. Hand 1973;5:209–13.

Roberts AP, Allan DB. Digital nerve injuries in orthopaedic surgeons. Injury 1988;19:233–34.

Schmitz RL, Keeley JL. Lipomas of the hand. Surgery 1957;42:696–700.

Shields RW, Jacobs IB. Median palmar digital neuropathy in a cheerleader. Arch Phys Med Rehabil 1986;67:824–26.

Siegel IM. Bowling-thumb neuroma. JAMA 1965;192:163.

Tyler G, Stein A. Aneurysm of a common digital artery: resection and vein graft. J Hand Surg 1988;13B:348–49.

Widder S, Shons AR. Carpal tunnel syndrome associated with extra tunnel vascular compression of the median nerve motor branch. J Hand Surg 1988;13A:926–27.

Yates SK, Yaworski R, Brown WF. Relative preservation of lumbrical versus thenar motor fibres in neurogenic disorders. J Neurol Neurosurg Psychiatry 1981;44:768–74.

Zweig J, Burns H. Compression of digital nerves by Pacinian corpuscles. A report of two cases. J Bone Joint Surg 1968;50A:999–1001.

19

Tumors of the Median Nerve

"The trouble about these tumors is that they are just common enough to come within the experience of almost all surgeons and rare enough to cause embarrassment in diagnosis and treatment" (Seddon 1972, 153). Peripheral nerve tumors of any nerve of the arm comprise less than 5% of all hand and arm tumors. Strickland and Steichen (1977) found only 6 nerve tumors in their series of 689 tumors of the hand and arm. Study of median nerve tumors is complicated both by their rarity and by the variety of synonyms that are used for related histologic types. Harkin and Reed (1969, 1983) provide a detailed pathologic review and discussion of the nomenclature.

NEURILEMOMA

Neurilemomas or schwannomas are the most common solitary nerve tumors. They are benign tumors that originate from Schwann cells, typically present as masses, and infrequently cause neurologic deficit or sensory symptoms (Brooks 1984). The tumor is usually discovered by palpation. In consistency and mobility the neurilemoma may be mistaken for a ganglion, but the neurilemoma is more likely to be tender; nonetheless, nerve tumors are so much rarer than ganglions that most tender subcutaneous masses are not nerve tumors. A classic but not invariable finding that favors the diagnosis of neurilemoma is a mass that is movable laterally but not longitudinally. In some cases, percussion of the tumor elicits distal paresthesias.

Neurilemomas of the median nerve may be found in the volar forearm, in the palm, or affecting a single digital nerve in the finger or distal palm (Phalen 1976; Rinaldi 1983; Ritt and Bos 1991). Among 50 patients with neurilemomas, Stout (1935) found seven arising from the palm, digital nerves, or median nerve. When the tumor occurs within the carpal tunnel, it may cause symptoms of carpal tunnel syndrome (Barre et al. 1987). Rarely, a patient has multiple neurilemomas (Lewis et al. 1981; Barre et al. 1987).

Neurilemomas are encapsulated and arise from a single nerve fascicle. They usually can be completely removed surgically without disturbing nerve continuity or function (Phalen 1976).

NEUROFIBROMA

Neurofibromas are benign tumors that arise from the perineurium and the endoneurium. They grow slowly and interdigitate with nerve fibers, so they are more likely than neurilemomas to cause pain, other sensory symptoms, or neurologic deficit.

Neurofibromas are most commonly cutaneous, rather than on main nerve trunks, and present either as an isolated finding or as part of von Reckling-hausen's neurofibromatosis. Whether as isolated tumors or as part of neurofibromatosis, neurofibromas in the median or digital nerves are even rarer than neurilemomas. When a neurofibroma involves the median nerve in the carpal tunnel, the symptoms may be those of an asymptomatic mass or of a progressive median neuropathy.

Surgical resection of neurofibromas usually requires nerve transection, often followed by nerve grafting to reestablish nerve continuity (Figure 19.1) (Rinaldi 1983). Successful microscopic excision of neurofibromas while maintaining nerve continuity is rare (Strickland and Steichen 1977).

NEUROFIBROMATOSIS

Median nerve tumors may occur in patients with either type 1 or type 2 neurofibromatosis (von Recklinghausen's disease). Tumors include median nerve neurofibromas, plexiform neurofibromas, and malignant peripheral nerve sheath tumors. The semantics are sometimes confusing, because the most common neurofibromas in patients with neurofibromatosis are small tumors that arise from cutaneous nerves in the dermis.

In patients with median nerve neurofibromas, the characteristics of the tumor are the same whether or not the patient has neurofibromatosis. The diagnosis of neurofibromatosis rests on cutaneous manifestations of the disease, on the genetic history, and on the presence of other nervous system tumors.

Plexiform neurofibromas are distinctive nerve tumors that are seen only in patients with neurofibromatosis (Harkin 1980). Multiple nerve fascicles are swollen and contain accumulations of Schwann cells, endoneurial cells, and primitive cells. The fascicular swelling creates a macroscopic "tangle of worms" appearance. For example, Brooks (1984) describes plexiform median nerve fibromas localized to the carpal tunnel in a 5-year-old boy, and extending along the nerve from axilla to elbow in a 17-year-old girl.

Both neurofibromas and plexiform neurofibromas may undergo malignant transformation. Neurofibromatosis is the most common setting for development of malignant peripheral nerve sheath tumors.

MALIGNANT PERIPHERAL NERVE SHEATH TUMORS

Most peripheral nerve sheath tumors are benign. Clinical clues to malignancy are spontaneous pain, swelling, and associated neurologic dysfunction.

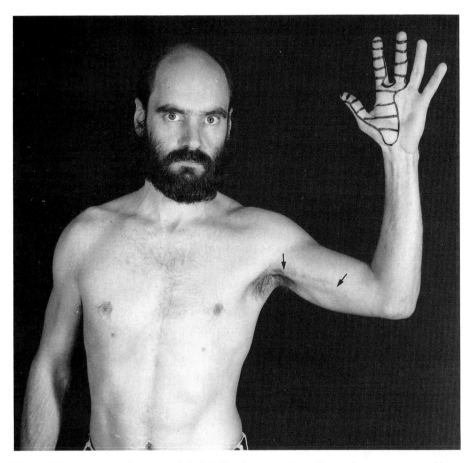

Figure 19.1 Pattern of sensory deficit following resection of a median nerve neurofibroma in the upper arm. The patient also had a profound postoperative median motor deficit.

However, most malignant peripheral nerve tumors present as painless masses (Das Gupta and Brasfield 1970). Malignant nerve sheath tumors may arise as solitary lesions or as malignant transformation of neurofibromas in patients with neurofibromatosis (Ducatman et al. 1986). Malignant transformation should be suspected when a neurofibroma shows accelerated growth. In a series of 31 malignant tumors of peripheral nerve, Vieta and Pack (1951) encountered 5 arising from the median nerve.

Treatment is by total excision. Even after excision, patients are at high risk for local recurrence or development of metastases (Rogalski and Louis 1991). Association with neurofibromatosis and tumor size greater than 5 cm are adverse prognostic signs (Ducatman et al. 1986).

FATTY NERVE TUMORS

Fatty tumors of the median nerve include isolated lipomas encapsulated within the nerve, infiltrative lipofibromatous hamartomas of the nerve, or macrodystrophia lipomatosa in which there is fatty infiltration of both the median nerve and of subcutaneous tissue of the hand. These are all distinguishable from median nerve compression by a lipoma external to the nerve (see Table 6.4).

Encapsulated lipomas are rarely found within the median nerve. They have been reported to occur in the nerve within the carpal tunnel or in the forearm (Watson-Jones 1900; Morley 1964; Rusko and Larsen 1981). The soft subcutaneous mass may be palpable for years before it causes paresthesias. At surgery the encapsulated tumor can be removed completely without damaging nerve fascicles, and microscopic examination shows no nerve fibers within the tumor capsule.

Lipofibromatous hamartomas of the median nerve are known by a number of synonyms: fibrolipomatous hamartoma, fibrofatty proliferation, fatty infiltration of nerve, and intraneural lipofibroma (Pulvertaft 1964; Yeoman 1964; Callison et al. 1968; Johnson and Bonfiglio 1969; Jamra and Rebeiz 1979; Kalisman and Dolich 1982; Louis et al. 1985; Houpt et al. 1989). The median nerve is the most common site of these hamartomas; similar hamartomas are extremely rare in other nerves (Silverman and Enzinger 1985). Some cases have been reported as median nerve lipomas, but histology does not show the typical encapsulation and excisability of a lipoma (Mikhail 1964; Friedlander et al. 1969). Lipofibromatous hamartomas have a predilection for the carpal tunnel, spreading distally into the palm and proximally into the forearm. The symptoms are those of a slowly growing palmar or forearm mass, often accompanied by symptoms of carpal tunnel syndrome. The symptoms often start in childhood, but some patients do not develop symptoms until their forties or fifties. X rays occasionally show calcification within the hamartoma (Louis et al. 1985). Figure 19.2 shows a magnetic resonance imaging (MRI) scan of a median nerve mass in the carpal tunnel; the MRI suggested median nerve fascicular enlargement and fatty infiltration; biopsy confirmed the fibroblastic nature of the proliferative tissue (Bodne et al. 1988).

At surgery a lipofibromatous hamartoma typically appears as a fusiform enlargement of nerve within the epineurium. If the epineurium is divided, the tumor is seen closely intertwined with nerve fascicles, so that microdissection of the tumor is usually impossible. Release of the flexor retinaculum is often sufficient treatment, at least for the symptoms of median neuropathy. Rowland (1977) followed a patient for 10 years following initial biopsy of a lipofibromatous hamartoma and noted regression of the tumor, but other patients have progressive or recurrent symptoms of median nerve compromise despite carpal tunnel release (Louis et al. 1985). The indications for tumor debulking or resection with nerve grafting in these patients with progressive symptoms are unclear.

Rarely, a lipofibromatous hamartoma is limited to a single digital nerve (Steentoft and Sollerman 1990). These tumors present as focal swelling of the

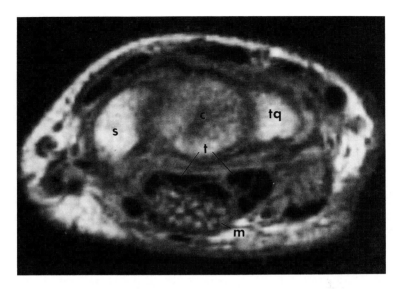

Figure 19.2 Reactive perineural fibroblastic proliferation of the median nerve. The axial magnetic resonance (MR) image of the wrist shows marked enlargement of the median nerve *(m)*. The perineural fibroblastic proliferation is so prominent that individual nerve fascicles can be identified. Sagittal images (not shown) confirmed fatty infiltration of the nerve as well. Scaphoid *(s)*, capitate *(c)*, triquetrum *(tq)*, and flexor tendons *(t)*. (Reproduced with permission of the authors and publisher from Bodne D, Quinn SF, Kloss J, Bolton T, Murray WT, Roberts W, Cochran C. Reactive perineural fibroblastic proliferation of the median nerve: MR characteristics. J Comput Assist Tomogr 1988;12:532–34.)

finger or distal palm with or without sensory disturbance. When only a digital nerve is involved, the tumor can occasionally be dissected free of the nerve with aid of the microscope (Kalisman and Dolich 1982).

Some patients have a combination of macrodactyly of one or more digits and lipofibromatous hamartoma of the corresponding digital nerve or of the median nerve (Hueston and Millroy 1968; Paletta and Rybka 1972; Frykman and Wood 1978; Silverman and Enzinger 1985). The combination is sometimes called macrodystrophia lipomatosa. At times fibrous rather than lipomatous change is the predominant histologic change in nerve (Moore 1942; Allende 1967). The macrodactyly is often congenital (Barsky 1967).

HEMANGIOMA

Hemangiomas of the median nerve are extremely rare; it is hard to find a handful of reported cases (Kojima et al. 1976; Peled et al. 1980; Kon and Vuursteen 1981; Prosser and Burke 1987). These tumors may present in childhood or adolescence with a visible, compressible soft tissue tumor or, when the hemangioma is within the carpal tunnel, with symptoms of carpal tunnel syndrome. Computed tomography (CT) scan of the tumor with contrast can confirm the vascular nature of the tumor (Feyerabend et al. 1990).

DIGITAL NERVE TUMORS

Two nerve tumors specifically involve the digital nerves. Dermal nerve sheath myxoma is a very rare benign tumor that probably originates from Schwann cells (Webb 1979; Blumberg and Adelaar 1989). It presents as a small digital mass. It can become painful or develop a Tinel's sign. Hyperplastic Pacinian corpuscles may also cause small, painful subcutaneous digital masses. Normal Pacinian corpuscles are sensory receptors for mechanical stimuli that are formed by concentrically arranged squamous epithelium derived from perineurium. On rare occasion they may become tender and hyperplastic, particularly after hand trauma, and present either as a single mass or as a string of masses (Sandzen and Baksic 1974). At times a hyperplastic Pacinian corpuscle can cause digital nerve compression, with resulting pain and paresthesia (Zweig and Burns 1968; Hart et al. 1971; Cameron 1976; Gama and Franca 1980; Jones and Eadie 1991). Surgical excision of the corpuscles often succeeds in relieving symptoms.

Kline et al. (1990) described glomus tumors originating in a digital nerve and associated with digital paresthesias. Symptoms may include sensitivity of the tip of the digit to gentle mechanical or cold stimulation, relief of pain by warm stimulation, or evident focal swelling of the digit (Ochoa et al. 1991, 28).

LOCALIZED HYPERTROPHIC NEUROPATHY

Localized hypertrophic neuropathy is an exceedingly rare cause of focal mononeuropathy (Mitsumoto et al. 1980; Phillips et al. 1991). Clinical presentation is usually insidious with painless motor deficit and little sensory change. Nerve biopsy shows focal onion bulb formation; it is intriguing whether to class this as a benign neoplasm. One of the reported cases involved the recurrent thenar motor branch of the median nerve (Mitsumoto et al. 1991). In another case, a patient with macrodactyly had onion bulb formation noted on biopsy of the localized hypertrophy of the median nerve in the carpal tunnel (Appenzeller and Kornfeld 1974).

METASTATIC TUMORS

Metastatic spread of tumor specifically to the median nerve is very rare. However, Mackay and Barua (1990) described a man who had undergone index finger amputation for well-differentiated squamous cell carcinoma. Three years later he developed carpal tunnel syndrome. At surgery the median nerve in the carpal tunnel was encased in squamous cell carcinoma. Metastasis of bronchogenic carcinoma to the anterior interosseous nerve has also been reported (Peters and Todd 1983).

INFECTION MISTAKEN FOR TUMOR

Two case reports illustrate an oddity: A mass lesion attached to nerve may be infectious rather than neoplastic. A painful 2-cm diameter, mobile nodule attached to the median nerve in the upper arm was thought to be a neurilemoma until pathologic examination showed that it was a cysticercus cyst (Nosanchuk et al. 1980). A 55-year-old woman, who presented with a forearm mass and a distal median neuropathy, was found at surgery to have a calcified mass adherent to the median nerve. A calcified guinea worm *(Dracunculus medinensis)* was identified under the nerve sheath (Balasubramanian and Ramamurthi 1965).

TUMOR IMAGING

MRI scanning, CT scanning, and ultrasound can aid in the diagnosis of median nerve tumors. The first characteristic of a nerve sheath tumor is localization of the tumor in or contiguous with a nerve. On MRI the tumors typically are intermediately or moderately bright on T1-weighted images, moderately bright on proton-density-weighted images, and bright on T2-weighted images (Stull et al. 1991). The signal is usually heterogeneous. This combination of findings is seen with neurilemomas, neurofibromas, and malignant nerve sheath tumors. Tumor margins are usually well defined; an irregular or indistinct margin may occur with malignant tumors, plexiform neurofibromas, or after nerve biopsy.

CT scanning can also be used to confirm the location of a soft tissue tumor in relation to peripheral nerve (Powers et al. 1983). At times CT appearance gives clues to tumor histology (Feyerabend et al. 1990). Neurilemomas appear as well-defined, hypodense masses and sometimes develop ring enhancement after administration of intravenous contrast; the tumor mass may appear inhomogeneous (Levine et al. 1987). Neurofibromas are similar in appearance but may be less well defined and occasionally contain areas of calcification. Lipomas and lipofibromatous hamartomas are distinguished by low CT numbers because of their fat content. Hemangiomas show rapid transient enhancement.

On high-resolution real-time ultrasound, the normal median nerve can be identified with an echogenic fibrillar texture (Fornage 1988). Relative immobility with joint movement helps distinguish it from flexor tendons, which have similar echogenicity. Nerve tumors, like other soft tissue tumors, appear as hypoechoic masses; usually their attachment to nerve is the only clue to their origin. Neurilemomas usually have more well-defined contours than neurofibromas. Neurilemomas may also show distal sound enhancement (Fornage 1988).

With the possible exception of lipomas and hemangiomas, CT and MRI findings will rarely be specific to tumor pathology. For example, they do not reliably distinguish neurofibromas and neurilemomas from malignant peripheral nerve sheath tumors.

CONCLUSION

Median nerve tumors should be considered whenever a patient presents with a mass along the course of the median nerve. The diagnosis should be particularly suspected in patients with neurofibromatosis or when the mass is accompanied by symptoms of median neuropathy. Even with modern imaging techniques, the final diagnosis is often not established prior to biopsy of the mass. Appropriate surgical management is determined by the tumor type and location and by the extent of associated neurologic deficit.

REFERENCES

Allende BT. Macrodactyly with enlarged median nerve associated with carpal tunnel syndrome. Plast Reconstr Surg 1967;39:578–82.

Appenzeller O, Kornfeld M. Macrodactyly and localized hypertrophic neuropathy. Neurology (Minneap) 1974;24:767–71.

Balasubramanian V, Ramamurthi B. An unusual location of guineaworm infestation. J Neurosurg 1965;23:537–38.

Barre PS, Shaffer JW, Carter JR, Lacey SH. Multiplicity of neurilemomas in the upper extremity. J Hand Surg 1987;12A:307–11.

Barsky AJ. Macrodactyly. J Bone Joint Surg 1967;49A:1255–66.

Blumberg AK, Adelaar RS. Nerve sheath myxoma of digital nerve. Cancer 1989;63:1215–18.

Bodne D, Quinn SF, Kloss J, Bolton T, Murray WT, Roberts W, Cochran C. Reactive perineural fibroblastic proliferation of the median nerve: MR characteristics. J Comput Assist Tomogr 1988;12:532–34.

Brooks D. Clinical presentation and treatment of peripheral nerve tumors. In: Dyck PJ, Thomas PK, Lambert EH, Bunge R, eds. Peripheral neuropathy. 2nd ed. Philadelphia: WB Saunders, 1984;2236–51.

Callison JR, Thoms OJ, White WL. Fibro-fatty proliferation of the median nerve. Plast Reconstr Surg 1968;42:403–13.

Cameron S. Two rare cases of nerve entrapment. J Bone Joint Surg 1976;58B:266.

Das Gupta TK, Brasfield RD. Solitary malignant schwannoma. Ann Surg 1970;171:419–28.

Ducatman BS, Scheithauer BW, Piepgras DG, Reiman HM, Ilstrup DM. Malignant peripheral nerve sheath tumors. Cancer 1986;57:2006–21.

Feyerabend T, Schmitt R, Lanz U, Warmuth-Metz M. CT morphology of benign median nerve tumors. Report of three cases and a review. Acta Radiol 1990;31:23–25.

Fornage BD. Peripheral nerves of the extremities: imaging with US. Radiology 1988;167:179–82.

Friedlander HL, Rosenberg NJ, Graubard DJ. Intraneural lipoma of the median nerve. J Bone Joint Surg 1969;51A:352–62.

Frykman GK, Wood VE. Peripheral nerve hamartoma with macrodactyly in the hand: report of three cases and review of the literature. J Hand Surg 1978;3:307–12.

Gama C, Franca LCM. Nerve compression by Pacinian corpuscles. J Hand Surg 1980;5:208–10.

Harkin JC. Differential diagnosis of peripheral nerve tumors. In: Omer GE Jr, Spinner M, eds. Management of peripheral nerve problems. Philadelphia: WB Saunders, 1980;657–68.

Harkin JC, Reed RJ. Tumors of the peripheral nervous system. Washington, DC: Armed Forces Institute of Pathology, 1969.

Harkin JC, Reed RJ. Tumors of the peripheral nervous system, supplement. Washington, DC: Armed Forces Institute of Pathology, 1983.

Hart WR, Thompson NW, Hildreth DH, Abell MR. Hyperplastic Pacinian corpuscles: a cause of digital pain. Surgery 1971;70:730–35.

Houpt P, Storm van Leeuwen JB, van den Bergen HA. Intraneural lipofibroma of the median nerve. J Hand Surg 1989;14A:706–9.

Hueston JT, Millroy P. Macrodactyly associated with hamartoma of major peripheral nerves. Aust NZ J Surg 1968;37:394–97.

Jamra FN, Rebeiz JJ. Lipofibroma of the median nerve. J Hand Surg 1979;4:160–63.

Johnson RJ, Bonfiglio M. Lipofibromatous hamartoma of the median nerve. J Bone Joint Surg 1969;51A:984–90.

Jones NF, Eadie P. Pacinian corpuscle hyperplasia in the hand. J Hand Surg 1991;16A:865–69.

Kalisman M, Dolich BH. Infiltrating lipoma of the proper digital nerves. J Hand Surg 1982;7:401–3.

Kline SC, Moore JR, deMente SH. Glomus tumor originating within a digital nerve. J Hand Surg 1990;15A:98–101.

Kojima T, Ide Y, Marumo E, Ishikawa E, Yamashita H. Haemangioma of median nerve causing carpal tunnel syndrome. Hand 1976;8:62–65.

Kon M, Vuursteen PJ. An intraneural hemangioma of a digital nerve—case report. J Hand Surg 1981;6:357–58.

Levine E, Huntrakoon M, Wetzel LH. Malignant nerve-sheath neoplasms in neurofibromatosis: distinction from benign tumors using imaging techniques. AJR 1987; 149:1059–64.

Lewis RC, Nannini LH, Cocke WM Jr. Multifocal neurilemomas of median and ulnar nerves of the same extremity—case report. J Hand Surg 1981;6:406–8.

Louis DS, Hankin FM, Greene TL, Dick HM. Lipofibromas of the median nerve: long-term follow-up of four cases. J Hand Surg 1985;10A:403–8.

Mackay IR, Barua JM. Perineural tumour spread: an unusual cause of carpal tunnel syndrome. J Hand Surg 1990;15B:104–5.

Mikhail IK. Median nerve lipoma in the hand. J Bone Joint Surg 1964;46B:726–30.

Mitsumoto H, Wilbourn AJ, Goren H. Perineuroma as the cause of localized hypertrophic neuropathy. Muscle Nerve 1980;3:403–12.

Mitsumoto H, Estes ML, Wilbourn AJ, Culver JE Jr. Localized hypertrophic neuropathy: perineuroma or perineural hyperplasia? Muscle Nerve 1991;14:906.

Moore BH. Macrodactyly and associated peripheral nerve changes. J Bone Joint Surg 1942;24:617–31.

Morley GH. Intraneural lipoma of the median nerve in the carpal tunnel. J Bone Joint Surg 1964;46B:734–35.

Nosanchuk JS, Agostini JC, Georgi M, Posso M. Pork tapeworm of cysticercus involving peripheral nerve. JAMA 1980;244:2191–92.

Ochoa JL, Marchettini P, Cline M. Lessons from human research on the pathophysiology of neuropathic pains in limbs. In: Wynn Parry CB, ed. Management of pain in the hand and wrist. Edinburgh: Churchill Livingstone, 1991;28–33.

Paletta FX, Rybka FJ. Treatment of hamartomas of the median nerve. Ann Surg 1972;176:217–22.

Peled I, Iosipovich Z, Rousso M, Wexler MR. Hemangioma of the median nerve. J Hand Surg 1980;5:363–65.

Peters WJ, Todd TR. Anterior interosseous nerve compression syndrome: from metastatic bronchogenic carcinoma to the forearm. Plast Reconstr Surg 1983;72:706–7.

Phalen GS. Neurilemmomas of the forearm and hand. Clin Orthop 1976;114:219–22.

Phillips LH, Persing JA, Vandenberg SR. Electrophysiological findings in localized hypertrophic mononeuropathy. Muscle Nerve 1991;14:335–41.

Powers SK, Norman D, Edwards MSB. Computerized tomography of peripheral nerve lesions. J Neurosurg 1983;59:131–36.

Prosser AJ, Burke FD. Haemangioma of the median nerve associated with Raynaud's phenomenon. J Hand Surg 1987;12B:227–228.

Pulvertaft RG. Unusual tumours of the median nerve. J Bone Joint Surg 1964;46B:731–33.

Rinaldi E. Neurilemomas and neurofibromas of the upper limb. J Hand Surg 1983;8:590–93.

Ritt MJPF, Bos KE. A very large neurilemmoma of the anterior interosseous nerve. J Hand Surg 1991;16B:98–100.

Rogalski RP, Louis DS. Neurofibrosarcomas of the upper extremity. J Hand Surg 1991;16A:873–76.

Rowland SA. Case report: ten year follow-up of lipofibroma of the median nerve in the palm. J Hand Surg 1977;2:316–17.

Rusko RA, Larsen RD. Intraneural lipoma of the median nerve—case report and literature review. J Hand Surg 1981;6:388–91.

Sandzen SC, Baksic RW. Pacinian hyperplasia. Hand 1974;6:273–74.

Seddon H. Surgical disorders of the peripheral nerves. Baltimore: Williams & Wilkins, 1972.

Silverman TA, Enzinger FM. Fibrolipomatous hamartoma of nerve. A clinicopathologic analysis of 26 cases. Am J Surg Pathol 1985;9:7–14.

Steentoft J, Sollerman C. Lipofibromatous hamartoma of a digital nerve. A case report. Acta Orthop Scand 1990;61:181–82.

Stout AP. The peripheral manifestations of the specific nerve sheath tumor (neurilemoma). AJC 1935;24:751–96.

Strickland JW, Steichen JB. Nerve tumors of the hand and forearm. J Hand Surg 1977; 2:285–91.

Stull MA, Moser JRP, Kransdorf MJ, Bogumill GP, Nelson MC. Magnetic resonance appearance of peripheral nerve sheath tumors. Skeletal Radiol 1991;20:9–14.

Vieta JO, Pack GT. Malignant neurilemomas of peripheral nerves. Am J Surg 1951;82:416–31.

Watson-Jones R. Encapsulated lipoma of the median nerve at the wrist. J Bone Joint Surg 1964;46B:736.

Webb JN. The histogenesis of nerve sheath myxoma: report of a case with electron microscopy. J Pathol 1979;127:35–37.

Yeoman PM. Fatty infiltration of the median nerve. J Bone Joint Surg 1964;46B:737–39.

Zweig J, Burns H. Compression of digital nerves by Pacinian corpuscles. A report of two cases. J Bone Joint Surg 1968;50A:999–1001.

Index